Essentials of Ophthalmology

For Medical School and Beyond

Second Edition

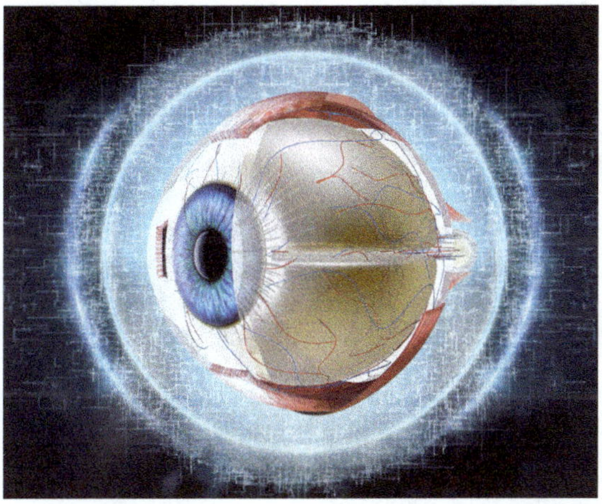

Essentials of Ophthalmology

For Medical School and Beyond

Second Edition

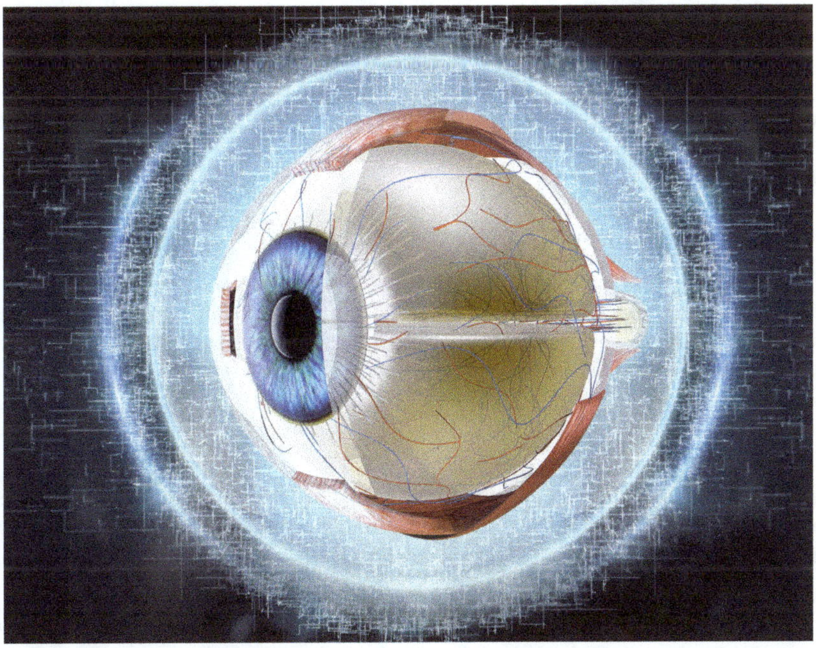

Editors

Ray Manotosh

Yuen Yew Sen

Victor Koh

National University Hospital, Singapore

World Scientific

NEW JERSEY • LONDON • SINGAPORE • BEIJING • SHANGHAI • HONG KONG • TAIPEI • CHENNAI

Published by

World Scientific Publishing Co. Pte. Ltd.
5 Toh Tuck Link, Singapore 596224
USA office: 27 Warren Street, Suite 401-402, Hackensack, NJ 07601
UK office: 57 Shelton Street, Covent Garden, London WC2H 9HE

British Library Cataloguing-in-Publication Data
A catalogue record for this book is available from the British Library.

ESSENTIALS OF OPHTHALMOLOGY
For Medical School and Beyond
Second Edition

ISBN 978-981-98-0354-5 (hardcover)
ISBN 978-981-98-0681-2 (paperback)
ISBN 978-981-98-0355-2 (ebook for institutions)
ISBN 978-981-98-0356-9 (ebook for individuals)

For any available supplementary material, please visit
https://www.worldscientific.com/worldscibooks/10.1142/14095#t=suppl

FOREWORD

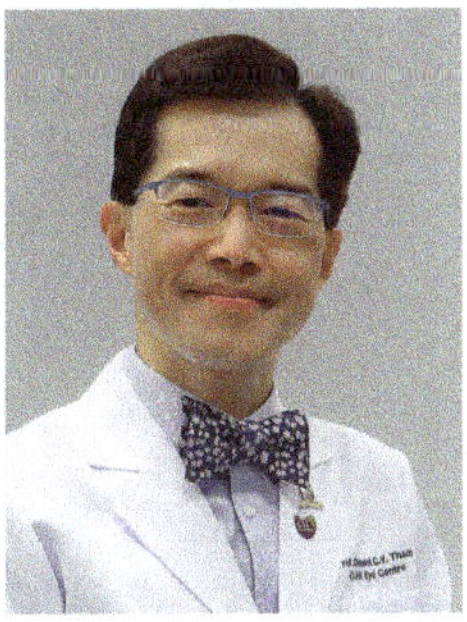

The study of ophthalmology is not just an academic pursuit, but a journey into understanding the profound impact of sight on our everyday lives. This textbook, *Essentials of Ophthalmology, Second Edition*, meticulously edited by A/Prof Ray Manotosh, A/Prof Victor Koh, and Asst Prof Yuen Yew Sen, represents a significant contribution to the educational resources available to undergraduate students in this fascinating field.

The authors, from the highly esteemed Department of Ophthalmology at the National University Hospital, bring together decades of clinical experience, research acumen, and a passion for teaching. Their collective expertise ensures that this book is not only comprehensive, but also practical, bridging the gap between theoretical knowledge and clinical applications.

In an era when the field of medicine is constantly expanding, *Essentials of Ophthalmology, Second Edition*, stands as a testament to the importance of solid undergraduate training. The editors and authors have succeeded in creating a resource that is both rigorous and accessible, making it an indispensable tool for students embarking on their journey into the world of ophthalmology.

As you delve into the pages of this textbook, you will find not only the essentials of ophthalmology, but also the inspiration to pursue excellence in this dynamic field. It is my sincere hope that this book will ignite a passion for ophthalmology in its readers, and provide them with a solid foundation of knowledge in their future professional pursuits.

I do highly commend A/Prof Ray, A/Prof Koh, Asst Prof Yuen, and all the contributing authors for their dedication to advancing the education of future ophthalmologists. This textbook is a reflection of their commitment to nurturing the next generation of clinicians, and I am confident it will be an invaluable asset to all who seek to understand the art and science of ophthalmology.

Clement C.Y. Tham
Chairman and S.H. Ho Professor of Ophthalmology & Visual Sciences,
The Chinese University of Hong Kong
Secretary General & CEO, Asia-Pacific Academy of Ophthalmology (APAO)
President, Asia-Pacific Glaucoma Society (APGS)
Chair, Academia Ophthalmologica Internationalis (AOI)
Immediate Past President, The College of Ophthalmologists of Hong Kong (COHK)
Immediate Past Treasurer, International Council of Ophthalmology (ICO)
September 2024

PREFACE

Ophthalmology has undergone significant advancements over the years, necessitating an evolution in the way we teach and learn. This second edition of *Essentials of Ophthalmology for Medical School and Beyond* is our response to the ever-changing landscape of eye care, aimed at providing readers with the most up-to-date knowledge.

Our primary objective with this edition is to offer medical students a resource that is both comprehensive and contextually relevant. In Singapore and across Asia, eye conditions such as myopia, angle-closure glaucoma, and polypoidal choroidal vasculopathy are particularly prevalent, and this text places the appropriate emphasis on these concerns. Furthermore, as the role of primary care physicians in managing these conditions continues to evolve, it is crucial to equip future doctors with robust ophthalmic knowledge.

The past decade has also seen a shift in medical education, with digital learning platforms becoming integral to the curriculum. While these platforms offer flexibility and accessibility, we believe that a textbook remains an invaluable tool for in-depth study and reference. This edition has been meticulously crafted to complement available digital resources, providing a solid foundation for both patient-centred learning and clinical practice.

The creation of this book has been a collective effort, driven by a deep commitment to education. My co-editors, Ray and Yew Sen, have demonstrated remarkable dedication in bringing together the contributions of our authors, ensuring that this book upholds the highest standards of academic rigour and practical relevance.

This textbook is more than just a compilation of facts and figures — it is a testament to the passion and dedication of the Department of Ophthalmology at the National University Hospital and the National University of Singapore. It reflects our unwavering commitment to the education of medical students, residents, and future eye care professionals. We are proud to share this knowledge, continuing the legacy of our mentors, and we hope this book will inspire and guide those who use it on their journey to become skilled and compassionate clinicians.

Victor Koh, MBBS, MMed (Ophth), MRCSEd, MSc, FAMS
Head & Senior Consultant
Department of Ophthalmology
National University Hospital

ACKNOWLEDGEMENTS

We extend our heartfelt gratitude to the National University Health System (NUHS), Singapore, for granting us the opportunity to contribute to the esteemed NUHS Textbook series.

Our deepest thanks go to all the contributors who devoted their valuable time to writing and revising this book; their efforts were indispensable in making this work a reality.

We are especially thankful to our mentors and seniors, Professor Paul Chew, Associate Professor Caroline Chee and Associate Professor Shantha Amrith for their constructive guidance. We wish to acknowledge the unwavering encouragement from Associate Professor Clement Tan, whose significant contributions enriched this book. We are profoundly grateful to Professor Clement Tham for graciously agreeing to write the Foreword.

Lastly, we are deeply indebted to Ms. Ivy Law, Senior Manager, Education, whose tireless efforts were crucial in bringing this publication. No words can fully express our gratitude for her dedication.

ABOUT THE EDITORS

Ray Manotosh

Ray Manotosh is currently a Senior Consultant and Head of the Division of Cornea and Refractive Surgery at the National University Health System, Singapore. His areas of specialisation include the cornea, external eye diseases, contact lenses, and refractive surgery. He also serves as an Associate Professor and Education Director of Ophthalmology at the Yong Loo Lin School of Medicine, National University of Singapore. Additionally, he is actively involved in the postgraduate residency program as core faculty at the National University Hospital, Singapore.

Associate Professor Ray completed his undergraduate training at the University of Calcutta, India, and his basic surgical training in ophthalmology at the prestigious All India Institute of Medical Sciences (AIIMS), New Delhi, India's premier medical institute. He then pursued advanced surgical training in cornea and external diseases at AIIMS in 1998 and became a Fellow of the Royal College of Surgeons of Edinburgh (UK) in Ophthalmology. Following his advanced surgical training, he joined the National University Hospital, Singapore, in 2002. In 2006, he received the NHG Excellence Award for Teaching. He has published extensively in peer-reviewed journals and has contributed to numerous textbook chapters.

Beyond his academic and professional pursuits, Dr Ray enjoys spending time with his family. He is passionate about oil painting and has exhibited his work. He has also published a fiction book, which he is extremely proud of.

Yuen Yew Sen

Yuen Yew Sen, an ASEAN scholar who graduated from the National University of Singapore (NUS), is currently an Assistant Professor at the Department of Ophthalmology, NUS and Consultant in the Department of Ophthalmology, National University Hospital (NUH). He is also the Director of Undergraduate Education for the National University of Singapore's Department of Ophthalmology and part of the Core Faculty for the National University Health System (NUHS) Ophthalmology residency programme, involved in training the next generation of ophthalmologists.

He has sub-specialty training in both Vitreoretinal Surgery and Uveitis (Ocular Inflammation) and is the recipient of the Ministry of Health — Health Manpower Development Plan (HMDP) award.

Apart from his clinical duties, he has been awarded the Junior Doctor Teaching Award and Young Teacher Award for his educational work. He has also been honoured to serve as an examiner and admissions interviewer for his alma mater, the NUS School of Medicine.

Victor Koh

Associate Professor Victor Koh is a Consultant Ophthalmologist and is currently Head of the Department of Ophthalmology at National University Hospital. His clinical expertise encompasses both adult and childhood glaucoma management, as well as complex cataract surgery. He graduated from the Yong Loo Lin School of Medicine at the National University of Singapore in 2007 and received specialist accreditation in 2016. His primary research focus is on developing disruptive medical devices for community-based ophthalmic diagnostics and innovative laser and implant solutions for refractory glaucoma. His practice and professional philosophy are deeply influenced by his mentors, including Prof. Paul Chew, A/Prof. Clement Tan, Adj. A/Prof. Loon Seng Chee, Prof. Aung Tin, Prof. Sir Peng Khaw, and Dr. Aliza Jap. Inspired by the guidance he received, he is dedicated to educating the next generation of doctors and medical students, ensuring the highest standards of patient care. He expresses his heartfelt gratitude to his wife and two sons, whose unwavering support has been invaluable throughout his training years and career.

LIST OF CONTRIBUTORS

Blanche Xiaohong Lim, MBBS, MMed (Ophth), FAMS
Consultant
Division of Orbit and Oculofacial Surgery
National University Hospital

Chai Hui Chen Charmaine, MBBS, MMed (Ophth), FAMS Senior Consultant
Division of Cornea & Refractive Surgery

Chan Hwei Wuen, MBBS, MMed (Ophth), FAMS, FRCOphth (UK)
Senior Consultant
Division of Vitreo-retina & Electrophysiology

Chen Ziyou David, MBBS, MMed (Ophth), FAMS
Consultant
Division of Cataract and Refractive Surgery
National University Hospital

Cheryl Ngo Shufen, MBBS, MMed (Ophth), FRCSEd (Ophth)
Visiting Consultant
Division of Paediatric Ophthalmology
National University Hospital

Chris Hong Long Lim BSc (Med), BMed, MD, MMed (Ophth), FAMS
Consultant
Division of Cornea and Refractive Surgery
National University Hospital

Clement Tan Woon Teck, MBBS, MMed (Ophth), FRCSEd, FAMS
Senior Consultant & Head, Division of Neuro-Ophthalmology
National University Hospital

Danial Bohan, BSc (Hons), MSc
Senior Optometrist
Division of Low Vision and Vision Rehabilitation
National University Hospital

Dawn Lim Ka-Ann, MBBS, MRCP (UK), MMed (Int.Med), MMed (Ophth), FAMS
Senior Consultant
Division of Ocular Inflammation & Glaucoma
National University Hospital

Gangadhara Sundar, DO, FRCSEd, FAMS Senior Consultant
Head, Division of Orbit & Oculofacial Surgery
National University Hospital

George Naveen Thomas, MBBS, MMed (Ophth)
Consultant, Division of Vitreo-retina
National University Hospital

Graham E Holder
Hong Leong Professor
Division of Electrophysiology
National University Hospital

Janice Lam Sing Harn MBBS, MMed (Ophth) FAMS
Consultant
Division of Paediatric Ophthalmology
National University Hospital

Jeyabal Preethi MBBS, MRCS(Edin), FRCOphth (London)
Resident Physician
Department of Ophthalmology
Ng Teng Fong General Hospital

Katherine Lun MB, BCH BAO, MMed (Ophth), FAMS
Consultant and Programme Director
Division of Glaucoma
National University Hospital

Koh Teck Chang Victor MBBS (S'pore), MMed (Ophth), MRCSEd, MSc, FAMS
Head & Senior Consultant, Department of Ophthalmology,
National University Hospital
Associate Professor, Department of Ophthalmology,
Yong Loo Lin School of Medicine,
National University of Singapore

Lin Hui'en Hazel Anne, MBBS, MMed (Ophth), FAMS
Senior Consultant
Division of Neuro-ophthalmology
National University Hospital

Lingam Gopal MBBS, MS, DNBE, MSC (Epidemiology)
Visiting Consultant
Division of Vitreo-retina
National University Hospital

Maryanne Chew Romero, MBBS, MMed (Ophth)
Associate Consultant
Division of Orbit and Oculofacial Surgery
Alexandra Hospital

Ray Manotosh, MBBS, MD (AIIMS), FRCSEd, FAMS
Senior Consultant & Head
Director Division of Cornea & Refractive Surgery
National University Hospital

Stephanie Ming Young, MBBS, MMed (Ophth), FRCOphth, FAMS
Visiting Consultant
Division of Orbit & Oculofacial Surgery
National University Hospital

Wong Meihua Wendy MBBS, MMed (Ophth), FRCOphth, FAMS
Consultant
Division of Medical Retina
National University Hospital

Yuen Yew Sen, MBBS, MMed (Ophth), FAMS Consultant and UG Program Director
Division of Vitreo-retina & Ocular Inflammation
National University Hospital

CONTENTS

Chapter 1

BASIC ANATOMY OF THE EYE, ADNEXA AND VISUAL PATHWAYS

Jeyabal Preethi, Koh Teck Chang Victor

1.1 Basic Anatomy

Learning Objective

Understand the basic anatomical structures of the globe.

Eyeball is an oblate spheroid-shaped structure. The external structure of the globe comprises the sclera (outermost layer), uveal tissue (middle layer) and retina (innermost layer). Refer to Fig. 1.1.

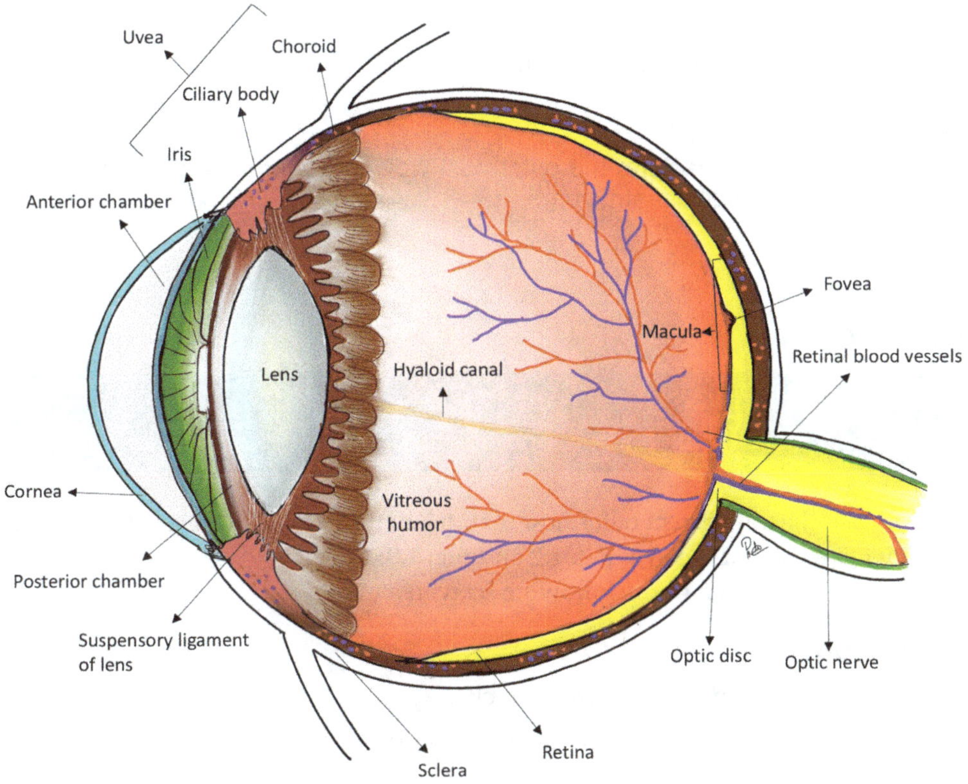

Fig. 1.1. Coronal section of the eyeball showing the various structures.

Sclera

- Strong and dense coat protecting the intraocular contents
- Anterior 1/6th — transparent cornea, posterior 5/6th opaque sclera. Junction is called the limbus
- Thickness:
  - Thickest posteriorly (1 mm) and gradually becomes thinner upon tracing anteriorly
  - Thinnest at the level of insertion of extraocular muscles
- Lamina cribrosa: sieve-like part of sclera through which optic nerve exits the globe

Uveal Tissue

- Supplies nutrition to various structures of the eyeball
- From anterior to posterior, it consists of the iris, ciliary body and choroid
- Functions:
  - Iris: Iris colour varies among different individuals depending on the amount of melanin. Controls the amount of light entering the eye
  - Ciliary body: aqueous humour production, accommodation
  - Choroid: supplies oxygen and nutrition to the outer layers of the retina

Retina

- See the sections below for more details

Take Home Message

The cornea and sclera form the outermost wall of the globe and a protective cover over the intraocular structures.

1.2 Cornea

Learning Objective

Understand the components and functions of the different layers of the cornea.

The cornea is the transparent outermost covering of the eye and is the most important refractive medium of the eye (Fig. 1.2 and Fig. 1.3).

Cornea is composed of the following 5 layers:

Epithelium

- 5 layers of cells and 50–60 microns thick
- Approximately 7 days for complete turnover of the corneal surface epithelium

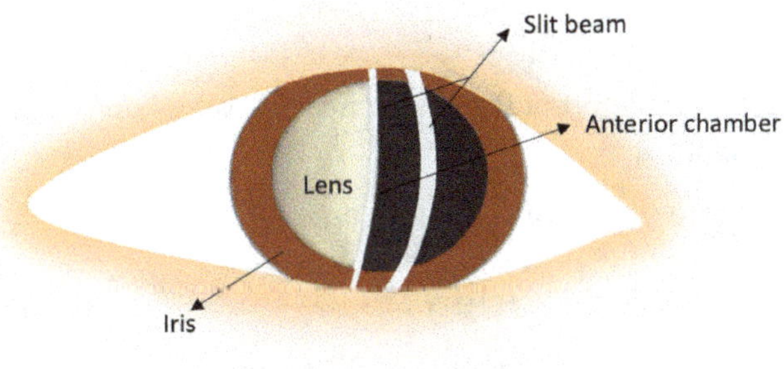

Fig. 1.2. Illustration of slit-lamp beam image of the anterior segment. The first broad slit beam corresponds to the cornea and the second narrow beam corresponds to the anterior surface of the lens.

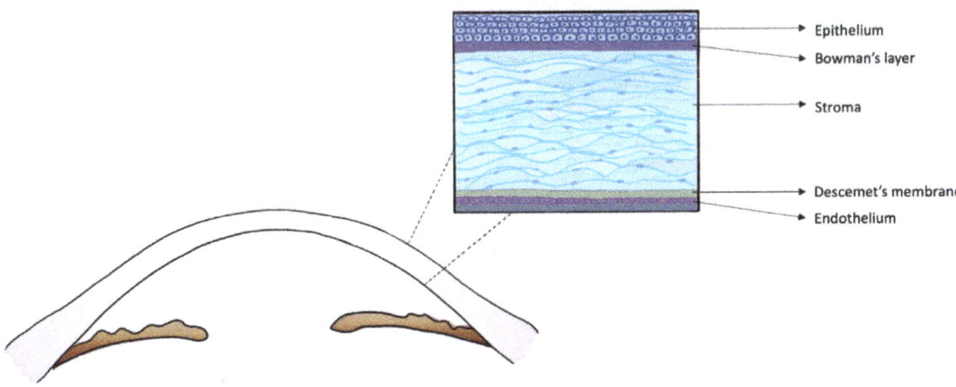

Fig. 1.3. Cross-section of the cornea and the 5 layers.

- Production of new cells occurs at the limbus and grow centripetally from the periphery towards the centre
- Nerve endings of sensory nerve fibres run between the epithelial cells

Bowman's Layer

- Acellular tough layer. 8–12 microns thick
- Cannot be restored after injury but replaced by scar tissue

Stroma

- Forms 90% of corneal thickness
- Multiple lamellae of compact collagen fibrils
- Uniform spacing of collagen fibrils maintains the transparency

Descemet's Membrane

- Basement membrane of the endothelium
- 10 microns thick

Endothelium

- Single layer of flattened cells
- Important in the transport of fluid, keeping the cornea dehydrated and transparent
- Does not regenerate
- Physiological rate of loss of cells with age

Nerve Supply of the Cornea

- From the ophthalmic division of the trigeminal nerve (mainly through the long ciliary nerves)
- Forms the annular plexus at the limbus
- Branches pass radially into the stroma
- Branches unite to form subepithelial plexus
- Terminal branches traverse the bowman membrane and form the intraepithelial plexus

Important Features of the Cornea

Avascular

- Receives its nutrients from diffusion from the aqueous humour and dissolved oxygen from the tear film

No lymphatic drainage

- Avascularity and the absence of immune cells in the cornea make it an immune-privileged site for grafting

Nerve plexus

- Naked nerve endings that run in the epithelium result in intense pain in the presence of a corneal abrasion

Limbal stem cells

- Found at the limbus and are important for the regeneration of new epithelial cells

Endothelial pump

- Corneal oedema occurs due to fluid entering the stroma, leading to a loss of the regularity of the stromal collagen fibrils
- This can occur due to insufficient endothelial cells or from dysfunction of the cells (e.g. trauma or acute rise in intraocular pressure)

Take Home Messages

- There are 5 distinct layers of the cornea, and each plays an important role in the overall function of the cornea.
- The cornea endothelium does not regenerate.

1.3 Anterior Chamber Angle

Learning Objectives

- The components and position of each part of the anterior chamber angle from a gonioscopic view.
- Understand the aqueous outflow dynamics and pathways.

The angle of the anterior chamber is made up of the Schwalbe's line, anterior and posterior trabecular meshwork, scleral spur and ciliary body. These structures are involved in the production and drainage of aqueous humour of the eye and maintenance of the intraocular pressure (Fig. 1.4 and Fig. 1.5).

The anterior segment is made up of the cornea, anterior chamber, iris, lens, ciliary body and the anterior part of the sclera. The anterior chamber is bound anteriorly by the cornea and posteriorly by the iris and pupil, while the posterior chamber is bound anteriorly by the iris and posteriorly by the ciliary body and lens. Aqueous humour fills both the anterior and posterior chambers.

Flow of Aqueous Humour

- Produced at the ciliary body (Fig. 1.6)
- Flows anterior to the lens and through the pupil
- 90% drain through the trabecular meshwork into the Schlemm's canal
- 10% drain via the uveo-scleral pathway

Function of Aqueous Humour

- Maintenance of intraocular pressure and structural form of the globe

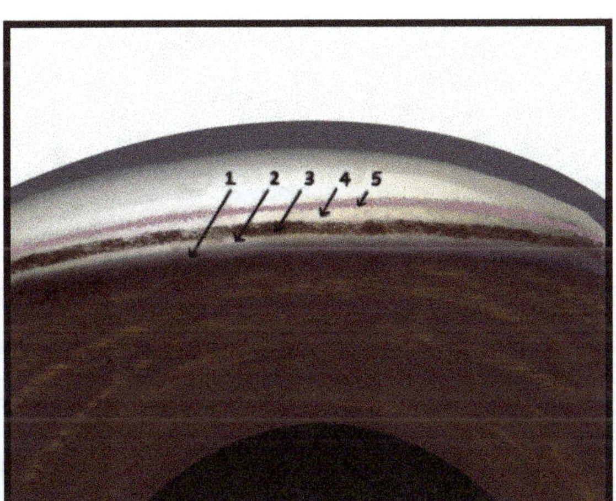

Fig. 1.4. Gonioscopic view of the anterior chamber angle.

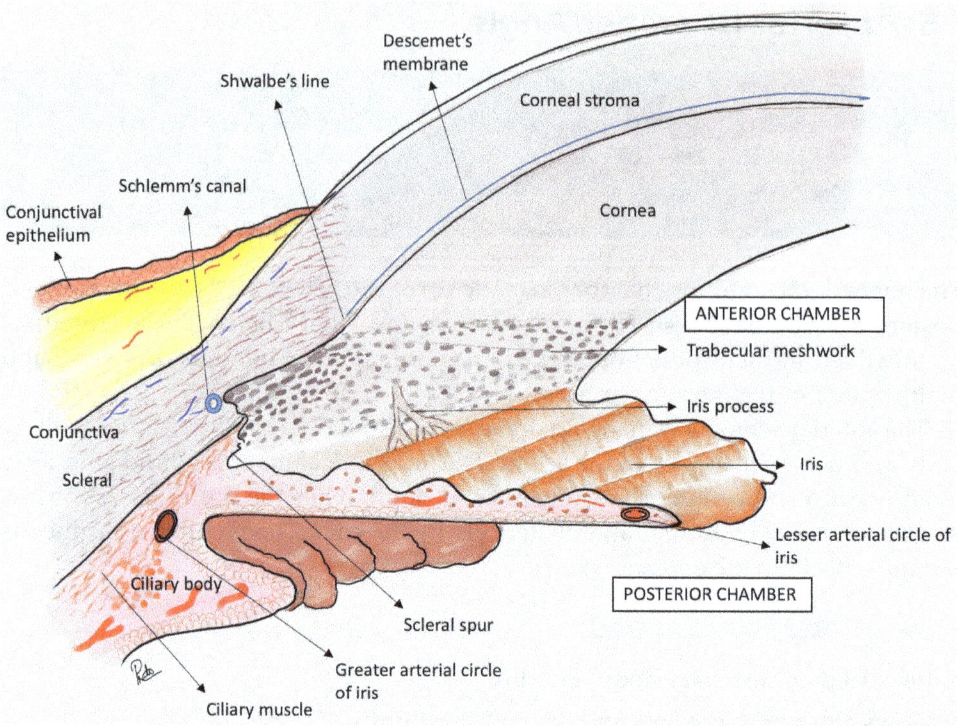

Fig. 1.5. Structures of the anterior chamber angle.

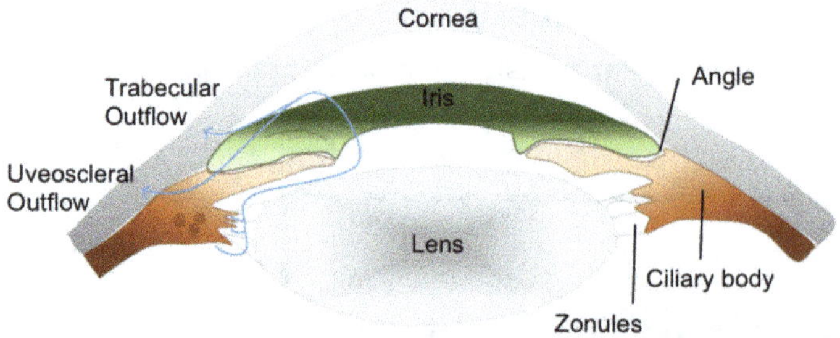

Fig. 1.6. Dynamics of the aqueous humour.

- Provide nutrition to surrounding tissues such as the posterior cornea, trabecular meshwork and lens
- For its refractive index

Take Home Messages

- The posterior trabecular meshwork is an important landmark in the gonioscopic view due to its function in aqueous outflow.
- Aqueous outflow from the eye is mainly via the trabecular meshwork and uveo-scleral pathway.

1.4 Vitreous

Learning Objective

Understand the composition and function of the vitreous gel.

- Viscous, gel-like fluid that is composed of 99% water mainly type II and some type IX collagen fibres, mucopolysaccharides and hyaluronic acid
- Volume 4 mL
- Functions:
  - Mechanical stabilisation of the volume of the globe
  - Shock absorption
  - Nutrition supply to lens and retina
- As we age, syneresis (liquefaction) occurs

Vitreous Base

- Portion of vitreous that is attached to the peripheral retina and pars plana
- It is 6 mm wide (straddling the ora serrata — 2 mm anterior and 4 mm posterior to it)
- The vitreous base is tightly adherent to the ora serrata

Vitreoretinal Junctions

- Firm attachment between the vitreous and retina at the level of the foot plate of Müller's cells at the internal limiting membrane.
- Locations of vitreoretinal junctions (Fig. 1.7):
  - Vitreous base — strongest
  - Margin of optic disc
  - Fovea
  - Back of lens
  - Areas of chorioretinal scars
  - Edges of lattice degeneration
- Blunt trauma may cause avulsion of the vitreous base, which may lead to tearing of the retina along its posterior border
- Posterior vitreous detachment is separation of the cortical vitreous from the retina anywhere posterior to the vitreous base

Take Home Messages

- The vitreous is a clear media that acts as a shock absorbent for the eye.
- There are firm adhesions between the vitreous and the retina, which might result in retinal tears or detachment.

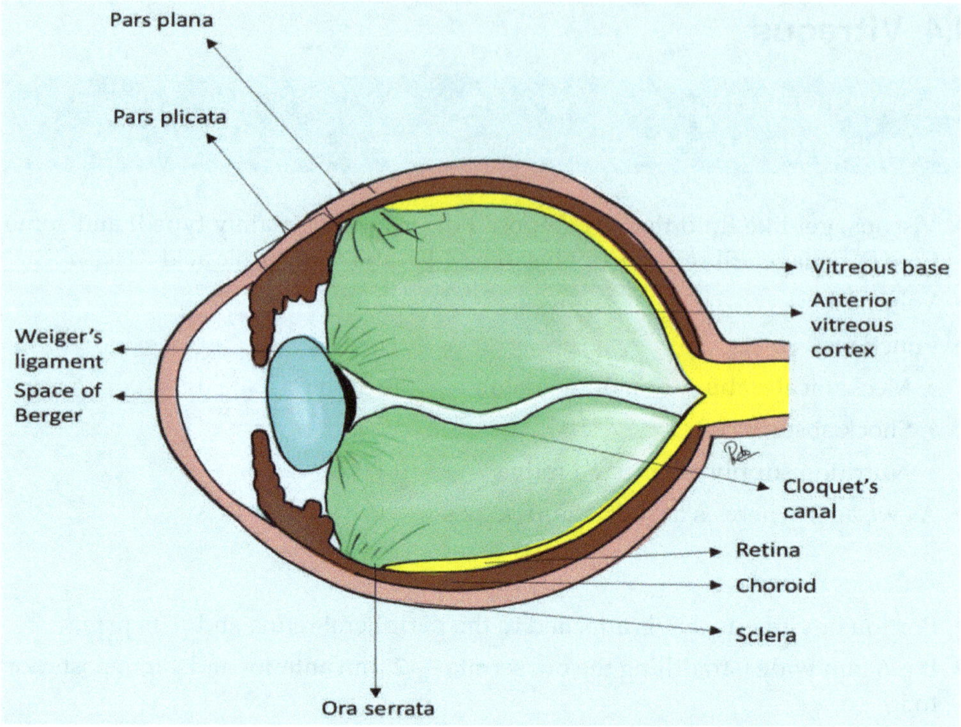

Fig.1.7. Vitreous anatomy and the vitreoretinal junctions.

1.5 Retina

Learning Objectives

- Identify the different layers of the retina and their boundaries.
- Understand the functions of the retina and how the different components contribute to vision.

- Retina forms the inner nervous coat of the eyeball
  - It extends from the optic disc posteriorly to the ora serrata anteriorly
- Retina is divided into posterior pole and peripheral retina by the equator
  - Equator is an imaginary circle drawn at the level of exit of the 4 vortex veins
- Optic disc
  - Circular area of approximately 1500 μm in diameter
  - Nerve fibres exit the retina through the lamina cribrosa to run into the optic nerve
  - Optic cup is a physiological depression seen in the disc. The central retinal artery and vein emerge through the centre of this cup
- Macula lutea
  - 5500 μm area located at the posterior pole temporal to the optic disc (Fig. 1.8)

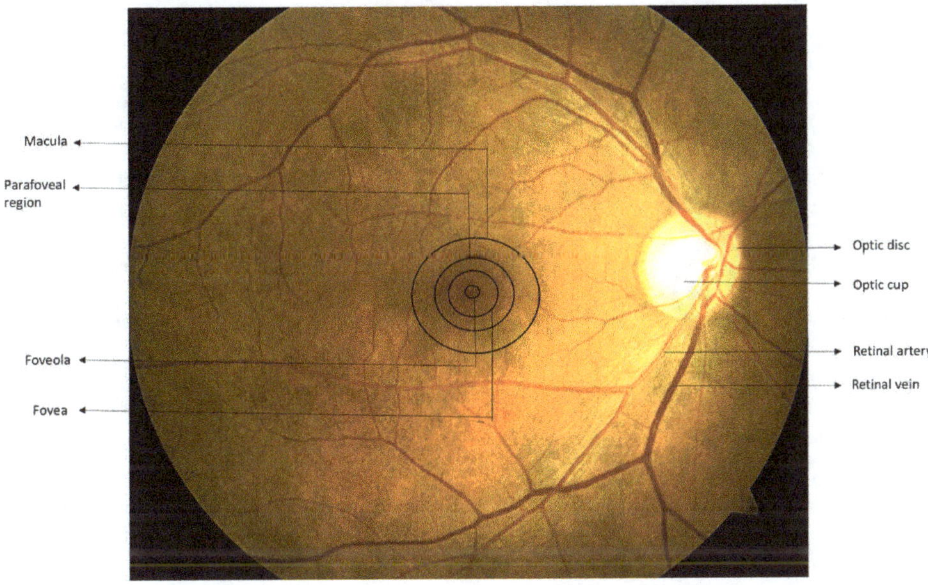

Fig.1.8. Fundus photograph showing the posterior pole and its important landmarks.

  - Fovea centralis is the central depressed part of the macula, about 1500 µm in diameter
  - Foveola is the central shiny pit, about 350 µm in diameter, located 2 disc diameter temporal to the optic disc and 1 mm below the horizontal meridian
  - Foveal avascular zone comprises the foveola and some area surrounding it (total of 800 µm in diameter) that is devoid of any retinal capillaries
- Ora serrata
  - Serrated peripheral margin forming the anterior boundary of the retina
  - Retina is attached firmly to the vitreous and choroid
  - Pars plana extends anteriorly from the ora serrata

Layers of Retina

Based on light microscopy, the retina is made up of 10 layers from outward to inwards (Fig. 1.9)

Pigment epithelium

- Outermost layer consisting of a single layer of cells containing pigment
- Firmly adherent to underlying basal lamina (Bruch's membrane) of the choroid
- Functions:
  - Absorptions of light, blood retinal barrier, visual pigment regeneration and synthesis, and removal of debris from photoreceptors by phagocytic action

Photoreceptor layer

- Layer of rods and cones (photoreceptors) arranged in a palisade manner

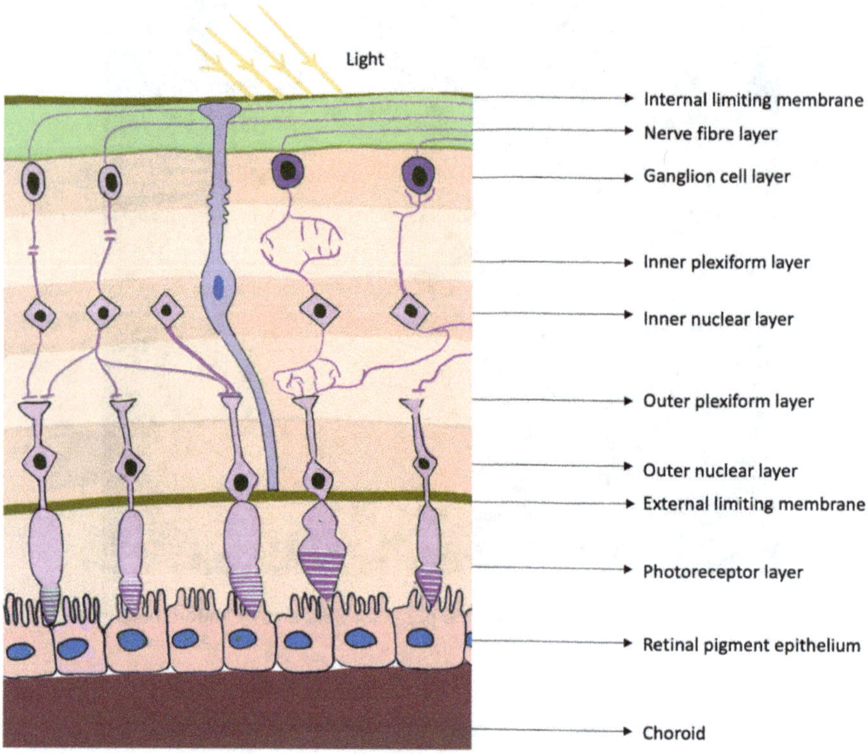

Fig. 1.9. Layers of the retina demonstrating various neuronal connections.

- Human eye consists of about 120 million rods and 6.5 million cones
- Functions:
  - Rods — night (scotopic) vision
  - Cones — daylight (photopic) vision and colour vision
- Rods and cones are the end-organs of vision that transform light energy into visual (nerve) impulse

External limiting membrane

- Junction between cell membrane of photoreceptors and Müller's cells
- The processes of rods and cones pass through this fenestrated membrane
- Functions:
  - Selective barrier for nutrients
  - Stabilisation of the transducing portion of photoreceptors

Outer nuclear layer

- Nuclei of rods and cones

Outer plexiform layer

- Connections of rod spherules and cone pedicle with dendrites of bipolar and horizontal cells

- Functions:
  - Transmission and amplification of electric potential
  - Functional barrier to diffusion of fluids and metabolites
- Clinical significance: Hard exudates, dot and blot haemorrhges are found in this layer

Inner nuclear layer

- Bipolar, horizontal and amacrine cell bodies
- Function: Numerous cells and extensive cellular connections of INL is essential for transduction and amplification of light signals
- Bipolar cells — first-order neurons. Relay information from photoreceptors to horizontal, amacrine and ganglion cells
- Horizontal cells — modulate and transform visual information received from photoreceptors
- Amacrine cells — modulate the electrical information reaching the ganglion cells

Inner plexiform layer

- Connections of axons of bipolar cells with dendrites of ganglion cells and processes of amacrine cells

Ganglion cell layer

- Cell bodies of ganglion cells (second-order neurons)
- Function: Transmission of signals from bipolar cells to lateral geniculate body

Nerve fibre layer

- Axons of ganglion cells
- Usually unmyelinated within the retina
- Clinical significance: Cotton wool spots (infarcts) and flame-shaped haemorrhages are found in this layer

Internal limiting membrane

- Innermost layer of retina separating it from the vitreous
- Basement membrane formed by the union of terminal expansions of Müller's cells

Structure of Fovea Centralis (Fig. 1.10)

- Fovea: 1500 μm central depression of inner retinal surface within the macula
- Corresponds to FAZ (foveal avascular zone)
- No rods. Cones are tightly packed and the other layers of the retina are thin
- Contains taller RPE cells and xanthophyll pigments
- Foveola: 350 μm avascular central area of fovea. Absence of ganglion cells and other nucleated cells.

Why is fovea dark?

RPE cells at the fovea are taller and thinner and contain more pigment granules, thereby giving a dark colour to this area as compared to the rest of the retina.

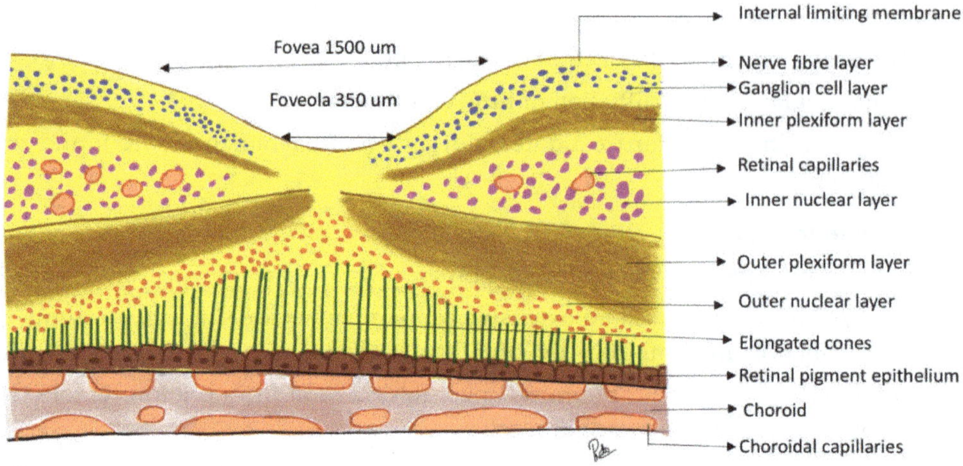

Fig. 1.10. Cross-section at the fovea. Note the difference in architecture of the layers at the fovea compared to rest of the retina.

Blood Supply of the Retina

- The central retinal artery is a branch of the ophthalmic artery. It is an end artery that enters the optic nerve nearly 1 cm behind the globe. After emerging from the centre of the optic cup, it divides into 4 branches (supero-nasal, supero-temporal, infero-nasal and infero-temporal).
- Retinal veins follow the pattern of arteries. They drain into the cavernous sinus either directly or via the superior ophthalmic vein.
- Inner 6 layers of the retina are supplied by the central retinal artery
- Outer 4 layers are supplied by choroidal vessels

Take Home Messages

- There are 10 layers of the retina and each layer plays a different function.
- Macula is further subdivided into 3 zones.
- The photoreceptors comprise cones and rods, and they are distributed differently in the retina.
- There is dual blood supply to the retinal layers.

1.6 Eyelid

Learning Objectives

- Understand the topographical and cross-sectional anatomy of the eyelid — blood and nerve supply.
- Learn the function of the eyelid.

Lamellae of the Upper Eyelid (Fig. 1.11 and Fig. 1.12)

Anterior: skin, orbicularis
Posterior: tarsus, levator aponeurosis, Müller's muscle, palpebral conjunctiva

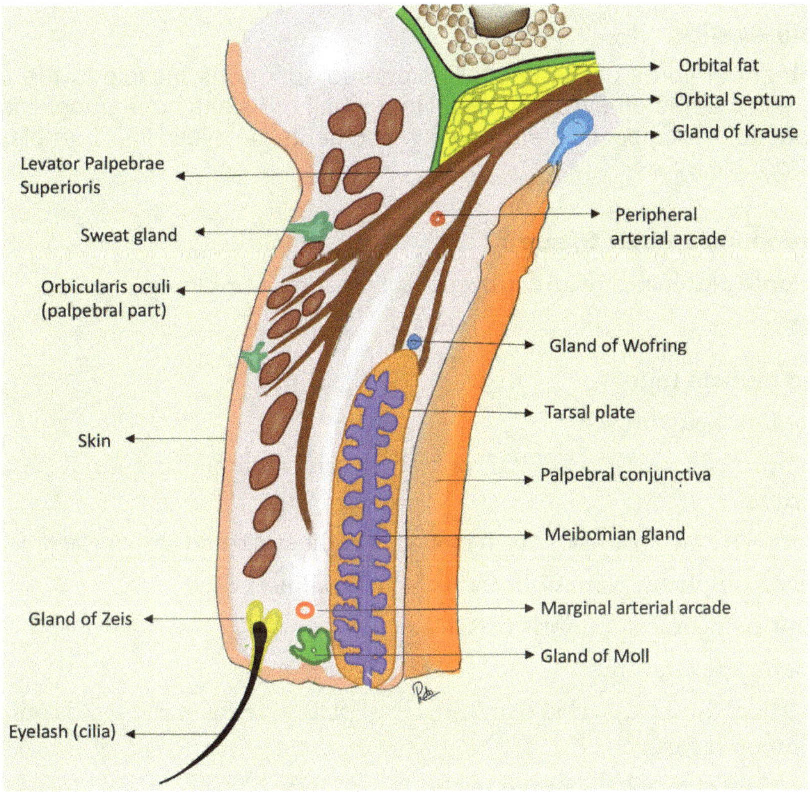

Fig. 1.11. Anatomy of the upper eyelid.

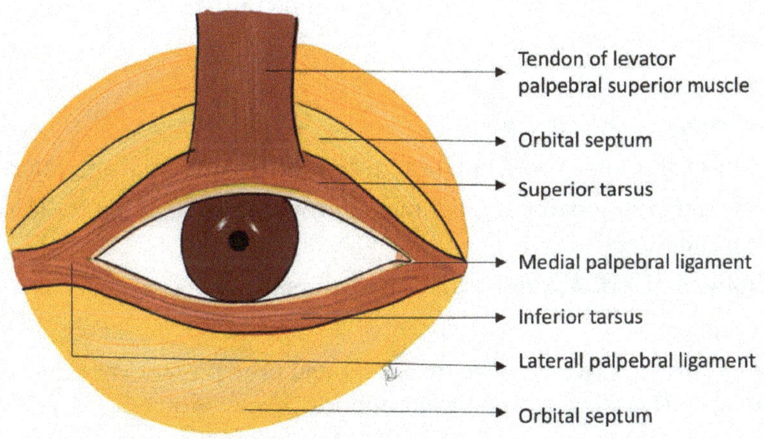

Fig. 1.12. Anatomy of the fibrous layer of the eyelid showing tarsal plates and orbital septum.

The following are the structures found in eyelids from superficial to deep:

Skin

- Thinnest in the body

Double eyelids

Attachment of fibres of the levator palpebrae superioris muscle to the upper eyelid skin creates an eyelid crease. Nearly half of Asians have upper lids with a low but defined upper lid crease, which segments the eyelid into 2 visible parts called "double eyelids".

Subcutaneous areolar tissue

- Very loose and hence readily distended by oedema or blood
- No fat

Striated muscle layer

- Orbicularis oculi muscle
  - Comprises 3 parts — orbital, palpebral (pretarsal and preseptal parts) and lacrimal.
  - Function: closure of eyelids, main protractor of the eyelid and acts as a lacrimal pump
  - Nerve supply: zygomatic branch of the facial nerve
- Levator palpebrae superioris (LPS)
  - Origin: apex of orbit
  - Insertion: (by 3 parts) skin of eyelid, tarsal plate anterior surface and conjunctiva of superior fornix
  - Function: elevates the upper eyelid
  - Nerve supply: oculomotor nerve

Fibrous layer

- Forms the structural framework of eyelids and consists of tarsal plate centrally and orbital septum peripherally
- Tarsal plate
  - Dense connective tissue layer
  - The upper and lower tarsal plates are connected at medial and lateral canthi
  - Medial and lateral palpebral ligaments provided attachment for tarsal plates with orbital margin
  - Meibomian glands are embedded in the tarsal plates
- Orbital septum
  - Forms a barrier between eyelid anteriorly and orbit posteriorly; prevents spread of infection/oedema/blood/inflammation
  - Attachments: periosteum of orbital margin and tarsal plates

Non-striated muscle layer

- Palpebral muscle of Müller: lies deep to the orbital septum
- Origin: upper lid — from fibres of the LPS muscle; lower lid — prolongation of the inferior rectus muscle
- Insertion: peripheral margin of tarsal plate
- Nerve supply: sympathetic fibres

Palpebral conjunctiva

- Inner lining of eyelids
- 3 parts: marginal, tarsal and orbital

Landmarks on Eyelid Margins (Anterior to Posterior)

- Lash line: 2 to 3 rows of nearly 100 lashes in upper lid and 50 lashes in lower lid
- Grey line: junction of anterior and posterior lamellae. Vascular watershed area
- Meibomian gland orifices: nearly 30 in upper lid and 20 in lower lid

Eyelid laceration repair

For full-thickness eyelid lacerations involving the lid margin, the proper technique of repair involving suturing of the tarsal plate(partial thickness), meimobian gland orifices, lash line and skin sequentially is essential for restoring the structural integrity of the eyelid.

Glands of Eyelids

Table 1.1 Glands of Eyelids

Gland	Location	Features
Meibomian/tarsal	Within tarsus	Opens at lid margin Oily layer of tear film
Glands of Zeis	Near lid margin Associated with cilia	Opens into follicles of eyelashes Lubricates cilia
Glands of Moll	Near lid margin	Lubricates cilia
Accessory lacrimal glands: Krause	Superior fornix	Basal tear secretion (aqueous)
Wolfring	Just above tarsus	
Sweat gland	Skin	Electrolyte balance
Goblet cells	Conjunctiva Plica Caruncle	Mucin secretion Corneal wetting

Blood Supply

Arterial supply

- Medial palpebral arteries (arising from a ophthalmic artery) and lateral palpebral arteries (arising from a lacrimal artery) form the marginal arterial arcade
- Another arcade (superior arterial arcade) is present in the upper lid. It lies near the upper border of the tarsus
- Anastomoses between the facial artery (derived from the external carotid) and palpebral arteries (derived from the internal carotid) are present at the medial and lateral aspect of eyelids

Venous drainage

Arranged in 2 plexus:

- Pre-tarsal: opening into subcutaneous veins
- Post-tarsal: drains into the ophthalmic vein

Lymphatics

Arranged in 2 sets:

- Pre-tarsal and post-tarsal
- Lateral ½ of lids drain into preauricular nodes and medial ½ drains into submandibular nodes

Nerve Supply

Motor

- Facial N — orbicularis muscle
- Oculomotor N — levator palpabrea superioris muscle
- Sympathetic fibres — Müller's muscle

Sensory

- Upper lid: branches of V1 of the trigeminal nerve (lacrimal, supraorbital and supratrochlear)
- Lower lid: branches of V2 of the trigeminal nerve (infratrochlear) along with branches of infraorbital (V1)

Take Home Messages

- The eyelid can be divided into the anterior and posterior lamellae.
- There are 3 distinct landmarks on the eyelid margins, which is relevant to eyelid laceration repair.

1.7 Orbit

Learning Objectives

- Understand the orbital wall boundaries and its bony parts.
- Learn the relationship of the orbital walls with the blood and nerve supply that enters/exits the orbit.

The bony orbits are pear/pyramid-shaped cavities sandwiched between the anterior cranial fossa and maxillary sinus; made up of 7 bones (Fig. 1.13).

Each orbit is about 30 mL in volume. One-fifth is occupied by the eyeball.

Floor

- Thin, triangular-shaped
- Formed primarily by the orbital plate of the maxilla with contributions from zygomatic and palatine bones
- Before puberty, these bones are not calcified and more prone to "trap-door" type fracture
- The infraorbital nerve traverses the floor in the infraorbital groove and descends anteriorly in the infraorbital canal. It exits the orbit via the infraorbital foramen just below the inferior orbital rim.

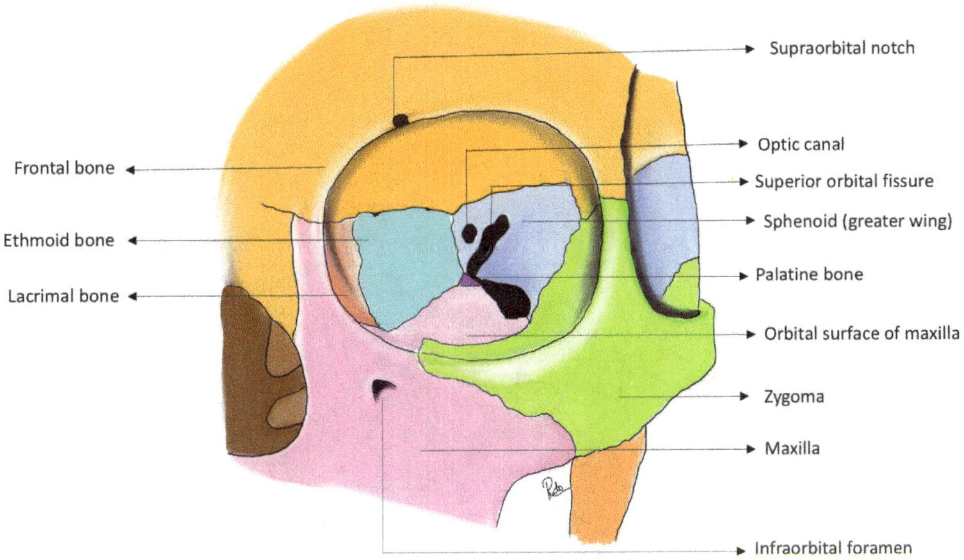

Fig. 1.13. Bony architecture of orbit. Note the various bones forming the different walls of the orbit.

- Easily involved in orbital blow-out fractures and easily invaded by a tumour of the maxillary sinus.

Lateral Wall

- Triangular; covers only the posterior half of the eyeball. Surgical approach to orbit via lateral orbitotomy is popular
- Formed by zygomatic bone anteriorly and greater wing of sphenoid posteriorly

Roof

- Formed by the orbital plate of the frontal bone and lesser wing of the sphenoid
- Separates orbit from anterior cranial fossa

Medial Wall

- Medial walls of 2 orbits are parallel to each other
- Thinnest of orbital walls (hence aka *lamina papyracea*) — frequently fractured
- Formed by maxilla, lacrimal, ethmoid and body of the sphenoid bone

Orbital Apex

Posterior convergence of 4 orbital walls. Consists of the following orifices: superior orbital fissure, inferior orbital fissure and optic canal. (Fig. 1.14.)

Optic Canal

- Transmits optic nerve and ophthalmic artery

Superior Orbital Fissure

- Slit between cranium and orbit, lying between greater and lesser wings of sphenoid bones

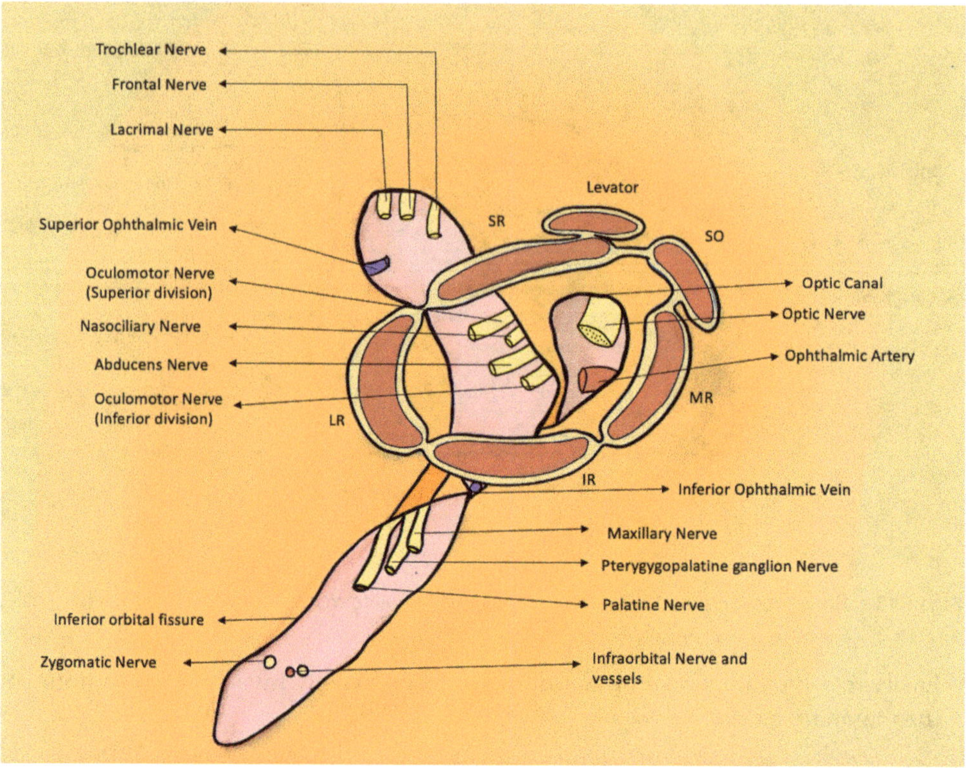

Fig. 1.14. Anatomy of superior and inferior orbital fissures. Note the various important structures traversing it.

- Lacrimal, frontal, trochlear nerve and superior ophthalmic vein pass through the superior orbital fissure above the tendinous ring
- Nasociliary, abducent and oculomotor nerve (superior and inferior divisions) pass inside the tendinous ring
- Inferior ophthalmic vein pass inferior to tendinous ring
- Inflammation of the Superior Orbital Fissure or Orbital apex may result in a multitude of signs like ophthalmoplegia and venous outflow obstruction

Inferior Orbital Fissure

- Slit between the greater wing of the sphenoid and the maxilla
- Connects the orbit to the pterygopalatine and infraorbital fossae
- Continuous with the infraorbital canal
- Transmits branches of the maxillary nerve, and an emissary vein connecting ophthalmic vein to pterygoid plexus

Orbital Fascia (Fig. 1.15)

- Thin connective tissue membrane lining various intraorbital structures
- Divided into fascia bulbi (Tenon's capsule), which envelopes the globe from the limbus to optic nerve, muscular sheaths, intermuscular septa, membranous expansion of muscles and ligament of Lockwood (thickened lower part in the form of a hammock or sling on which the globe sits)

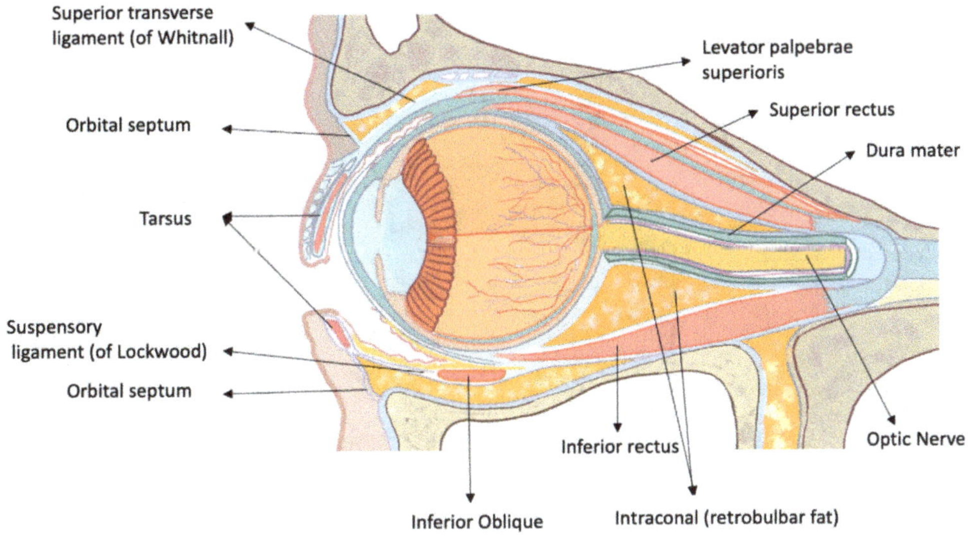

Fig. 1.15. Orbital fascia: Sagittal section of orbit showing orbital fascial architecture in relation to different structures.

Take Home Messages

- The orbit comprises 4 walls arranged in a pyramidal fashion and has 2 main orifices — optic canal and orbital fissure.
- The medial wall and floor of the orbit are thin and are prone to fractures in trauma.
- The orbital apex region has to accommodate multiple structures, including the recti muscles, cranial nerves and large orbital vessels.

1.8 Lacrimal System

Learning Objective

Understand the lacrimal drainage pathway of the eye.

Lacrimal Gland

- Almond-shaped gland located in the orbital part of the frontal bone. Lateral expansion of levator aponeurosis divides it into orbital and palpebral lobes.
- Exocrine glands producing serous secretions
- About 12 lacrimal ducts pass through the palpebral lobe and empty into the conjunctival fornix

Puncta (Fig. 1.16)

- 2 in number: upper and lower
- Located at the junction of the lash-bearing lateral 5/6th (pars cilia) and the medial non-ciliated 1/6th (pars lacrimalis), at the posterior edge of the lid margin about 6 mm from the medial canthus, lower slightly more temporal
- Slightly inverted against globe. Examined by everting the eyelid

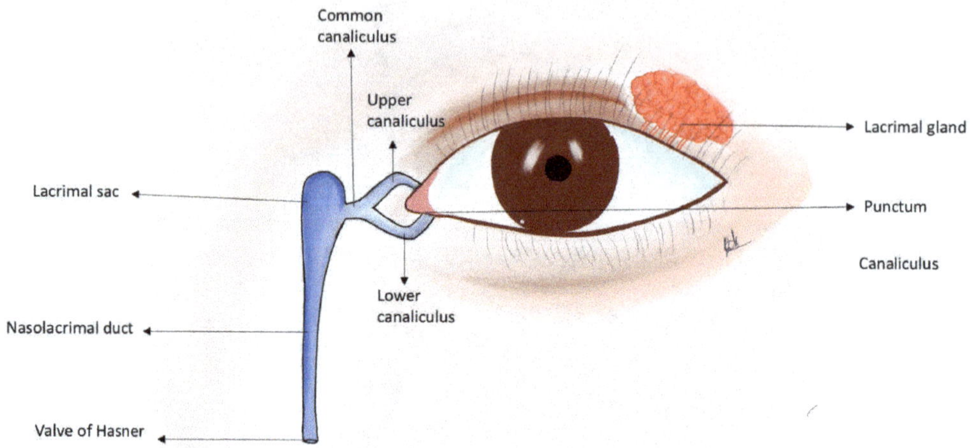

Fig. 1.16. Anatomy of the lacrimal system.

Canaliculi

- 10 mm long (2 mm vertical segment [ampulla] and 8 mm horizontal portion parallel to the lid margin)
- Combine to form a single canaliculus in 90% of individuals
- Reflux from the lacrimal sac to the canaliculus is prevented by valve of Rosenmuller

Nasolacrimal Sac

- 10–12 mm long
- Lies between the anterior and posterior medial canthal tendon, lodged in the lacrimal fossa in between the anterior and posterior lacrimal crests
- Lies lateral to middle meatus of the nose, separated by the lacrimal bone and frontal process of maxilla

Nasolacrimal Duct

- 12–18 mm long inferior continuation of the lacrimal sac
- Lies within the lacrimal canal formed by the maxillary and lacrimal bones, passing inferiorly, posteriorly and laterally
- Opens into the ipsilateral inferior meatus. Opening is covered by a partial fold of mucosa called valve of Hasner

Physiology

- Tears are secreted by the main and accessory lacrimal gland, pass along the ocular surface and enter the upper and lower canaliculi by capillary action and suction
- When eyelids close, ampullae are compressed by pretarsal orbicularis oculi, horizontal canaliculi are shortened and compressed, puncta closed and moved

medially, resisting reflux. Also, by the contraction of the lacrimal part of the orbicularis oculi, positive pressure is created, forcing tears down the nasolacrimal duct into the nose, mediated by connective tissue fibres around the sac

- When eyelids open, negative pressure is created as the canaliculi and sac expand, drawing tears from the canaliculi into the sac

Take Home Message

Tears drain from the puncta through the canaliculi and into the nasolacrimal sac/duct.

1.9 Visual Pathway

Learning Objectives

- Learn the visual pathway from the optic nerve up to the visual cortex.
- The relationship of the optic chiasm with the intracranial structures.
- Familiarise with reflex pupillary pathways.

Visual Pathway Comprises Optic nerve, optic chiasm, optic tract, lateral geniculate body, optic radiations and visual cortex. Image from the temporal part of the visual field falls on the nasal retina and vice versa for each eye.

Optic nerve (Fig. 1.17)

- 47–50 mm in length.
- Distal continuation of the nerve fiber layer of retina consisting of axon of ganglion cells

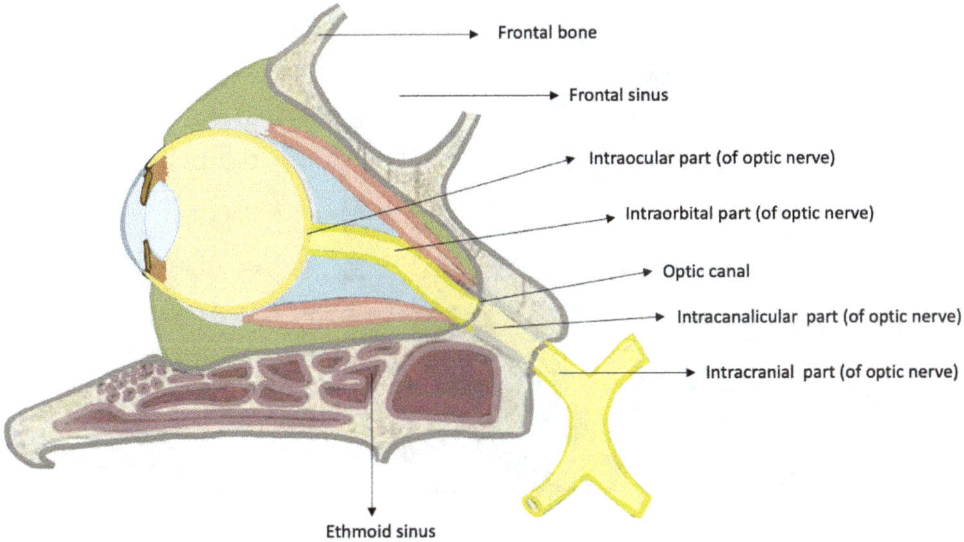

Fig. 1.17. Parts of the optic nerve.

- Parts of the optic nerve:
  - Intraocular part (1 mm): Starts from the optic disc and pierces the choroid and sclera (lamina cribrosa)
  - Intraorbital part (25 mm-longest): Extends posteriorly until optic foramina, where it is surrounded by Annulus of Zinn (refer to Fig. 1.14). Optic nerve is myelinated posterior to the lamina cribrosa. Central Retina Artery enters and the central Retinal Vein exits the dural sheath here
  - Intracanalicular part (5 mm): Within the optic canal, the nerve is closely related to the ophthalmic artery, which lies inferolaterally initially and later crosses obliquely over it to lie medially
  - Intracranial part (10 mm): Travels upwards, backwards and medially to reach the optic chiasm

Optic chiasm (Fig. 1.18)

- Location — Over the tuberculum and diaphragm sellae. Hence, visual field defects are seen in patients with pituitary tumour having suprasellar extension
- Important relations
  - Superiorly: floor of 3rd ventricle, lamina terminalis and anterior communicating artery
  - Inferiorly: diaphragma sellae

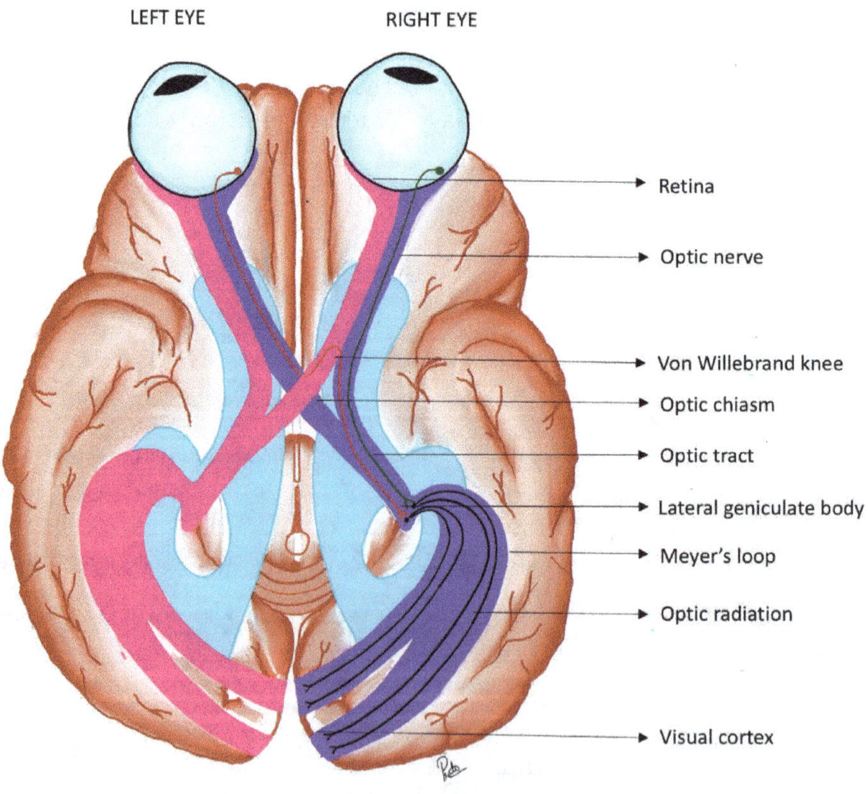

Fig. 1.18. Anatomy of the visual pathway.

  - Anteriorly: anterior cerebral artery
  - Posteriorly: tuber cinereum (base of pituitary stalk), mammillary bodies
  - Laterally: internal carotid artery and cavernous sinus
- Optic nerve fibres from the nasal retina undergo decussation at the optic chiasm
- Wilbrand knee: small anterior loop of nerve fibres from nasal retinal that travel a short distance in the contralateral prechiasmatic optic nerve after decussation at the chiasm

Optic tract

- Cylindrical bundle of nerve fibres extending outwards and backwards from the posterolateral aspect of optic chiasm to lateral geniculate body (LGB)
- Contains fibres from temporal retina of the ipsilateral eye and nasal retina of the contralateral eye
- The pupillary reflex fibres pass on to the pretectal nucleus, bypassing the LGB

Lateral geniculate body

- Oval structures at termination of the optic tract
- Consists of 6 layers of neurons
- Layers 2, 3 and 5 receive fibres from the temporal retina of the ipsilateral eye and layers 1, 4 and 6 receive fibres from the nasal retina of the opposite eye
- Second-order neurons relay in LGB

Optic radiations

- Third-order neurons of the visual pathway
- Extends from LGB to the visual cortex passing forward initially, then laterally and then spreads out like a fan, forming medullary optic lamina
- Superior fibres subserving the inferior visual field traverse posteriorly through the parietal lobe
- Inferior fibres subserving the superior visual field sweep anteroinferiorly in Meyer's loop and traverse through the temporal lobe

Visual cortex

- Located at the medial aspect of each occipital lobe, in the area above and below the calcarine fissure
- 2 divisions:
  - Primary visual cortex/visuosensory area: striate area 17
  - Secondary visual cortex/visuopsychic area: peristriate area 18 and parastriate area 19

Blood Supply of the Visual Pathway

Except the orbital part of the optic nerve, which is supplied by an axial system derived from the central retinal artery, the remainder of the visual pathway is supplied by a pial network of vessels. The pial plexus gets contribution from different arteries at different levels of the visual pathway, as shown in Fig. 1.19.

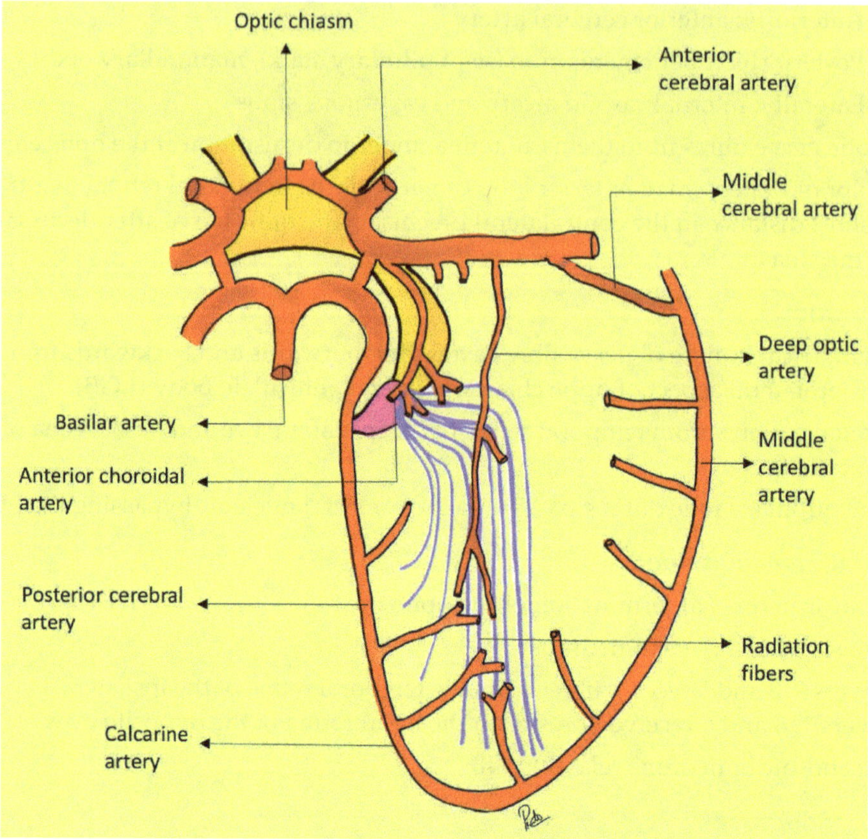

Fig. 1.19. Blood supply to the various parts of visual pathway.

Blood Supply of the Optic Nerve (Fig. 1.20)

- Prelaminar portion: Centripetal branches from peripapillary choroidal vessels
- Lamina cribrosa: Short posterior ciliary arteries that form the circle of Zinn. No significant anastomoses with branches of the central retinal artery
- Retrolaminar: Mainly by centripetal branches from the pial plexus and also from branches of the central retinal artery

Pupillary Reflex

Shining light in one eye causes constriction of pupils in both eyes. Constriction of the pupil in the eye where light is shone is called direct light reflex and constriction of the pupil in the fellow eye is called consensual (indirect) light reflex

Pathway (Fig. 1.21)

- Afferent fibres travel along the optic nerve and extend from the retina to the pretectal nucleus in the mid-brain at the level of superior colliculus
- At the optic chiasm, fibres from the nasal retina decussate to the optic tract on the opposite side and terminate in the contralateral pretectal nucleus. Fibres from the temporal retina remain uncrossed and terminate in the ipsilateral pretectal nucleus

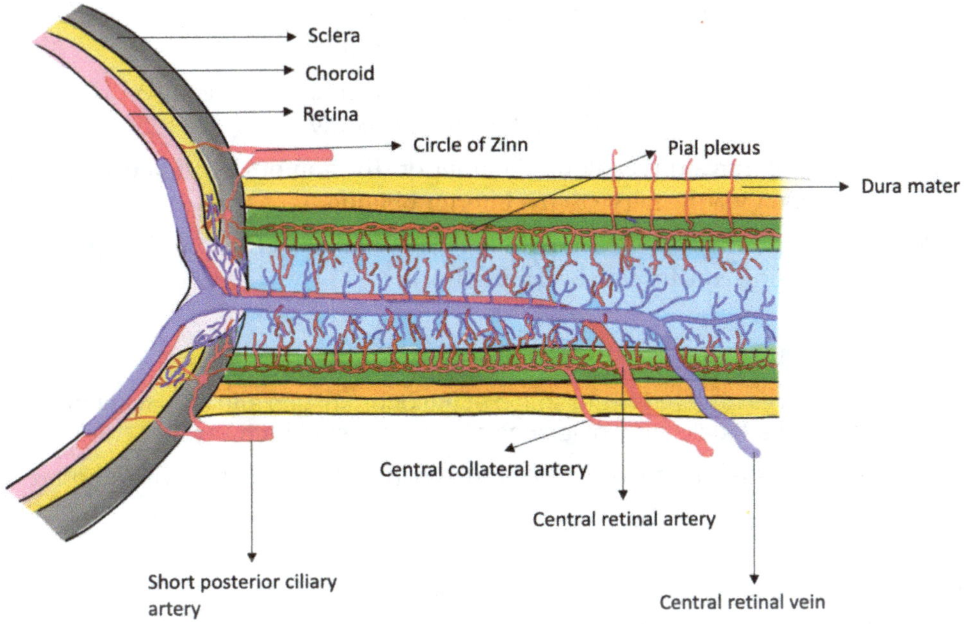

Fig. 1.20. The sheath and vascular supply to the intraocular and intraorbital portions of the optic nerve.

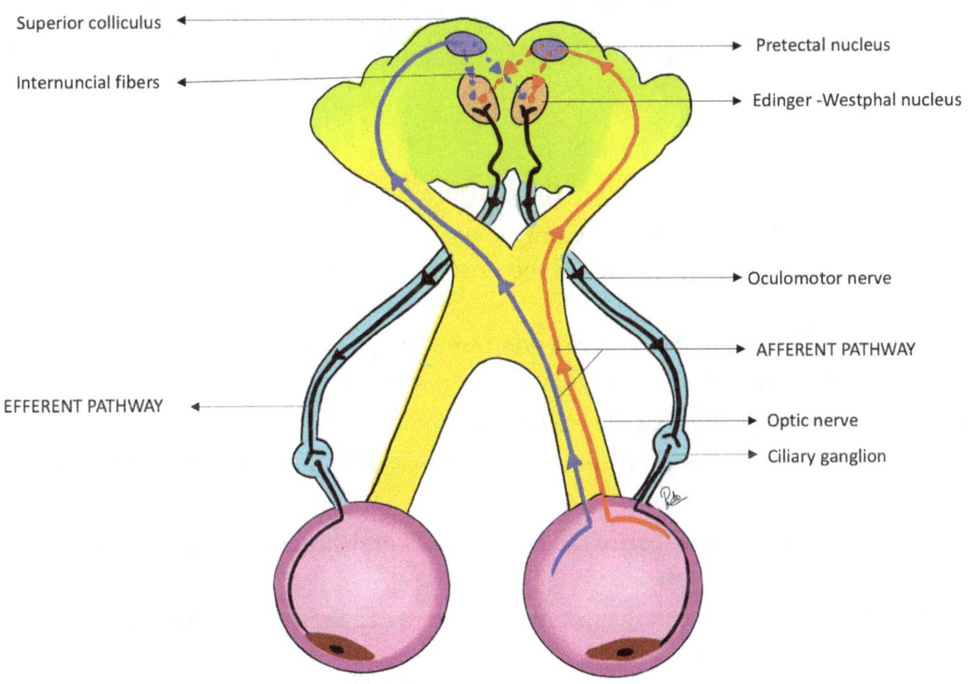

Fig. 1.21. Pupillary reflex pathway.

- Each pretectal nucleus is connected with Edinger-Westphal nuclei of both sides via internuncial fibres. (This forms the basis of consensual response.)
- Parasympathetic fibres arising from Edinger-Westphal nucleus travel along the oculomotor nerve (CN III) to form the efferent pathway
- Pre-ganglionic fibres travel along the inferior division of CN III and reach the ciliary ganglion via the nerve to the inferior oblique
- Post-ganglionic fibres travel via short ciliary nerves to supply the sphincter pupillae, causing constriction of the pupil

Take Home Messages

- The nerve fibres undergo decussation at the optic chiasm and it is an important landmark in the localisation of lesions along the visual pathway.
- The visual fields are represented differently in the retina and at the visual cortex.

1.10 Selected Cranial Nerves Related to Ophthalmology

Learning Objectives

- Understand the pathway and function of the oculomotor, trochlear and abducens nerve.
- Learn the components and their relationship within the cavernous sinus.

Oculomotor Nerve (Cranial Nerve 3) (Fig. 1.22)

- Oculomotor nuclei are found in the mid-brain adjacent to the superior colliculi
- Passes anteriorly through the red nucleus and emerges on the ventral side of the mid-brain, where it lies between the posterior cerebral artery and the superior cerebellar artery
- Then, it lies parallel to the posterior communicating artery (PCA), hence aneurysms of PCA may compress the nerve, causing paresis
- Runs in the lateral wall of the cavernous sinus
- Divides into superior and inferior branches before entering the orbit via the superior orbital fissure
- All extraocular muscles except the lateral rectus and superior oblique are supplied by the oculomotor nerve
- Inferior branch carries parasympathetic supply to the ciliary ganglion

Trochlear Nerve (Cranial Nerve 4) (Fig. 1.23)

- Trochlear nerve nuclei are found in the mid-brain at the level of the inferior colliculus
- After emerging from the nucleus, the fibres undergo decussation before exiting from the dorsal aspect of the brainstem (hence supplying the contralateral superior oblique muscle because of the decussation)

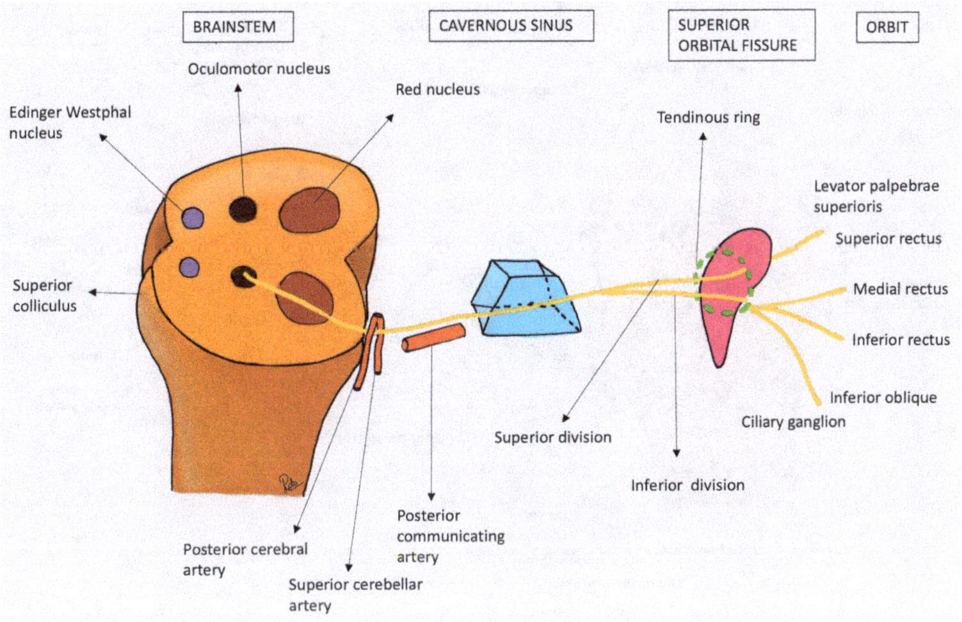

Fig. 1.22. Pictorial description of course of the oculomotor nerve.

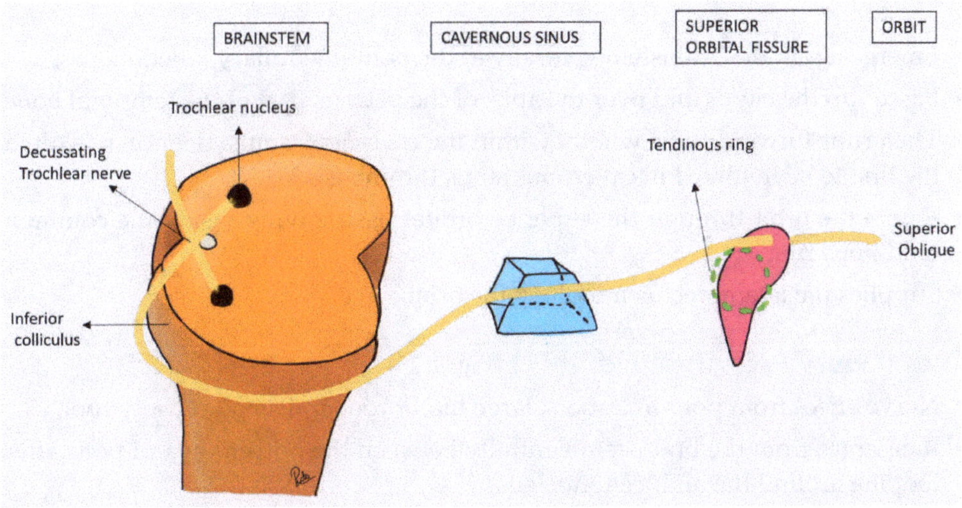

Fig. 1.23. Pictorial description of course of the trochlear nerve.

- It turns around the cerebral peduncles to enter the lateral wall of the cavernous sinus
- Enters the orbit through the superior orbital fissure lying outside the tendinous ring
- The trochlear nerve innervates the superior oblique muscle

Abducens Nerve (Cranial Nerve 6) (Fig. 1.24)

- Nucleus lies at the level of the pons, ventral to the floor of the fourth ventricle. Facial nerve passes over it, forming the facial colliculus

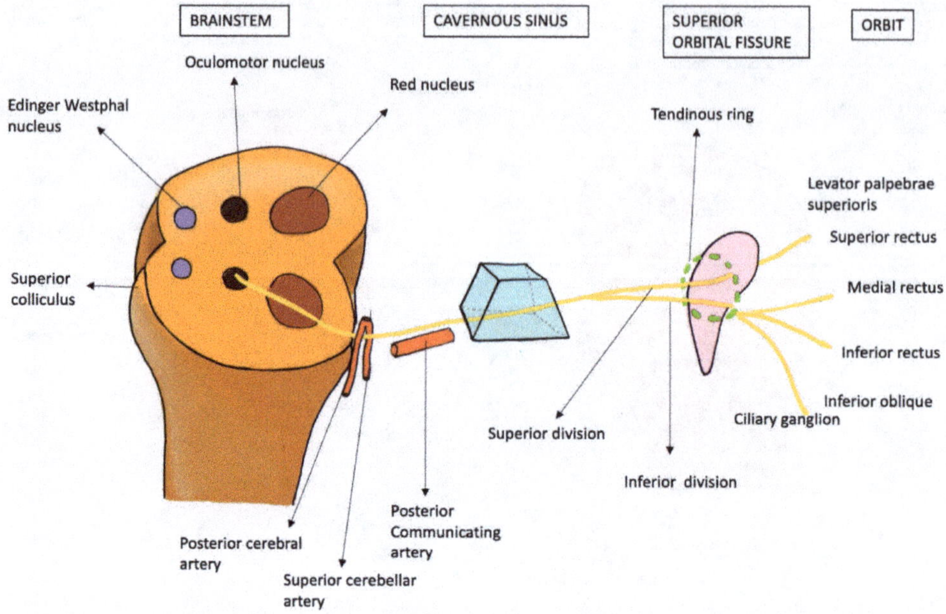

Fig. 1.24. Pictorial description of course of the abducens nerve.

- Emerges from the brainstem ventrally at the pontomedullary junction
- Passes up the clivus and over the apex of the petrous part of the temporal bone
- Then runs forward to lie wholly within the cavernous sinus. (Hence, it is often the first to be involved in cavernous sinus thrombosis.)
- Enters the orbit through the superior orbital fissure lying inside the common tendinous ring
- Supplies the lateral rectus muscle in the orbit

Facial Nerve (Cranial Nerve 7) (Fig. 1.25)

- Nerve arises from pons as 2 roots: large motor root and small sensory root
- It emerges from the brainstem ventrally between the mid-brain and pons after looping around the abducent nucleus
- 2 roots travel through the internal acoustic meatus
- After leaving the meatus, enters the z-shaped facial canal
- Within the facial canal:
  - The 2 roots fuse
  - Nerve forms geniculate ganglion
  - The nerve gives rise to the greater petrosal nerve, nerve to stapedius and chorda tympani
- Exits the facial canal through the stylomastoid foramen

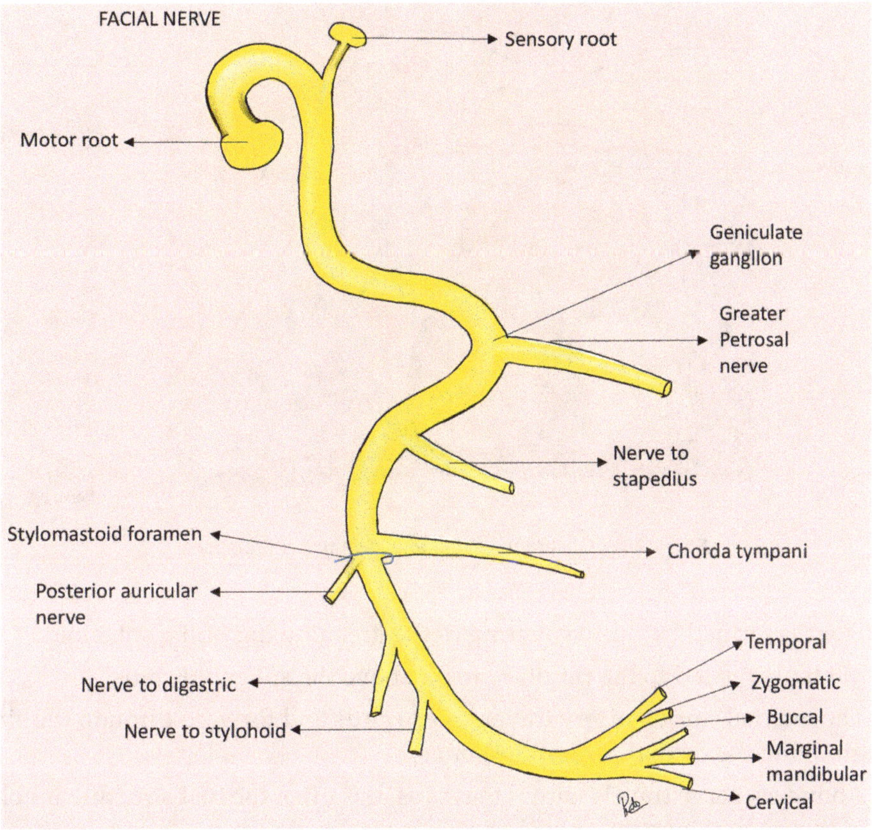

Fig. 1.25. Pictorial description of the course of the facial nerve and its various branches.

- Turns superiorly and runs anterior to the outer ear. Gives rise to the posterior auricular nerve, nerve to digastric and stylohyoid
- Within the parotid gland, the nerve terminates by splitting into 5 terminal motor branches:
  - Temporal — supplies frontalis, orbicularis oculi and corrugator supercilii
  - Zygomatic — supplies orbicularis oculi
  - Buccal — supplies orbicularis oculi, buccinator and zygomaticus
  - Marginal mandibular — supplies mentalis
  - Cervical — supplies platysma

Cavernous Sinus

- Cavernous sinuses are located on either side of the body of the sphenoid bone

  Important contents and relations of the cavernous sinus (Fig. 1.26):
  - Extends from the superior orbital fissure anteriorly to the apex of the petrous part of the temporal bone posteriorly

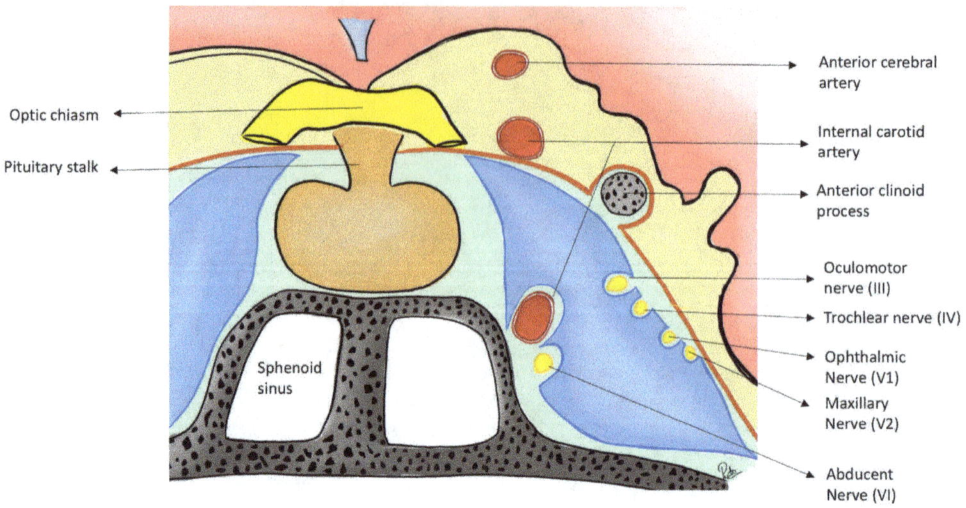

Fig. 1.26. Cavernous sinus and its important relations.

– Floor is formed by dural covering of the greater wing of the sphenoid
– Medially related to the pituitary fossa above the sphenoid sinus
– The internal carotid artery traverses upwards and forward through the sinus, grooving the medial wall of the sinus
– Abducens nerve travels within the sinus. It is often the first structure involved in cavernous sinus thrombosis
– The lateral wall encloses the oculomotor nerve, trochlear nerve and the first 2 divisions of the trigeminal nerve
– Tributaries of the cavernous sinus:
  ▪ Superior ophthalmic vein
  ▪ Inferior ophthalmic vein
  ▪ Superficial middle cerebral veins
  ▪ Inferior cerebral veins
  ▪ Sphenoparietal sinus
– Drainage of the cavernous sinus is via the superior and inferior petrosal sinus as well as the venous plexus around the internal carotid artery and emissary veins through the skull base foramina
– Interconnections exist between the right and left cavernous sinuses. Hence, infection of one side can spread and manifest in the opposite side

Take Home Messages

- All extraocular muscles except the lateral rectus and superior oblique are supplied by the oculomotor nerve.
- The trochlear nerve innervates the superior oblique muscle.
- The abducens nerve supplies the lateral rectus muscle.
- Infection in the cavernous sinus can spread to the opposite side.

References

1. American Academy of Ophthalmology — *Fundamentals and Principles of Ophthalmology.*
2. Snell R. *Clinical Anatomy of the Eye.*

Chapter 2

CORNEA AND EXTERNAL EYE DISEASES

Chai Hui Chen Charmaine, Ray Manotosh

2.1 Basic Anterior Segment Examination

Learning Objectives

- Recognising and understanding common corneal pathologies.
- Recognising normal and pathological slit-lamp examination findings.
- Ability to incorporate clinical findings with various common pathological cornea and external eye conditions.

Anterior segment examination can be performed grossly with the use of a torch light or direct ophthalmoscope. However, a detailed examination would require the proficient use of the slit-lamp biomicroscope (Fig. 2.1). A good understanding of the anterior segment anatomy is essential for the identification of the various structures seen the slit-lamp biomicroscope (Fig. 2.2).

Slit-lamp Examination Findings Based on Anatomy

Table 2.1. Slit-lamp Examination Findings Based on Anatomy

	Findings to Look Out For
Conjunctival	Injection Nodules/growth (pinguecula, pterygium)
Cornea	Epithelial erosions/abrasions scars Infiltrates cornea oedema Cornea vascularisation
Anterior chamber	Anterior chamber depth Anterior chamber reaction — cells, flare Keratic precipitates
Iris	Nodules atrophy Synechiae (peripheral anterior synechiae, posterior synechiae) Vascularisation Abnormal pupil (corectopia, polycoria)

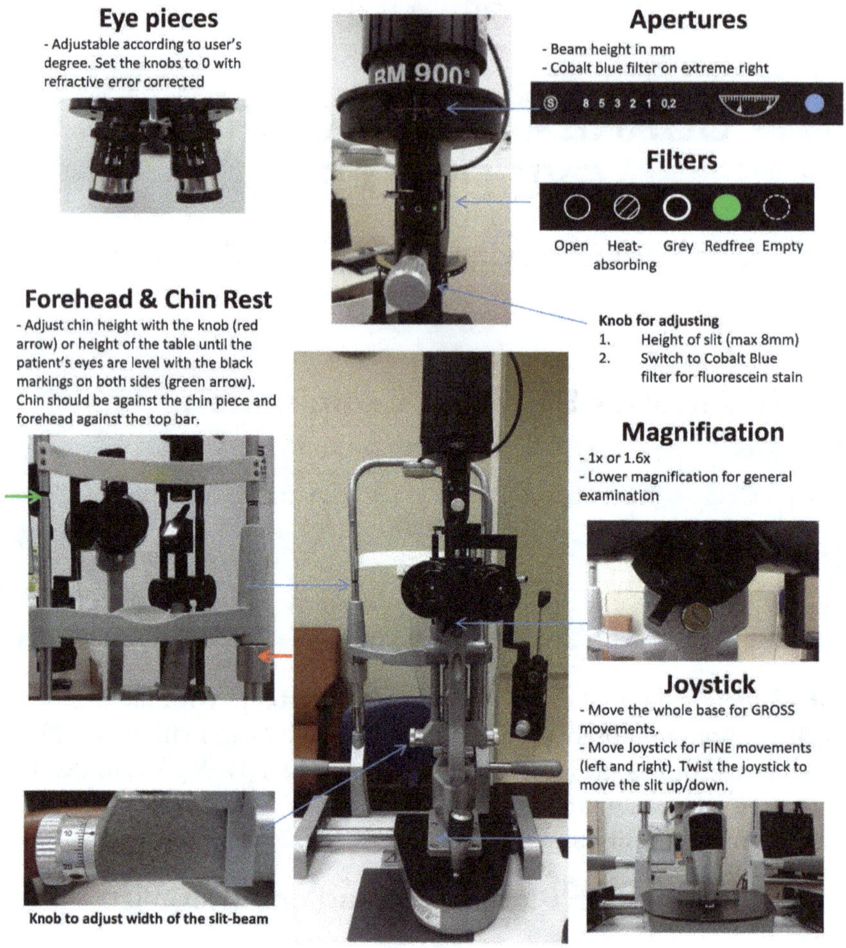

Fig. 2.1. Basic components of the slit-lamp biomicroscope.

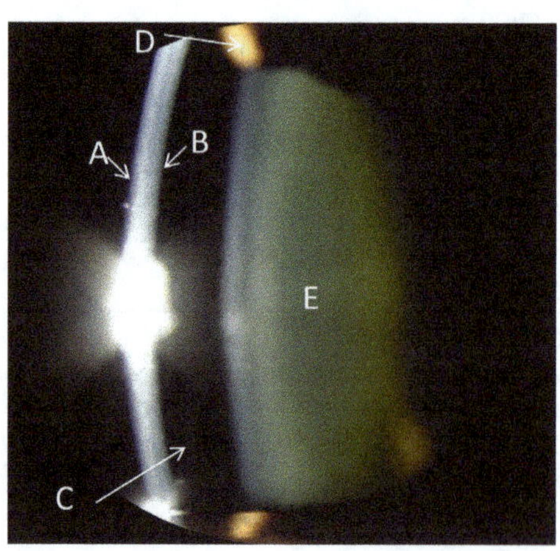

Fig. 2.2. Slit-beam image of the anterior segment demonstrating: (A) anterior corneal surface, (B) posterior corneal surface, (C) anterior chamber, (D) iris, and (E) cataract.

What are the Causes of a Red Eye?

Table 2.2. What are the Causes of a Red Eye?

	Ocular Causes	Extraocular Causes
Infective causes	Conjunctivitis Infective keratitis Endophthalmitis	Orbital cellulitis
Non-infective causes	Corneal abrasion Allergic conjunctivitis Blepharoconjunctivitis Marginal keratitis Uveitis Acute primary angle closure Episcleritis Scleritis Dry eyes Subconjunctival haemorrhage	Thyroid eye disease Carotid-cavernous sinus Fistula

What are the Uses of Fluorescein Stain?

- Checking of intraocular pressure with Goldmann applanation tonometry
- Fluorescein dye disappearance test
- Stains epithelial defects and epitheliopathy
- To check for "tear break-up time"
- Reduction in tear break-up time seen in dry eyes
- To check for wound leak ("Seidel's" test)
- Hard contact lens fitting

What Causes a Diffusely Hazy Cornea?

- Raised intraocular pressure (e.g. acute primary angle closure)
- Bullous keratopathy from endothelial failure

Hazy cornea can be identified based on the inability to check the iris details and the pupil margin. Comparison with the fellow eye can be made in unilateral cases.

What are the Causes of Focal Corneal Opacity?

- Infective keratitis
- Marginal keratitis
- Shield ulcer
- Corneal scar
  - Characterised by a quiescent eye — white conjunctiva, no surrounding corneal haze and no associated epithelial defect

Take Home Messages

- Not all red eyes are caused by viral conjunctivitis.
- Not all corneal opacities are infective in origin.

2.2 Subconjunctival Haemorrhage

Learning Objectives

- Recognise the appearance of subconjunctival haemorrhage.
- Management of subconjunctival haemorrhage.

What is a Subconjunctival Haemorrhage?

- Occurs due to a rupture of the conjunctival vessels
- Results in a homogenous red patch on the conjunctiva (Fig. 2.3)

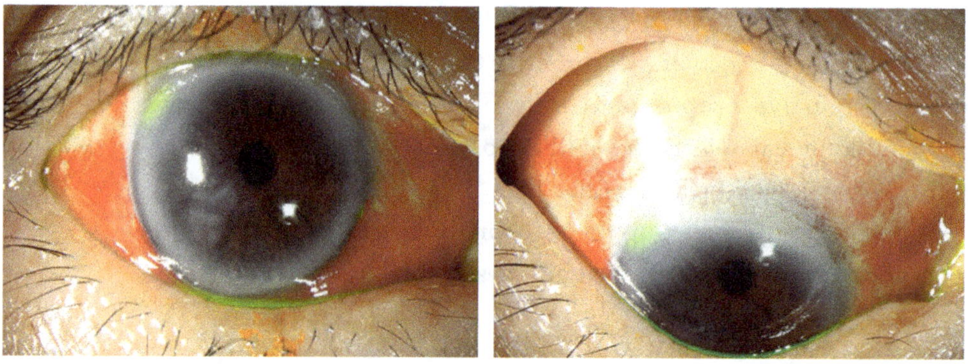

(A) (B)

Fig. 2.3. Demonstrating subconjunctival haemorrhage of the eye at post-operative day 1 after a cataract surgery.

What are the Risk Factors for this Occurring?

- Trauma
- Blood thinners (e.g. aspirin, warfarin, clopidogrel)
- Hypertension
- Valsalva manoeuvre (e.g. constipation, coughing)

What is the Typical History?

- Sudden onset of red eye
- Painless
- No associated blurring of vision
- May have associated risk factors

What History or Clinical Finding are You Concerned About?

- Trauma
  - Will need to exclude underlying scleral involvement
- Unable to see the posterior extent of subconjunctival haemorrhage
  - Need to rule out retrobulbar haemorrhage

How Would You Manage the Patient?

- Conservative
  - Reassurance. Majority are managed conservatively and will resolve in 1–2 weeks spontaneously.
- Further management is dependent on the presence of other ocular injuries

In a patient with no risk factors and recurrent subconjunctival haemorrhage, consider working up for haematological abnormalities.

Take Home Message

Subconjunctival haemorrhage is very common, and it is important to rule out severe trauma.

2.3 Corneal Infections

Learning Objectives

- Recognise the signs and symptoms of infective keratitis.
- Understanding the acute management of infective keratitis.

Infective keratitis can result from various types of organisms, including viral, bacterial, fungal, and parasitic. Viral, fungal and parasitic infections tend to occur more commonly in immunosuppressed individuals, while bacterial infections occur in those with other pre-existing risk factors. Contact lens use, ocular contact with contaminated water or solution, corneal trauma and prolonged topical steroid use are the main risk factors for many of these infections.

Table 2.3. Examples of Various Aetiological Causes of Infective Keratitis

Viral	Herpes simplex virus 1 Herpes simplex virus 2 Varicella zoster virus
Bacterial	*Pseudomonas aeruginosa* *Staphylococcus aureus* *Streptococcus* species Atypical bacteria (e.g. *Mycobacterium* species)
Fungal	*Candida* species *Fusarium* species
Parasitic	*Microsporidia* *Acanthamoeba* species

Herpetic Keratitis

What is Herpetic Keratitis?

- Herpetic infection of the cornea
- Can affect various layers of the cornea
- Primarily caused by herpes simplex virus 1 (more commonly) and 2
- Virus can remain dormant in the trigeminal nerve and manifest with frequent reactivation
- Ocular manifestations are the result of ocular inflammation, viral activity, or both

What are the Symptoms that the Patient May Present With?

- Red eye
- Pain or ocular irritation
- Tearing
- Photophobia

What are the Clinical Signs?

- Reduced corneal sensation
- Conjunctival injection
- Epithelial keratitis may present with dendritic or geographic ulcers, which will stain with fluorescein (Fig. 2.4 and Fig. 2.5)
  - Dendritic ulcers are seen typically as branching lesions with terminal bulbs
  - Multiple dendritic ulcers coalesce to form a geographic ulcer
- Stromal infiltration and corneal oedema may be present in stromal keratitis
- Anterior chamber reaction may be present in herpetic keratouveitis or endothelitis

> Healing corneal abrasions can present as "pseudo-dendrites" and are frequently misdiagnosed as herpetic epithelial keratitis.

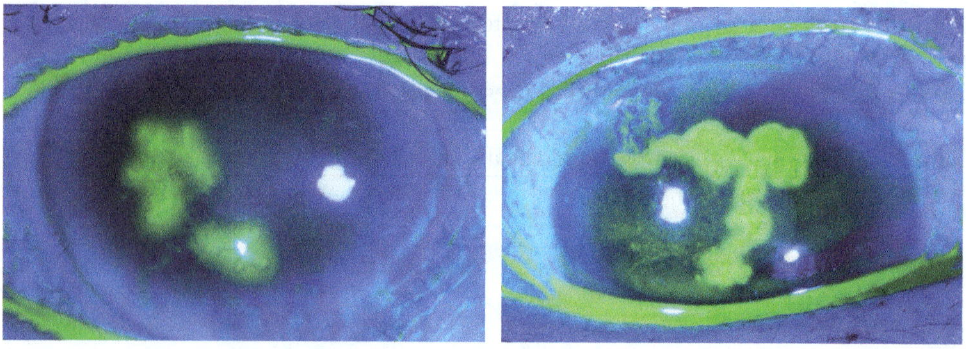

(A) (B)

Fig. 2.4. Photographs demonstrating epithelial keratitis with a dendritic ulcer seen in (A) and a geographic ulcer seen in (B).

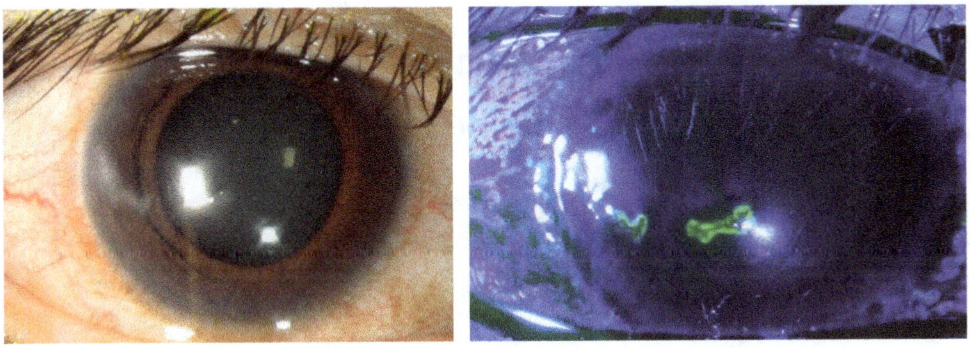

(A) (B)

Fig. 2.5. Photographs demonstrating dendritic ulcer before (A) and after (B) fluorescein staining.

What are the Risk Factors for this Condition?

- Reduced host immunity (e.g. HIV, organ transplant recipient, pregnancy)
- Long-term immunosuppression (e.g. systemic or topical steroids)
- Recent ocular surgery

How Do We Manage These Patients?

- Depends on the level of corneal involvement
- Patients are generally started on antiviral treatment such as topical acyclovir
- In the presence of stromal/endothelial keratitis, topical steroids must be added
- Oral acyclovir may be started in immunocompromised patients or children with HSV keratitis
- Oral acyclovir 400 mg twice a day can be started for long-term prophylactic treatment of recurrent herpetic keratitis

Topical steroids should be avoided in the presence of epithelial keratitis.

What are the Possible Long-term Complications?

- Recurrence
- Neurotrophic keratopathy with persistent epithelial defect or ulcer
- Stromal scarring
  - Resulting in high irregular astigmatism
  - Dense scarring may require treatment with a corneal transplant

What are the Other Ocular Manifestations of Herpes Simplex Virus?

- Blepharitis
- Acute anterior uveitis
- Retinitis
- Cranial nerve palsies

HSV blepharitis can present as a focal area of vesicular rash over the eyelid. This does not follow a dermatomal pattern, as seen in HZO.

Herpes Zoster Ophthalmicus

What is Herpes Zoster Ophthalmicus?

- Caused by reactivation of the varicella-zoster virus
- Manifests as a painful vesicular rash along the ophthalmic division (V1) of the trigeminal nerve distribution
- Vesicles or pustules eventually crust and heal within 2–6 weeks

What are the Important Examination Findings?

- Vesicular or pustular rash seen along the V1 dermatome distribution (some may be crusting)
- Look for involvement of the tip of the nose
- Check corneal sensation
- Visual acuity
- Intraocular pressure
  - Raised intraocular pressure may occur secondary to ocular inflammation
- Slit-lamp examination:
  - Conjunctival injection
  - Stain the cornea to look for dendritic lesions
    i. Typically, without terminal bulbs and without central ulceration
  - Anterior chamber reaction seen in keratouveitis
- Dilated fundus examination looking for posterior segment involvement

What is Hutchinson's Sign? (Fig. 2.6)

- This is when there is involvement of the tip of the nose
- Indicates involvement of the nasociliary branch of V1 of the trigeminal nerve
- This increases the risk of corneal involvement (50–76% chance of ocular complications)

What are Some of the Risk Factors?

- Advanced age
- Psychological stress
- Immunosuppressed state (e.g. systemic steroids)
- Immunocompromised patient (e.g. HIV, malignancies)

How Would You Manage the Patient?

- Isolate the patient
- Start oral acyclovir 800 mg 5 times a day for 2 weeks

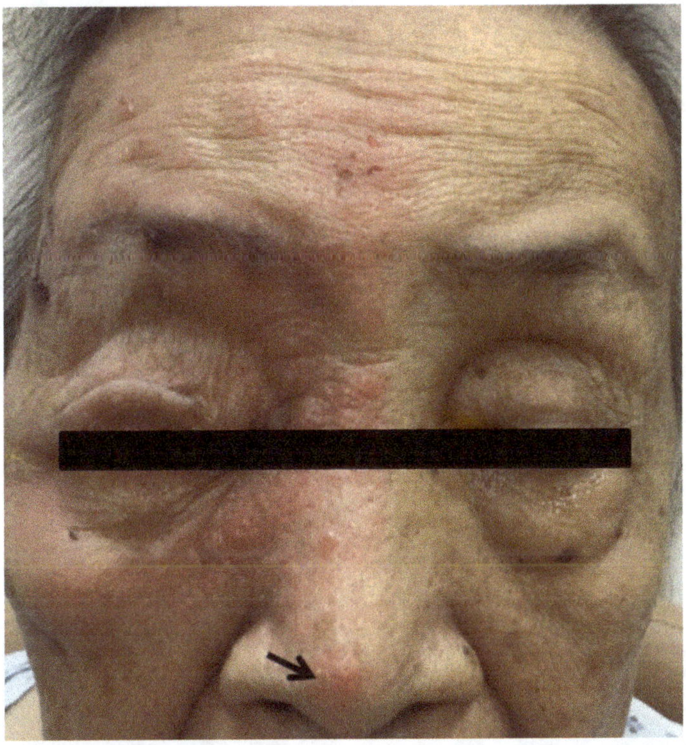

Fig. 2.6. Photograph showing a vesicular rash on the right side of the face along the V1 distribution. Hutchinson's sign is positive (shown by arrow).

- Start acyclovir ointment to the eye 5 times a day if there is corneal involvement
- Topical antibiotic cream to skin lesions to reduce the risk of a secondary bacterial infection
- May require steroid eyedrops if there is associated ocular inflammation

When there are multiple dermatomal involvement or multiple recurrences, always consider an immunocompromised state. Further blood investigations may be warranted.

What are the Possible Long-term Complications?

- Neurotrophic keratopathy due to impaired corneal innervation
- Post-herpetic neuralgia (10–17%)

Bacterial Keratitis

What are the Common Organisms for Bacterial Keratitis?

- *Pseudomonas aeruginosa*
- *Staphylococcus*
- *Streptococcus*

What are the Risk Factors?

- Contact lens — poor contact lens hygiene, overnight contact lens wear, contaminated contact lens solution
- Trauma
- Contaminated water contact with the eye

What are the Other Organisms that can Cause a Corneal Ulcer?

- Viral (e.g. herpetic)
- Fungal (e.g. *Fusarium, Candida*)
- Atypical organisms — *Mycobacterium, Acanthoameba*

What are the Clinical Signs? (Fig. 2.7)

- Conjunctival injection
- Corneal infiltrate
- Epithelial defect

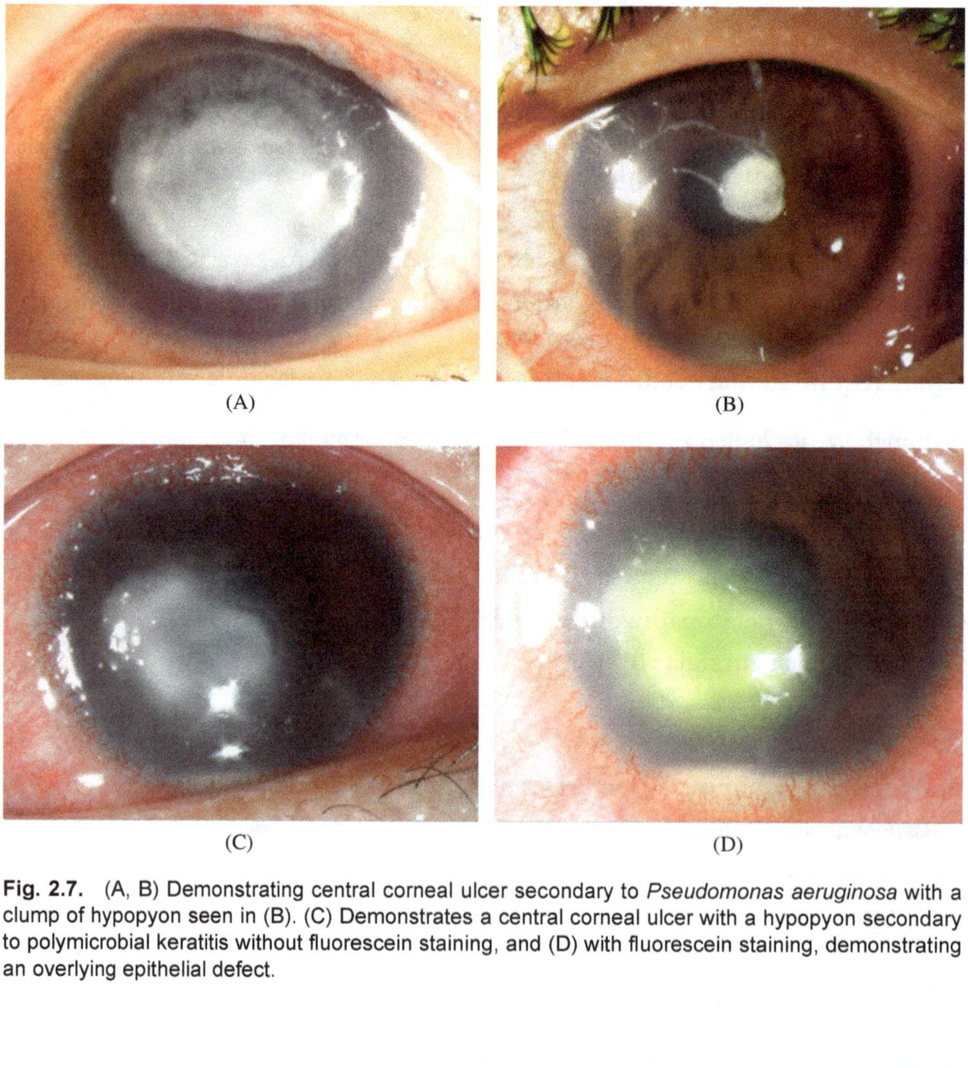

(A) (B) (C) (D)

Fig. 2.7. (A, B) Demonstrating central corneal ulcer secondary to *Pseudomonas aeruginosa* with a clump of hypopyon seen in (B). (C) Demonstrates a central corneal ulcer with a hypopyon secondary to polymicrobial keratitis without fluorescein staining, and (D) with fluorescein staining, demonstrating an overlying epithelial defect.

- Hypopyon
- Anterior chamber reaction

How Would You Manage the Patient?

- Corneal scraping to send for gram stain, fungal smear, fungal culture, aerobic and anaerobic culture
- May consider sending the contact lens/solution for culture
- Start hourly fortified topical cefazolin 50 mg/mL and topical gentamicin 14 mg/mL
- Topical cycloplegia

What are the Possible Complications?

- Corneal melt and perforation
- Corneal scar

Take Home Messages

- Contact lens wear, contaminated water or solution, ocular trauma and prolonged use of topical steroids are the main risk factors for infective keratitis.
- Early diagnosis and targeted treatment are important to reduce sight-threatening complications and scarring.
- Topical steroids should be avoided in the initial treatment of infective keratitis.

Fungal Keratitis

Learning Objectives

- Predisposing factors
- Aetiological organisms
- Clinical features
- How to make a diagnosis?
- How does it differ from bacterial keratitis?
- How to manage fungal keratitis

Fungal keratitis, also known as mycotic keratitis, is one of the major causes of microbial keratitis that often results in corneal blindness. Fungi are generally considered as opportunistic pathogens and rarely invade an intact cornea. However, it becomes pathogenic when the affected individuals are exposed to certain predisposing factors. It is more prevalent in developing countries with tropical and sub-tropical climates. The prevalence of this highly damaging corneal infection could be as high as 20–60% of all culture positive cases in these countries. The affected individuals are frequently young agricultural workers of low socio-economic status.

Predisposing Factors

- Young male outdoor workers
- Minor ocular injury with organic matter
- Immunosuppression

- Use of topical steroids
- Contact lens wearer
- Ocular surface diseases

Aetiological Organisms

Organisms causing fungal keratitis can be broadly classified into filamentous and non-filamentous fungi. Examples:

- Filamentous fungi: *Aspergillus, Fusarium, Curvularia*
- Non-filamentous: Yeast, *Candida, Cryptococcus*

Clinical Features

Good history-taking is the utmost important step in the evaluation of a case of suspected fungal keratitis. It usually has an insidious onset and a protracted clinical course. It is essential to ask the patient about exposure to possible risk factors such as trauma, systemic diseases and use of contact lenses. One of the striking features that differentiates fungal keratitis from other forms of infectious keratitis is a relative lack of photophobia.

Symptoms

- Eye irritation and pain (less than bacterial keratitis)
- Blurring of vision associated with redness of the eye
- Photophobia (less than bacterial keratitis)
- Tearing and discharge

Signs (Fig. 2.8)

- Conjunctival injection
- Corneal stromal infiltrate with dry elevated and occasionally feathery margins
- Satellite lesions
- Endothelial plaque
- Fixed hypopyon (hypopyon doesn't change position with different postures)
- Clinical variation is usually related to causative fungal species

Diagnosis

Initial diagnosis is based on clinical signs, which is valuable in terms of initiating the treatment. However, diagnosis must be confirmed by microbiological laboratory tests. Corneal scraping and testing the sample by various methods remain the mainstay of diagnosis.

- Direct microscopy
- KOH wet mount test (70–90% sensitivity)

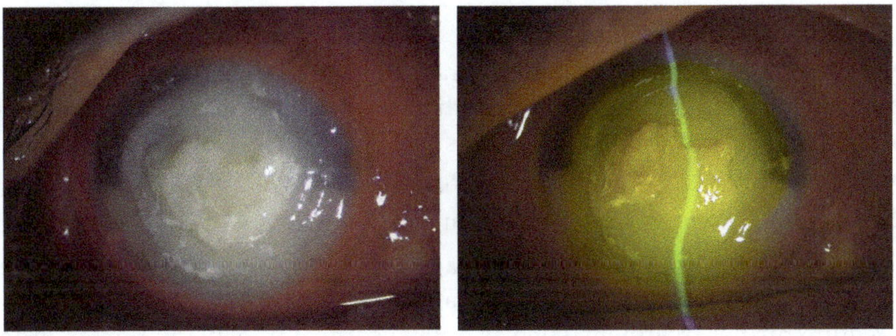

(A) (B)

Fig. 2.8. Fungal keratitis with dry elevated corneal lesion and Hypopyon (A). The same cornea with fluorescein staining (B).
PC : Dr Shivani Joshi

- Staining methods: Gram stain and Giemsa stain
- Fungal culture (Selective culture media: Sabouraud's Dextrose Agar media)
- Corneal biopsy
- Confocal microscopy: allows direct viewing of fungal elements in the patient's eye

Management

Medical:

Use of topical antifungal medications is considered the primary modality of treatment

- Natamycin 5% eye drop: First line of treatment
- Topical Amphotericin B (0.15%): Treatment of choice for *Candida* infection and also when not responding to Natamycin
- Topical Voriconazole 1%: Not commercially available but can be reconstituted in pharmacy
- Other Azole: Econazole 1%, Fluconazole 2%

Systemic antifungals are indicated in large fungal keratitis associated with:

- Limbal involvement
- Scleritis
- Endophthalmitis

Systemic antifungals, such as oral Voriconazole 200 mg twice daily or oral Ketoconazole 600 mg daily, must be continued for 6 to 8 weeks if indicated.

Surgical

Surgical treatment is only indicated in refractory cases that fail to respond well with adequate topical and/or oral antifungal therapy or when the infections threaten to perforate the cornea. Different modalities are:

- Intrastromal injection of antifungals (e.g. Voriconazole): In refractory cases
- Therapeutic corneal transplantation: In very thin cornea or corneal perforation

Once infections are resolved by treatment the patient is likely to develop significant corneal scarring, which may affect the visual outcome. These patients may require further treatment, such as optical corneal transplantation, in order to improve vision.

What are the Complications?

- Fungal endophthalmitis
- Corneal perforation

Take Home Messages

- Organic injury to the eye, use of topical steroids, immunosuppression and wearing contact lenses are the common risk factors for fungal keratitis.
- Unlike bacterial keratitis, fungal keratitis generally has a protracted course.
- Topical antifungals are the mainstay of management.
- Infections take a longer time to resolve in view of poor ocular penetration of ocular antifungals.

2.4 Conjunctivitis

Learning Objectives

- Recognising and understanding the various causes of conjunctivitis.
- Management of the various causes of conjunctivitis.

Conjunctivitis is an inflammation of the conjunctiva, which can be due to various causes. It is important to recognise the diagnosis as this has direct implications on the management of the patient. For example, failing to recognise an episode of allergic conjunctivitis can result in delayed treatment and recurrent flares.

Allergic Conjunctivitis

What are the Types of Allergic Conjunctivitis?

- Seasonal/perennial conjunctivitis
- Atopic keratoconjunctivitis (AKC)
- Vernal keratoconjunctivitis (VKC)

What are the Differences between the Various Types of Allergic Conjunctivitis?

Table 2.4. Types of Allergic Conjunctivitis

	Seasonal	VKC	AKC
Epidemiology		Typically aged 5–20 years old. Predominantly in male.	Teenage to 50 years old. Chronic course with periodic acute exacerbations.
Hypersensitivity reaction	Type 1	Type 1 and 4	Type 4
Associations	May have other atopy	May not have history of atopy. Keratoconus (from rubbing).	High association with atopic dermatitis and asthma. Increased risk with positive family history. Keratoconus. Anterior/posterior subcapsular cataracts.
Symptoms	Seasonal symptoms from environmental allergens (pollens, animal dander). Rapid symptoms after exposure (short lived and episodic).	Seasonal variation. Environmental allergen may incite acute exacerbation.	Disease year-round. Relapses and remits without seasonal correlation.
Examination findings	Generally, no corneal involvement	Limbal and palpebral form. Giant papillae of **only superior tarsal conjunctival**. Limbal (Horner Trantas dots). Corneal vernal plaques or shield (Togby's) ulcer.	Papillary hypertrophy of **superior and inferior** tarsal conjunctival, with an increased risk of eyelid thickening and scarring.

What is a Typical History?

- Intense itch
- Intermittent red eyes
- Lid swelling
- Thick ropy mucoid discharge

What are the Clinical Signs? (Fig. 2.9)

- Conjunctival chemosis
- Conjunctival injection
- Epithelial erosions or epithelial defect
- Papillae or cobblestone papillae
- Horner Trantas dots or limbitis
- Shield ulcer

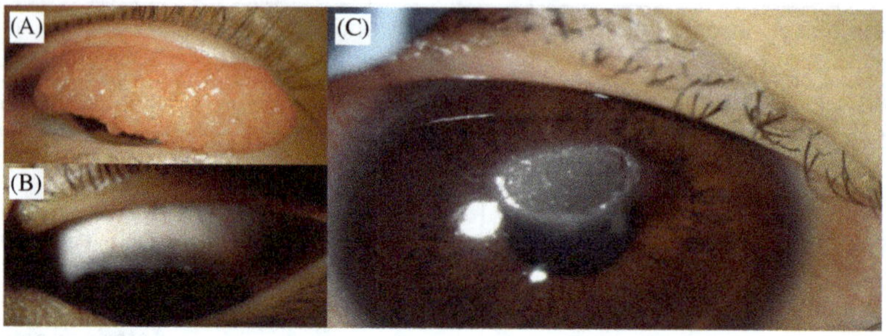

Fig. 2.9. Demonstrating various clinical signs seen in vernal keratoconjunctivitis, such as (A) cobblestone papillae, (B) limbitis, and (C) shield ulcer.

What are the Chronic Eye Changes that can Occur with Untreated VKC or AKC? (Fig. 2.10)

- Loss of eyelashes
- Conjunctival scarring
- Corneal neovascularisation
- Corneal ulcer
- Corneal scarring
- Keratoconus

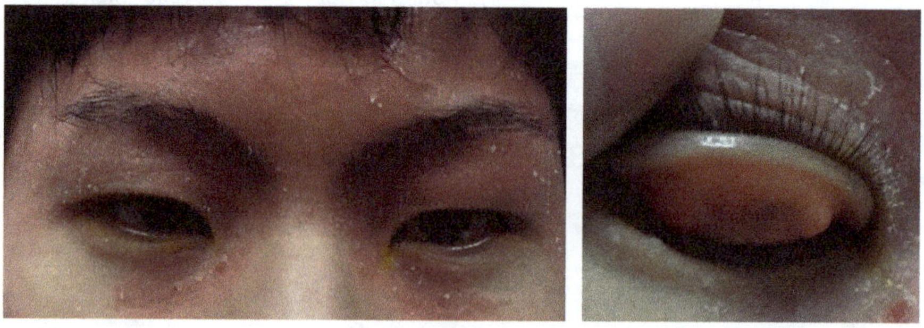

(A) (B)

Fig. 2.10. Demonstrating a case of atopic keratoconjunctivitis with (A) periocular dermatitis, and (B) papillae seen upon lid eversion.

What are Shield Ulcers?

- Sterile ulcers or plaques are macro-erosions that form due to the accumulation of fibrin and mucous
- Typically located at the upper 2/3 of the cornea

Shield ulcers are not infective in nature. Unlike infective keratitis, treatment will require the use of topical steroids while preventing secondary infection with topical antibiotics.

What are the Risk Factors?

- Atopic history of asthma, allergic rhinitis or eczema
- Young, male

What May Exacerbate Symptoms?

- House dust mites
- Dander
- Contact lens
- Dry eyes

How Would You Manage this Patient?

- Systemic management
  - Allergen avoidance
  - Skin prick test
  - Control of other allergies
- Ocular management
  - Topical mast cell stabilizers
  - Topical antihistamines
  - Topical lubricants
  - Cold compress
  - Topical steroids
  - Topical immunomodulators — cyclosporin, tacrolimus
  - Systemic steroids in severe cases
  - Supratarsal injection of steroids for recalcitrant cases

Viral Conjunctivitis

What is the Most Common Causative Virus?

- Adenovirus

What History Does the Patient Present With? (Fig. 2.11)

- Sequential red eyes
- Sticky discharge
- Tearing

- Other history — recent upper respiratory tract infection, lymphadenopathy, contact history

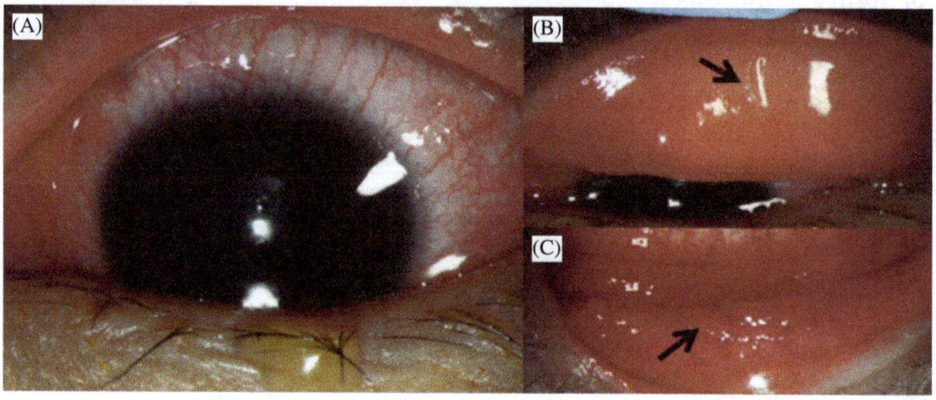

Fig. 2.11. Demonstrating various clinical signs seen in viral conjunctivitis, such as (A) diffuse conjunctival injection, (B) pseudomembrane seen on upper lid eversion, and (C) follicular conjunctival reaction on lower lid eversion.

What are the Clinical Findings?

- Conjunctival injection
- Conjunctival follicular reaction
- Pseudomembranes seen on lid eversion
- Check for corneal involvement — punctate epitheliopathy, epithelial defect

What are the Other Causes of Conjunctivitis?

- Bacterial conjunctivitis
  - Consider if extensive purulent discharge
  - Multiple sexual partners
- Allergic conjunctivitis
  - Chronic intermittent history of red eyes
  - Associated with itch predominantly
  - Background of other atopies
- Toxic conjunctivitis
  - Chronic use of topical eyedrops

How Would You Manage the Patient?

- Topical lubricants
- Generally self-limiting over 1–2 weeks
- Advise patient to practice good hand hygiene as viral conjunctivitis is highly contagious

What are the Possible Complications?

- Corneal epitheliopathy or epithelial defect
- Nummular keratitis (Fig. 2.12)

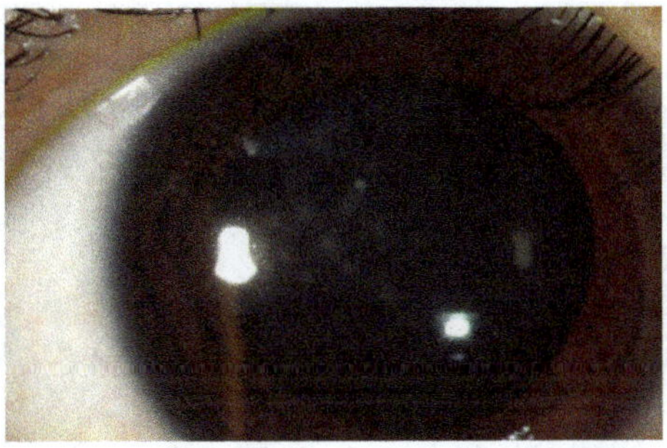

Fig. 2.12. A case of nummular keratitis seen after an acute episode of viral conjunctivitis.

Take Home Messages

- Not every red eye is viral conjunctivitis!
- Take a detailed history, particularly the presence of known atopy.
- There are various types of allergic conjunctivitis, depending on their presentation. However, the principle of management is similar.

2.5 Corneal Transplant

Learning Objectives

- Basic understanding of indications for a corneal transplant.
- Recognising the presence of a corneal transplant graft.

Corneal transplants have evolved over the years, from primarily performing full thickness graft to replacing only the diseased part of the cornea through performing a partial thickness keratoplasty. However, this involves overcoming a greater learning curve.

Comparable visual outcomes can be achieved after a lamellar keratoplasty, with improvement in graft survival, reduced rejection rates and post-operative glaucoma reported after a penetrating keratoplasty. Posterior lamellar keratoplasty allows for faster visual recovery, with a reduced risk of sight-threatening intraoperative complications such as suprachoroidal haemorrhage.

What are the Types of Corneal Transplants? (Fig. 2.13)

- Full thickness
  - Penetrating keratoplasty
- Partial thickness
  - Anterior lamellar keratoplasty
  - Endothelial keratoplasty
- Corneal patch graft

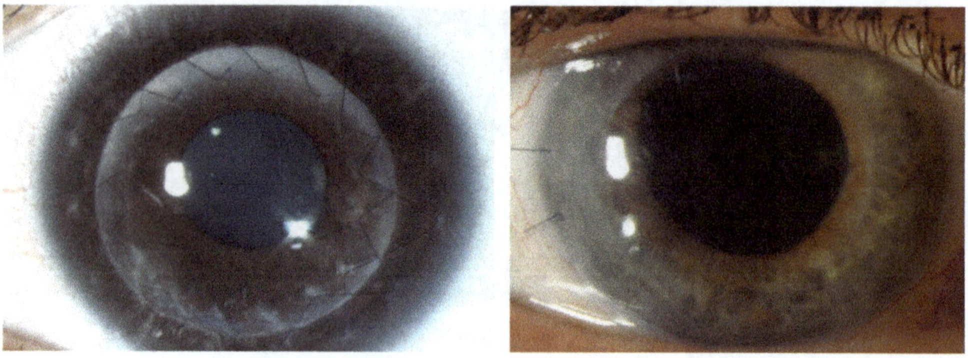

(A) (B)

Fig. 2.13. Of an eye post-corneal transplant: (A) After deep anterior lamellar keratoplasty, and (B) after endothelial keratoplasty.

What are the Common Indications for a Corneal Transplant?

- Optical indications
  - Corneal scar
  - Keratoconus
  - Bullous keratopathy
  - Corneal dystrophy
- Tectonic indication
  - Corneal perforation
- Therapeutic indication
  - Severe infective keratitis refractory to medical treatment

What are the Possible Complications of a Corneal Transplant?

- Glaucoma
- Infection
- Graft rejection
- Graft failure

Take Home Messages

- Different types of corneal transplants are performed depending on the location of the pathology.
- Penetrating keratoplasty → full thickness corneal scar.
- Endothelial keratoplasty → bullous keratopathy.
- Anterior lamellar keratoplasty → keratoconus, corneal scars.

2.6 Pterygium

Learning Objectives

- Recognising a pterygium and understanding the clinical consequences of the condition.
- Understanding common differentials, such as a pseudopterygium and a pinguecula (Fig. 2.14).

Pterygium is a fibrovascular, wing-shaped growth of the conjunctiva over the cornea. It is typically located at the interpalpebral region (3- and 9 o'clock) position and is degenerative in nature (Fig. 2.15).

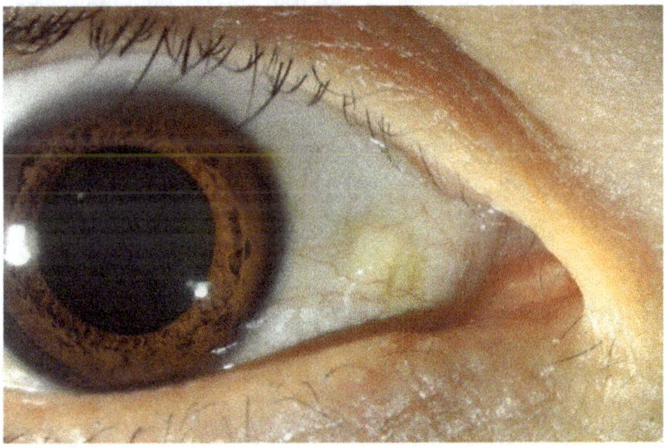

Fig. 2.14. Nasal pinguecula seen as a raised yellow-white conjunctival lesion. This is similarly secondary to UV exposure.

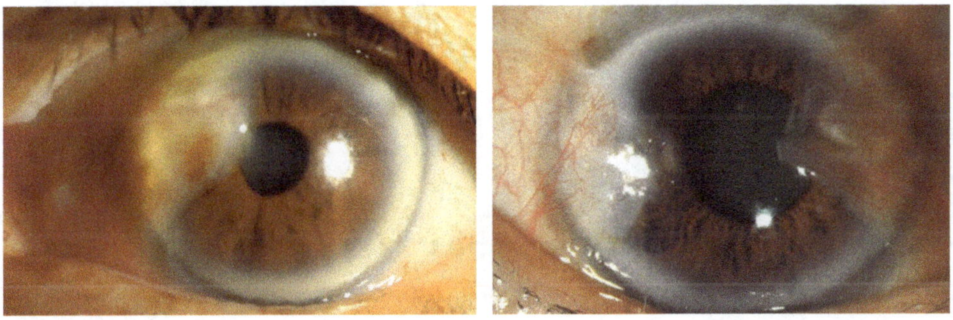

(A) (B)

Fig. 2.15. Demonstrating (A) Nasal pterygium, and a (B) Double-headed pterygium.

Suspect a pseudopterygium in the presence of a unilateral lesion NOT located at the interpalpebral region. This may be due to a previous insult (e.g. chemical injury) or chronic ocular inflammation (Fig. 2.16).

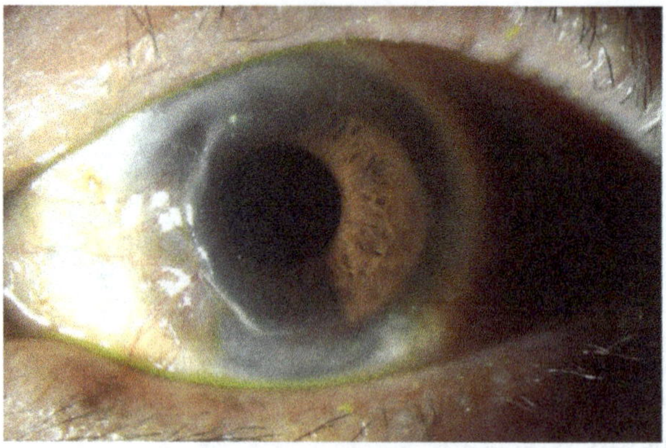

Fig. 2.16. Pseudopterygium seen in a patient with chronic peripheral ulcerative keratitis.

What are the Risk Factors?

- Sunlight exposure (main risk factor)
- Dry eyes
- Dust exposure

What are the Clinical Consequences?

- Majority asymptomatic
- Dry eyes-related symptoms from irregular ocular surface
- Induced corneal astigmatism
- Obstruction of visual axis
- Cosmesis

What are Indications for Surgery?

- Visual axis is involved
- High astigmatism
- Cosmesis

How Would You Manage the Patient?

- Most pterygiums can be treated conservatively. Sunglasses can be worn to reduce sunlight exposure
- Surgery is performed if clinically significant. Patient can undergo pterygium excision with conjunctival autograft

In a patient with a significant pterygium and a concomitant cataract, the pterygium is usually removed first to reduce the induced astigmatism before planning for cataract surgery.

Take Home Message

Pterygium is a common degenerative condition and may be managed conservatively if it is not causing any symptoms.

2.7 Episcleritis and Scleritis

Learning Objectives

- Recognising the difference between episcleritis and scleritis.
- Understanding the necessary investigations and management in these cases.

Episcleritis is an inflammation of the superficial episcleral vessels of the eye. On the other hand, scleritis involves inflammation of the deeper scleral vessels. It is important to differentiate between the two conditions as episcleritis is generally benign, while scleritis requires further systemic investigations. It is necessary to rule out autoimmune conditions in these cases, which may require subsequent systemic treatment.

What are the Types of Episcleritis and Scleritis?

Table 2.5. Episcleritis and Scleritis

Episcleritis	Scleritis

• Diffuse
• Sectoral
• Nodular
	• Anterior
	  ▪ Non-necrotising
	    i. Diffuse
	    ii. Nodular
	  ▪ Necrotising
	    i. Inflammatory
	    ii. Non-inflammatory (Scleromalacia perforans)
	• Posterior

What History Would the Patient Present With?

- Red eye
- Scleritis can present as an eye pain that is worse with eye movements and may wake the patient up at night
- May have a history of previous episodes
- History of autoimmune conditions
- Typically, no discharge or infective symptoms

What are the Clinical Findings?

- Episcleritis
  - Diffuse, sectoral or nodular injection
  - Episcleral vessels seen mobile over underlying scleral
  - May have an anterior chamber reaction
- Scleritis
  - Bluish-red violaceous hue (best seen under daylight) (Fig. 2.17)
  - Scleral tenderness
  - May have anterior chamber reaction

- Look for signs of previous ocular surgery (e.g. previous pterygium excision or corneal wound)
    i. Surgically induced necrotising scleritis
- Dilate the fundus to check for posterior segment inflammation (e.g. choroidal folds, disc swelling, serous retinal detachment)

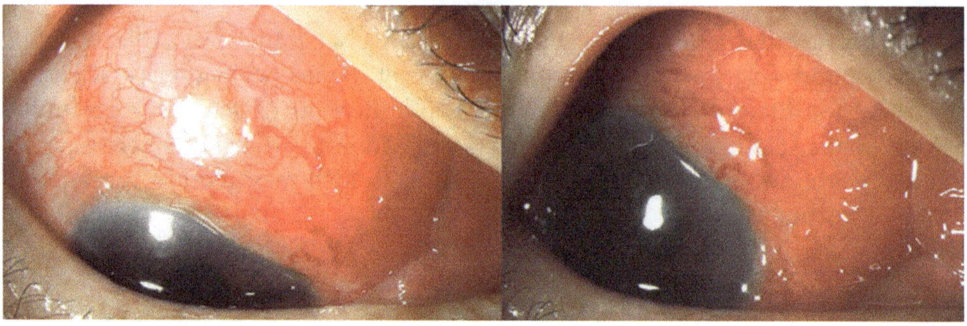

Fig. 2.17. Demonstrating a case of nodular scleritis.

What is the Clinical Test to Differentiate between Episcleritis and Scleritis?

- Phenylephrine 2.5% is used to blanch the overlying conjunctival and episcleral vessels (Fig. 2.18)
- Absence of blanching of the deep scleral vessels is seen in scleritis

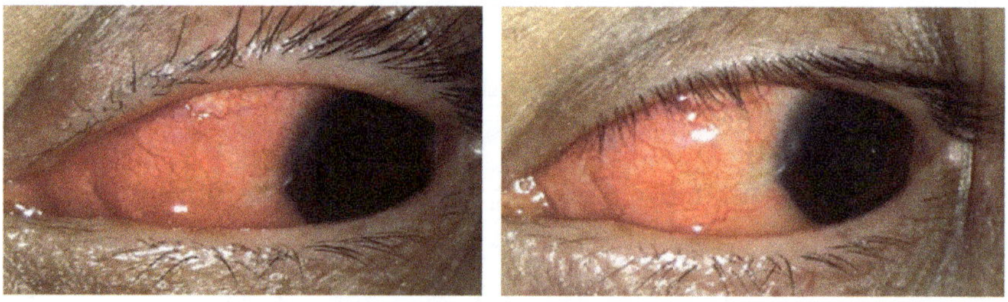

(A) (B)

Fig. 2.18. Demonstrating a case of scleritis (A) before, and (B) after, phenylephrine 2.5% instillation. There is the absence of blanching of the deep scleral vessels.

What Investigations Would You Perform?

- Episcleritis
    - Mostly idiopathic
    - Systemic evaluation only necessary in recurrent episodes

- Scleritis
  - B scan ultrasonography to look for "T sign" due to fluid in subtenon space
  - Systemic workup to rule out infective and autoimmune conditions
    i. Full blood count, erythrocyte sedimentation rate, rheumatoid factor, anti-nuclear antibody, lupus screen, anti-neutrophil cytoplasmic antibody and urine microscopy (looking for haematuria)
    ii. Chest X-ray, Mantoux test, syphilis screen

How Would You Manage the Patient?

- Episcleritis — topical NSAIDs or topical steroids
- Anterior scleritis
  - Topical NSAIDs and oral NSAIDS
  - May consider oral steroids
  - Necrotising scleritis may require pulse intravenous steroid treatment
- Posterior scleritis — systemic steroids

What are the Possible Complications of Scleritis?

- Necrotising anterior scleritis can present with scleral thinning and perforation
- Raised intraocular pressure
- Serous retinal detachment

Take Home Messages

- It is important to differentiate episcleritis and scleritis since scleritis requires further investigations and systemic treatment.
- Scleritis can lead to sight-threatening complications and requires early diagnosis and treatment.

2.8 Anterior Segment Trauma

Learning Objectives

- Recognising and understanding various types of anterior segment trauma.
- Understanding the acute management of types of ocular trauma.

Ocular trauma can be either sharp or blunt in nature. Depending on the mechanism, the location and the severity of the injury, there are various acute and long-term implications to the management of the patient. The Birmingham Eye Trauma Terminology system (BETT) provides a classification of the various types of ocular injuries, and the ocular trauma score allows us to prognosticate the injury (Fig. 2.19).

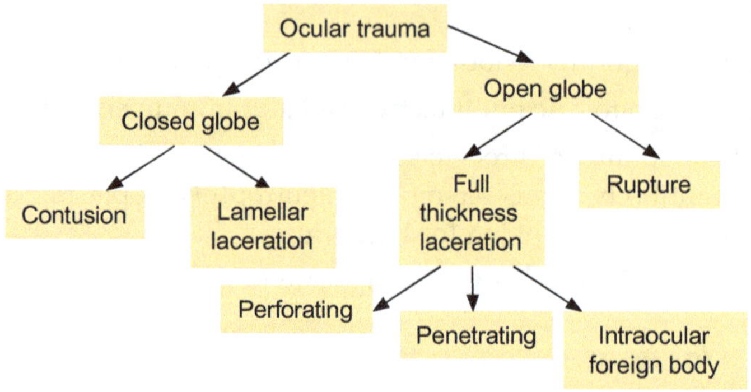

Fig. 2.19. Birmingham Eye Trauma Terminology system.

Table 2.6. Prognostication Factors in the Ocular Trauma Score

• Presenting visual acuity • Presence of i. Globe rupture ii. Endophthalmitis iii. Perforating injury iv. Retinal detachment v. Relative afferent pupillary defect

Corneal Abrasion

What is a Typical History?

- Preceding trauma
- Pain and tearing
- Inability to open the eye
- Red eye

What are the Clinical Signs?

- Corneal epithelial defect that fluoresces under cobalt blue light when fluorescein stain is applied to the eye (Fig. 2.20)
- Important to rule out secondary infection
- Look for corneal infiltrates and cellular activity

How Would You Manage the Patient?

- Lubricants
- Preservative-free artificial teardrops
- Ointment (e.g. Duratears)
- Topical antibiotics to prevent secondary infection

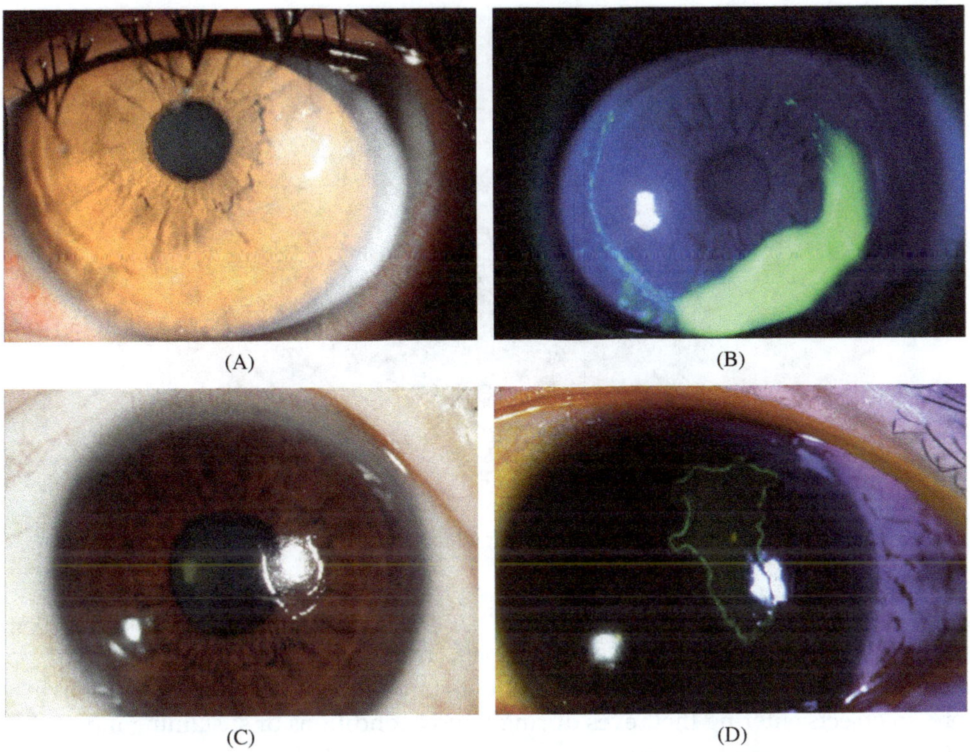

Fig. 2.20. Demonstrating a corneal abrasion, seen without fluorescein staining (A and C) and with fluorescein staining under cobalt blue light (B and D), respectively.

A drop of topical tetracaine prior to examination will make the patient more comfortable. DO NOT discharge the patient with tetracaine drops as that can cause epithelial toxicity instead.

What are the Potential Long-term Complications?

- Corneal scar
- Recurrent corneal abrasion

Foreign Body in Cornea and External Eye

Learning Objectives

- Recognise symptoms and signs of a foreign body in the external eye.
- Understanding the acute management, including the technique of removing the corneal foreign body.

Foreign body in the eye is one of the most common ophthalmic injuries. Although it is most frequently embedded at the superficial cornea (Fig. 2.21), it can also be impacted in other parts of the eye, such as the bulbar, forniceal or even tarsal

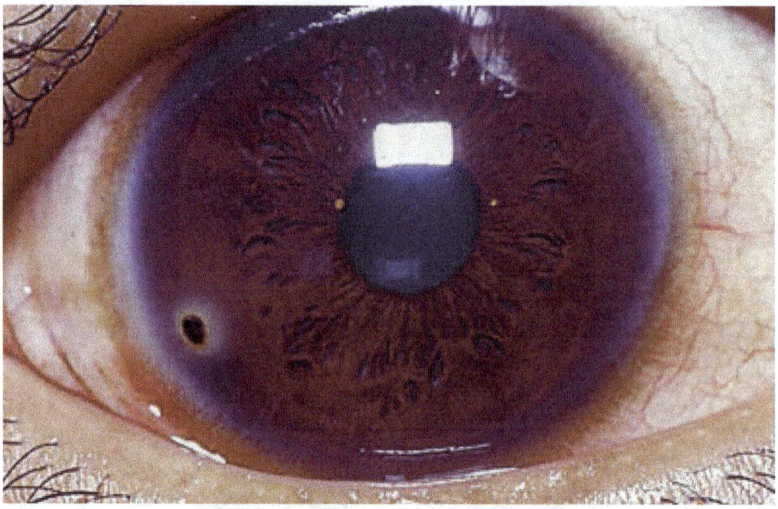

Fig. 2.21. Metallic foreign body in cornea

conjunctiva. High-velocity particles may enter deep into the eye and may cause devastating visual consequences. However, an intraocular foreign body will be discussed in the appropriate chapter. Patients frequently report incidents involving foreign objects entering their eyes during windy conditions or sustaining industrial injuries while engaged in activities such as grinding or hammering, particularly when not wearing any eye protection. A linear corneal abrasion might indicate the presence of a subtarsal foreign body. An iron foreign body within the cornea typically results in the formation of a rust ring encircling it.

What are the Symptoms?

- Photophobia and tearing
- Gritty sensation
- Pain
- Redness
- Blurring of vision

Diagnosis

- Examine under slit-lamp biomicroscope
- Scan the ocular surface, including conjunctival fornices
- Evert the eyelids
- Look for the potential route of entry (in case of an intraocular foreign body)
- Rule out multiple foreign bodies
- Stain the cornea with fluorescein (look for linear abrasion)

How Do You Manage Foreign Body in External Eye?

- Make sure there is no intraocular foreign body
- Loose foreign body may be irrigated away with normal saline

- Embedded foreign body must be removed manually
- Use lubricants
- Consider topical prophylactic antibiotics if there is a chance of infection after the removal of the foreign body

How Do You Remove Corneal Foreign Body?

- Anaesthetise the eye with topical anaesthetics
- Make sure the patient sits comfortably in a slit lamp
- Use a 27 G needle in an insulin syringe or a foreign body spud to remove the foreign body
- In case of a deep corneal foreign body, instil a drop of topical fluorescein for possible leakage of aqueous (Siedel's test)

Take Home Message

- Meticulous history-taking, especially the mechanism of foreign body entry, is extremely important
- Always rule out any intraocular foreign body
- For a corneal foreign body, always evert the eyelids to look at the tarsal conjunctiva
- If ordering an imaging to rule out an intraocular foreign body, never order an MRI

Corneal Laceration

What are the Common Mechanisms of Injury?

- Rupture
- Blunt trauma (e.g. golf ball injury)
- High-pressure injury (e.g. hydraulic-injection injury)
- Laceration (Fig. 2.22)
- High-velocity injury (e.g. grinding metal) — suspect an intraocular foreign body if an entry wound is seen
- Sharp injury (e.g. scissors, wires, hammering of nail)

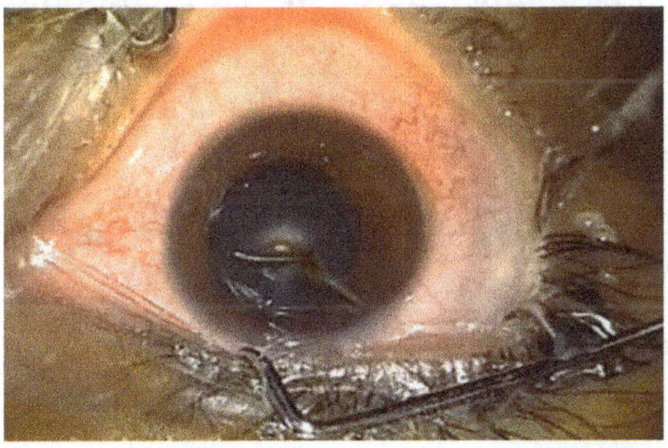

Fig. 2.22. Demonstrating an ocular-penetrating injury secondary to a foreign body. The foreign body is seen lodged within the cornea.

What is Your Immediate Management?

- Ensure the patient is haemodynamically stable — ensure "Airway, Breathing, Circulation" intact
- Keep the patient "Nil by mouth"
- IM tetanus
- IV ciprofloxacin
- Keep an eye shield on
- Do not touch the eye further as that may lead to further damage of intraocular structures and worsen the prognosis
- Refer to ophthalmology for subsequent assessment and surgical repair of corneal laceration and associated injuries

> Do not pull out a foreign body lodged within the laceration in an open globe injury. This should be done in a controlled manner in the operating theatre.

What Investigations Will You Perform?

- Arrange for CT orbits (1 mm fine cuts) to rule out an intraocular foreign body

What are the Poor Prognostic Factors in Ocular Trauma?

- Poor presenting visual acuity
- Presence of relative afferent papillary defect
- Retinal detachment
- Globe rupture
- Endophthalmitis
- Perforating injury

Chemical Injury

What are the Types of Chemical Injuries and How Do They Differ in Severity?

Alkaline injury

- More damaging as it saponifies lipids of cell membranes, penetrating deeper and more rapidly

Acidic injury

- Generally less damaging

What are the Important Clinical Findings That Would Determine Severity and the Prognosis of the Injury?

- Extent of corneal abrasion
- Corneal haziness and clarity of iris details
- Extent of conjunctival involvement
- Limbal ischaemia (Fig. 2.23)

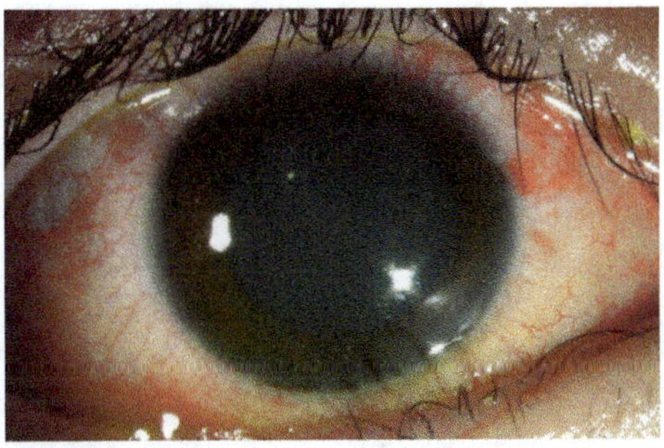

Fig. 2.23. Demonstrating a total corneal abrasion after an alkaline splash injury. Limbal ischaemia is seen from the 3–8 o'clock position.

How Would You Manage the Patient Acutely?

- Remove the inciting factor
- Irrigate the eye immediately with at least 1 litre of normal saline. Check the pH (ensure pH 7) and irrigate further if necessary
- Evert the lids to remove gross debris
- Promote re-epithelialisation
- Generous amount of lubricants with hourly preservative-free eyedrops and ointments
- May require the use of bandage contact lens or amniotic membrane transplant in the presence of a persistent epithelial defect
- Reduce ocular inflammation with a short course of topical steroids (not more than 10 days)
- Topical antibiotics to prevent secondary infection
- Treat any associated complications, such as an acute rise in intra-ocular pressure

What are the Long-term Complications?

- Persistent inflammation
- Persistent epithelial defect or recurrent epithelial breakdown
- Glaucoma
- Lid abnormalities (e.g. trichiasis, distichiasis, entropion)
- Cataract

Hyphaema

What is a Hyphaema?

- Fluid level of blood seen in the anterior chamber (Fig. 2.24)
- Due to a rupture of the iris or angle vessels

What Important History Would You Take from the Patient?

- Trauma (e.g. shuttlecock injury, punched)
- Ischaemic risk factors (e.g. DM, HTN)

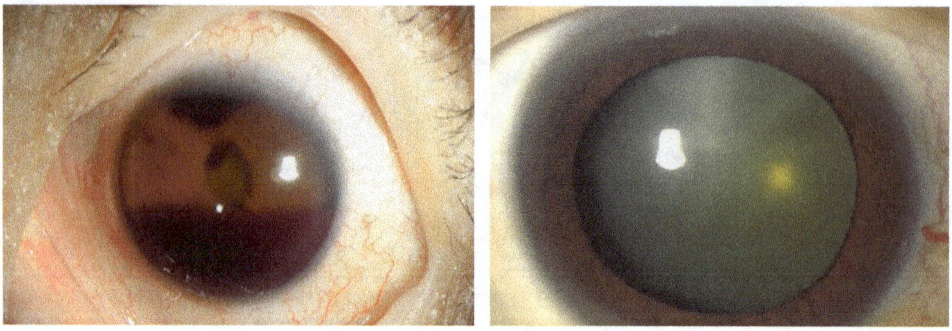

(A) (B)

Fig. 2.24. (A) Hyphaema as demonstrated by a dark red fluid level. (B) Shows iris neovascularisation in a patient secondary to proliferative diabetic retinopathy.

- Ocular history (e.g. recent surgery, chronic retinal detachment)
- History of haematological malignancies

What are the Risk Factors?

- Trauma
- Risk of iris neovascularisation (3 most important)
  - Proliferative diabetic retinopathy
  - Central retinal vein occlusion
  - Ocular ischaemic syndrome

What are the Important Clinical Findings?

- Loss of vision
- Raised intraocular pressure
- Level of the hyphaema (for monitoring)
- Look for iris neovascularisation and perform gonioscopy
- Dilated fundus examination looking for retinopathy
- In the presence of trauma, rule out other trauma-related injury

How Would You Manage the Patient?

- Management dependent on underlying aetiology
- Trauma-related
  - Complete rest in bed
  - Sleep 45° to allow blood to settle inferiorly
  - Topical steroid
  - Topical cycloplegia
  - Topical anti-glaucoma medications if raised intraocular pressure
  - Monitor the patient closely for re-bleeding, raised intraocular pressure or corneal blood staining
- Non-trauma related
  - Manage underlying medical condition

What are the Complications of a Trauma-related Hyphaema?

- Raised intraocular pressure
- Corneal blood staining
- Long-term risk of angle recession glaucoma

Take Home Messages

- Ocular trauma requires early and prompt treatment to maximise visual prognosis.
- Long-term monitoring or prolonged visual rehabilitation may be required for many of these patients.

References

1. Borderie VM, Sandali O, Bullet J, *et al.* (2012) Long-term results of deep anterior lamellar versus penetrating keratoplasty. *Ophthalmology* **119(2)**:249–255.
2. Han DC, Mehta JS, Por YM, *et al.* (2009) Comparison of outcomes of lamellar keratoplasty and penetrating keratoplasty in keratoconus. *AJ Ophthalmology* **148(5)**:744–751.e1.
3. Lee WB, Jacobs DS, Musch DC, *et al.* (2009) Descemet's stripping endothelial keratoplasty: Safety and outcomes: A report by the American Academy of Ophthalmology. *Ophthalmology* **116(9)**:1818–1830.
4. Awad R, Ghaith AA, Awad K, *et al.* (2024) Fungal keratitis: Diagnosis, management, and recent advances. *Clin Ophthalmol* **18**: 85–106.
5. Kuhn F, Morris R, Witherspoon CD, *et al.* (1996) A standardised classification of ocular trauma. Graefe's archive for clinical and experimental ophthalmology. *Albrecht von Graefes Archiv fur klinische und experimentelle Ophthalmologie* **234(6)**:399–403.
6. Kuhn F, Morris R, Witherspoon CD, *et al.* (2004) The Birmingham Eye Trauma Terminology system (BETT). *Journal francais d'ophtalmologie* **27(2)**:206–210.
7. Scott R. (2015) The Ocular Trauma Score. *Community Eye Health* **28(91)**:44–45.

Chapter 3

CATARACT

Chris Hong Long Lim, Chen Ziyou David

Learning Objectives

- Recognise different types of cataracts and their associated clinical implications.
- Understand the principles behind the management of cataracts.

A cataract refers to the clouding or opacification of the native crystalline lens. The lens is an important structure that focuses light on the retina. Loss of media clarity can alter light transmission and impact a patient's visual quality. Cataracts are the number one cause of preventable blindness globally and require surgical management when visually significant. Most cataracts develop gradually and contribute to a decline in vision with progression. Patients may report a range of symptoms, including blurred vision not correctable with glasses, decline in vision in low-lighting environments, glare, haloes and ghosting of images or double vision. Cataracts are typically classified according to the anatomical component that is affected (Fig. 3.1). The Lens Opacities Classification System III (LOCS III) classifies cataracts according to their anatomical location and density.

3.1 Senile Cataract

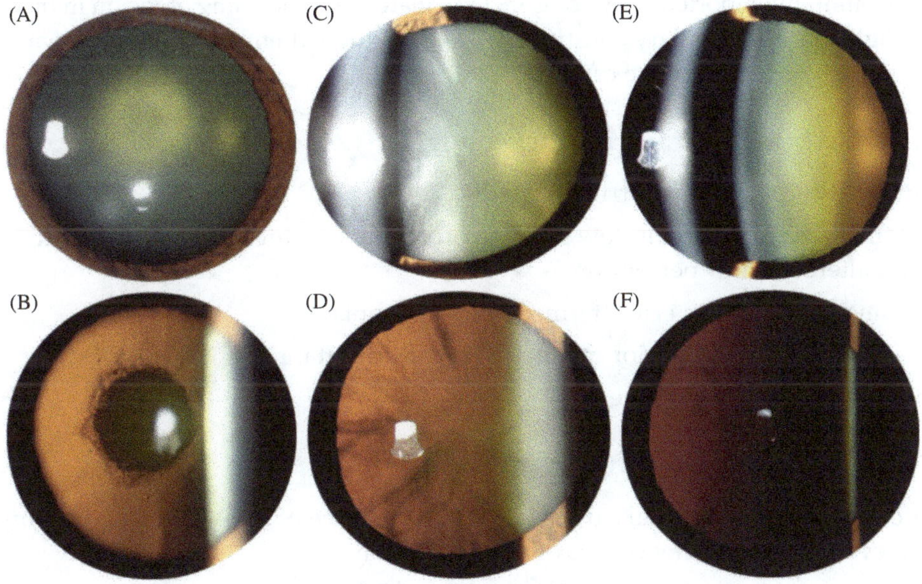

Fig. 3.1. Demonstrating posterior subcapsular cataract (A,B), cortical cataract (C,D), and nuclear sclerotic cataract (E,F).

What are the Risk Factors for Cataract Development?

- Congenital
- Age-related
- Drug-related (e.g. steroid use, chemotherapeutic agents)
- Intraocular inflammation or surgeries
- Metabolic
- Radiation-related (e.g. UV exposure, radiotherapy to the head and neck)
- Traumatic

What are the Common Types of Cataracts?

- Nuclear sclerotic cataract
  - Nuclear sclerosis refers to hardening of the central portion of the crystalline lens. The lens takes on an increasingly brownish hue as this progresses. These structural changes can lead to a change in refractive power, with the resultant myopic shift bringing about "second sight" and momentarily improved unaided vision.
- Cortical cataract
  - Cortical cataracts occur due to opacification of lens fibres surrounding the nucleus. These usually occur in the peripheries but can extend to the centre of the lens and involve the visual axis. Patients typically report presence of glare from bright lights in conditions of dim lighting conditions (pupils are larger in dim lighting).
- Posterior subcapsular cataract
  - Posterior subcapsular cataracts form within the posterior cortical layer of the crystalline lens. Patients may experience rapid onset of visual disturbance. Commonly reported symptoms include glare and worsening of vision in bright lights due to pupillary constriction, thus forcing patients to look out of part of the lens affected by the cataract.

What is the Typical Presenting History?

- Progressive, painless blurring of vision
- Difficulty with vision in low light environments, reduced contrast sensitivity, and altered colour perception
- Change in refractive error (termed "index myopia")
- Glare (especially posterior capsular and cortical cataracts)
- Change in refractive power

What are the Important Examination Findings?

- Relative afferent pupillary defect (RAPD): Presence of a RAPD should prompt an evaluation for other causes of reduced vision
- Best corrected visual acuity (BCVA): Reduced BCVA attributable to a cataractous lens is an indication for surgery

- Red reflex: This can be altered and dulled with any form of media opacity
- Intraocular pressure (IOP): Raised IOP may occur due to a variety of reasons attributable to the lens, including angle closure and/or glaucoma secondary to a lens effect.
- Slit-lamp examination: This is the main workhorse in the ophthalmic setting and is used to assess the type and density of cataract while excluding other possible pathology that might account for patients' decreased presenting visual acuity and portend a poor visual prognosis. This includes the presence of corneal, retinal or optic nerve pathology. Other important features to be assessed include factors that pose a challenge during surgery (e.g. shallow anterior chamber, poorly dilating pupil) or as part of post-operative recovery (e.g. corneal endothelial dystrophies).

When Will You Offer Cataract Surgery?

- Visually significant cataract
    - Generally taken to be a BCVA measured on a Snellen's chart of 6/12 or worse
    - Significant and debilitating visual symptoms such as glare
    - Decisions around surgery ought to be individualised, with discussions centred around the patient's visual needs. The abovementioned criteria only serve as a guide
- Secondary complications of cataract
    - Narrow angles, lens mechanism-related glaucoma, lens subluxation
- Anisometropia
    - Differences in refractive error between both eyes that may result in aniseikonia (difference in perceived image size) and poor tolerance of binocular vision

Learning Objectives

- Understand the different management options for cataracts.
- Understand common surgical complications in cataract surgery.
- Be familiar with different types of intraocular lenses available in cataract surgery.

Consider the following before offering surgery to a patient:

- Indications for cataract surgery
- Functional impact of the cataract
    - Occupation
    - Hobbies
- Visual prognosis
- Patient's visual requirements
- Is this a regular or complex case? What is the best surgical approach?
- Is the patient fit for surgery?

3.2 Principles of Management

What are the Management Options for Cataract Surgeries?

- Spectacle correction
  - This option may be offered to patients with early cataracts and reasonable correctable vision (e.g. BCVA better or equal to 6/9)
  - Early cataracts may cause a change in refractive error (e.g. index myopia), which could be relieved with glasses alone
- Cataract surgery
  - This is the definitive way to remove a cataract from the eye
  - Cataract surgery is the most performed ophthalmic surgery in the world

What are the Common Indications for Cataract Surgery?

- Significant visual impairment which is not adequately relieved by glasses alone
- Visually symptomatic anisometropia between both eyes
- Significant risk of angle closure glaucoma

What are the Different Types of Cataract Surgeries?

- Phacoemulsification (Fig. 3.2)
  - This is the most commonly performed surgery for cataract removal

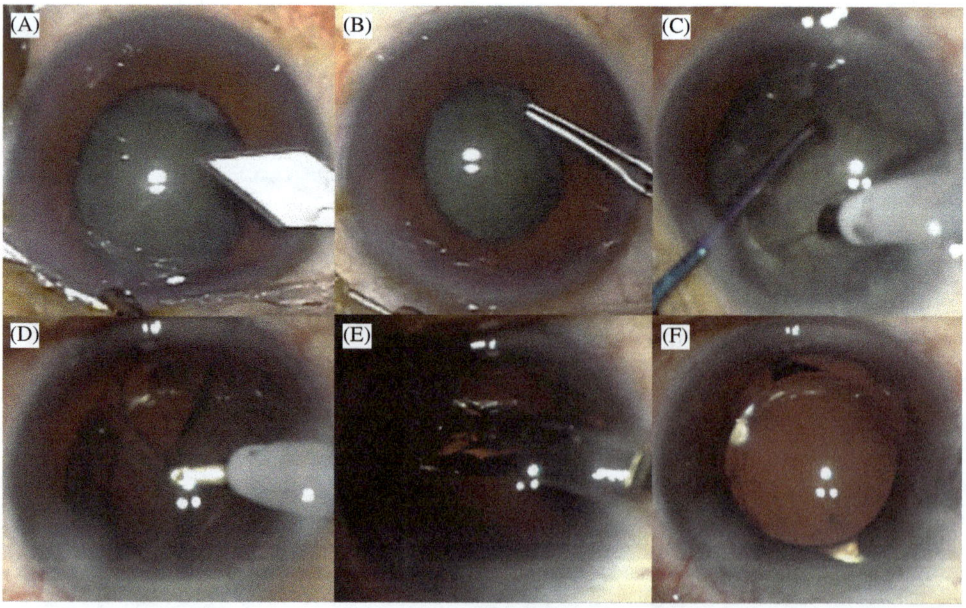

Fig. 3.2. Showing the steps of phacoemulsification, including (A) wound creation, (B) capsulorhexis, (C) phacoemulsification of lens material, (D) removal of soft lens material using an irrigation/aspiration probe, (E) implantation of a foldable intraocular lens, and the final image of the (F) completed surgery.

  - An ultrasonic probe delivers energy to break up and emulsify the cataract through a small (2–3 mm) wound. A foldable intraocular lens (IOL) is subsequently inserted through the small wound.
  - A femtosecond laser may be used to assist parts of the surgery (wound creation, capsulorhexis, or lens fragmentation)
- Extracapsular cataract extraction (ECCE)
  - A large incision (~10 mm) is created and the entire cataractous lens is delivered as a whole while leaving the capsular bag intact
  - The IOL is placed within the capsular bag
  - Sutures (10-0 nylon) are needed to close the large corneal wound
- Manual small incision cataract surgery (MSICS)
  - This is a small incision form of ECCE
  - A self-sealing scleral tunnel (2–3 mm) is created to facilitate the delivery of the entire cataract
  - MSICS is a low-cost surgery and is primarily performed in the developing world
- Intracapsular cataract extraction (ICCE)
  - A large incision (~10 mm) is created and the entire cataract is delivered together with the capsular bag
  - The IOL has to be placed in either the anterior chamber or be scleral-fixated
  - ICCE is not routinely performed for cataract surgery in the world

What are the Main Types of Intraocular Lenses?

- An intraocular lens (IOL) is inserted during cataract surgery to replace the crystalline lens after its removal
- The IOL can provide refractive error correction for the eye at the same time of cataract surgery; the different types of IOLs available are summarised in Table 3.1 below

Table 3.1. Types of Intraocular Lenses

Type of IOL	Description
1) Monofocal IOL	• Provides refractive error correction for one distance • Commonly, the goal of monofocal IOL is to provide good uncorrected distance vision (i.e. emmetropia) • Eyes with monofocal IOLs targeting emmetropia will require reading glasses for near work
2) Multifocal IOL	• Provides refractive error correction for distance, intermediate, and near visions, thus providing spectacle freedom • However, current multifocal IOLs can have side effects such as reduced contrast, glares and haloes • Multifocal IOLs are not suitable for eyes with other ocular pathology (e.g. advanced glaucoma, diabetic retinopathy, etc.)
3) Extended depth of focus (EDOF) IOL	• Provides good uncorrected distance and intermediate visions when targeted for emmetropia • EDOF IOLs produce less side effects when compared to multifocal IOLs

- Astigmatism correction could also be provided through IOLs; these are called toric IOLs (e.g. a monofocal IOL with astigmatism correction is called a toric monofocal IOL)

What are some Known Complications of Phacoemulsification?

- Intraoperative complications
  - Posterior capsular rupture
  - Dropped nucleus or nuclear fragment
  - Zonulysis
  - Iris trauma
  - Descemet membrane detachment
  - Suprachoroidal haemorrhage (rare but potentially blinding complication)
- Post-operative complications
  - Raised intraocular pressure from retained viscoelastic
  - Pseudophakic bullous keratopathy
  - Retained lens material
  - Posterior capsule opacification
  - Cystoid macular oedema
  - Endophthalmitis (rare but potentially blinding complication)

What are the Risk Factors for a Complicated Cataract Surgery?

- Patient factors
  - Uncooperative patient: dementia, excessive head movements, excessive lid squeezing
  - Challenging facial anatomy: deep set eyes, high nose bridge, prominent brow
- Ocular factors
  - Advanced cataract: dense cataract, brunescent cataract, white cataract
  - Pre-existing zonulysis: subluxated cataract
  - Narrow angles
  - Small pupil
  - Floppy iris (seen in patients on α_{1a} adrenergic antagonists such as tamsulosin, prazosin, and terazosin)
- Surgical factors
  - Inexperienced surgeon
  - Machine errors

Take Home Messages

- The mainstay of treatment for a visually significant cataract is cataract surgery.
- Everyone will eventually develop cataracts, but surgical indication is dependent on various other factors and the individual's visual needs.

Reference

1. Chylack LT Jr., Wolfe JK, Singer DM, *et al.* (1993) The Lens Opacities Classification System III. The Longitudinal Study of Cataract Study Group. *Arch Ophthal* (Chicago, Ill : 1960) **111(6)**:831–6.

Chapter 4

GLAUCOMA

Koh Teck Chang Victor, Katherine Lun

4.1 Definition and Classification

Learning Objectives

- Learn the definition of glaucoma
- To understand the various classifications of glaucoma

What is Glaucoma?

Glaucoma is a type of optic neuropathy characterised by progressive visual field loss in a patient with characteristic optic disc changes with corresponding visual field defects. Intraocular pressure is the main modifiable risk factor.

How Do You Classify Glaucoma?

Glaucoma can be classified into:

1) Open vs. Closed Angles (Table 4.1.)
2) Primary vs. Secondary (Table 4.1.)
3) Infantile/Childhood vs. adult onset

Table 4.1. Classification of Glaucoma

Open		Closed	
Primary	**Secondary**	**Primary**	**Secondary**
Primary Open Angle Glaucoma (POAG) (include Normal Tension Glaucoma (NTG))	- Trauma - Steroid-induced - Pseudoexfoliation - Pigment dispersion - Neovascular/Uveitic (in the absence of peripheral anterior synechiae (PAS)	Primary Angle Closure Glaucoma (PACG)	- Lens-related: Subluxed cataract, Intumescent cataract - Neovascular/ Uveitic (when PAS is present)

4.2 Primary Angle Closure Disease

Learning Objectives

- To learn the characteristics of primary angle closure glaucoma and its clinical features.
- To recognise acute angle closure and its immediate management.

What are the Various Subtypes of Primary Angle Closure Disease?

Primary angle closure disease can be differentiated according to gonioscopic findings, presence of raised IOP and evidence of glaucoma damage (Table 4.2).

Table 4.2. Showing the Characteristics of Various Primary Angle Closure Diseases

	Angle	IOP (Intraocular Pressure)	Glaucoma Damage	Remarks
PACS (Primary Angle Closure Suspect)	≥180 degrees of iridotrabecular contact (ITC) (determined by gonioscopy — see Section 4.4)	Not raised	Nil	No PAS on gonioscopy
PAC (Primary Angle Closure)	≥180 degrees of ITC May have PAS	May be raised	Nil	
PACG (Primary Angle Closure Glaucoma)	≥180 degrees of ITC Usually with PAS	Raised	Yes	

Who is at Risk of Developing Primary Angle Closure Glaucoma?

Risk of developing PACG can be divided into both systemic and ocular factors.

- Systemic risk factors
  - Older age
  - Female gender
  - Ethnicity: East Asian and Inuit
  - Genetics: 3–5 times greater risk of developing PACG with A positive family history of first-degree relatives

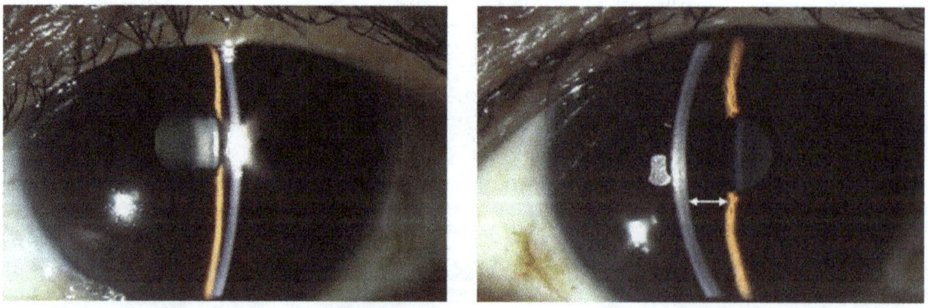

Fig. 4.1. (Left) Showing shallow anterior chamber depth and a deeper anterior chamber depth. (Right) Note the difference in distance between the two light beams (white double-headed arrow), which is used to estimate the anterior chamber depth.

- Ocular risk factors
    - Shallow anterior chamber depth (Figure 4.1)
    - Shorter axial length or hyperopia
    - Increased lens vault: Thick lens and/or anteriorly positioned lens

How is the Anterior Chamber Angle Assessed?

All patients referred for glaucoma evaluation require a standardised anterior chamber angle assessment.

- The anterior chamber angle can be assessed either clinically (with gonioscopy) or with anterior segment imaging (e.g. anterior segment optical coherence tomography and ultrasound biomicroscopy). This will be covered in detail in Section 4.4.
- Gonioscopy is still the current gold standard

How Do You Manage Eyes with Narrow Angles?

i. Management needs to be individualised depending on:
   1. Aetiology of the angle closure (primary or secondary)
   2. Stage of angle closure
   3. Mechanism of angle closure
   4. Adequacy of the preceding treatment

ii. The primary aim is to achieve an open angle with an acceptable target IOP with minimal side effects of treatment

iii. For PACS, the options include:
   1. Conservative monitoring with adequate education on symptoms and signs of acute primary angle closure (APAC) (See Table 4.3 on the summarised findings of the landmark ZAP study)
   2. Laser peripheral iridotomy (LPI) (Fig. 4.2)
      a. The most common mechanism of angle closure is pupil block
      b. LPI serves to eliminate pupil block and is an effective prophylaxis against an acute angle closure attack
   3. Other considerations for performing LPI in patients with PACS include:
      a. Require frequent dilated fundus examination (e.g. in diabetics)
      b. Using drugs that cause pupillary dilation (antidepressants, anticholinergics)
      c. Poorly educated patients or patients with reduced awareness who cannot identify symptoms of APAC
      d. Patients who are noncompliant or have difficulty accessing ophthalmic care during an APAC episode
      e. Fellow eye had APAC attack
      f. Only one functioning eye (monocular)
   4. Early Cataract Surgery (See Table 4.3 on the summarised findings of the landmark EAGLE study)

Table 4.3. Summarising Two Landmark Studies in Angle Closure Disease

	Zhongshan Angle Closure Prevention (ZAP) Study	**Effectiveness of Early Lens Extraction for the Treatment of Primary Angle-Closure Glaucoma (EAGLE) Study**
Aim	To evaluate the effectiveness of prophylactic LPI in preventing PAC and PACG in individuals with anatomically narrow angles.	To investigate the outcomes of clear lens extraction compared to standard LPI in patients with PACG and PAC.
Findings	Cumulative risk of progression was relatively low in the community-based PACS population over 14 years. Prophylactic LPI showed a modest effect in preventing angle closure disease. Prophylactic LPI should be reserved for those at the highest risk of primary angle closure glaucoma.	Compared to LPI and medical treatment, in patients with PAC (IOP >30 mmHg) and PACG (IOP >21 mmHg), early lens extraction was associated with better quality of life, lower IOP, less medication and the need for glaucoma interventions. Clear lens extraction was also more cost-effective than LPI in these groups of patients.

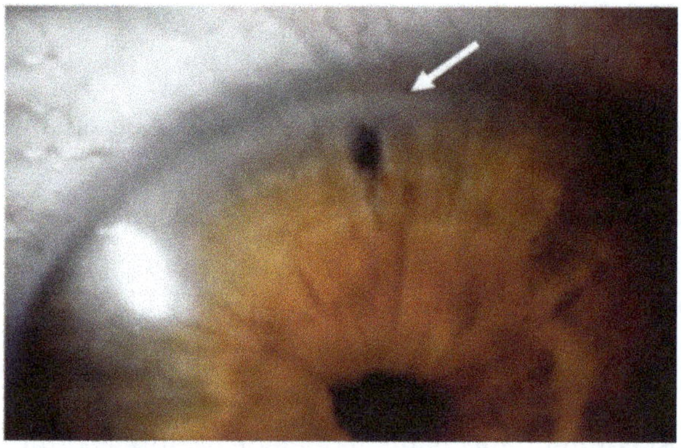

Fig. 4.2. Photograph showing a patent peripheral iridotomy (white arrow).

iv. For eyes with angle closure and raised IOP, i.e. PAC:
   1. Perform LPI or consider early cataract surgery (see EAGLE and ZAP study, Table 4.3)
   2. If target IOP is not reached, the patient should be started on topical IOP-lowering drugs

v. For PACG, the patient's IOP should be optimised based on the age, severity of glaucoma and presenting IOP. The target IOP should be reached in a step-wise approach (see Section 4.5)
   1. Medical therapy
   2. Laser
   3. Surgical intervention

Clinical Case Study

What is the Diagnosis? (Fig. 4.3)

Acute primary angle closure (APAC)

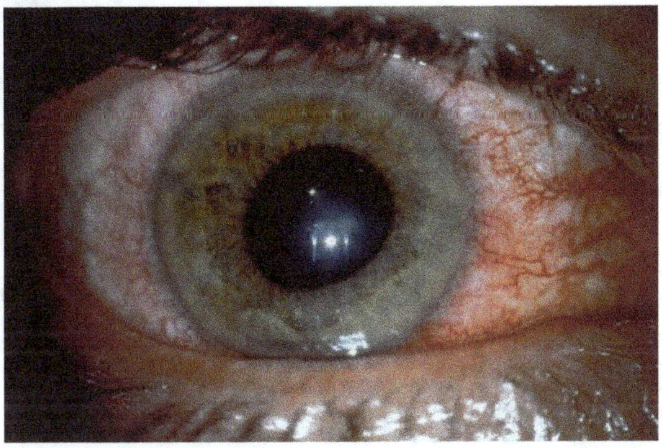

Fig. 4.3. A 70-year-old Chinese female presented with acute red and painful right eye.

This is a common EOPT question because APAC is an ocular emergency with significant visual morbidity if the diagnosis is missed in the primary eye care setting.

Differential Diagnoses

1. Acute anterior uveitis
2. Endophthalmitis
3. Scleritis

What are the Risk Factors of APAC?

The risk factors for APAC can be divided into systemic and ocular (Table 4.4)

Table 4.4. Risk Factors for APAC

Systemic	Ocular
Older age	Hypermetropia or shorter axial length
Chinese and Inuit race	Shallow anterior chamber depth
Female	Anterior lens vault
Family history of angle closure	Thicker peripheral iris

What are the Symptoms and Signs of APAC?

The typical symptoms of APAC are:

- Acute onset and unilateral
    - Eye redness and pain
    - Frontal headache
    - Blurring of vision
- Nausea and vomiting
- Preceding intermittent glares and haloes

The common signs of APAC include (in order of deceasing importance):

1. **Shallow anterior chamber depth** (note how close the two vertical beams of lights are to each other).	**Fig. 4.4** 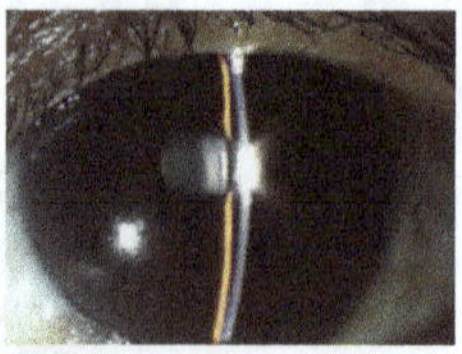
2. Gonioscopy showing **closed angle in both eyes** (note that the typical angle structures are obscured by the anterior bowing of the peripheral iris).	**Fig. 4.5** 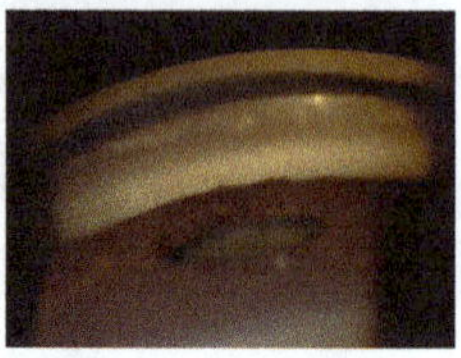
3. **Raised intraocular pressure**, which is measured using the Goldmann applanation tonometry.	
4. **Mid-dilated pupil**, which is non-reactive due to iris ischaemia from the raised intraocular pressure.	**Fig. 4.6** 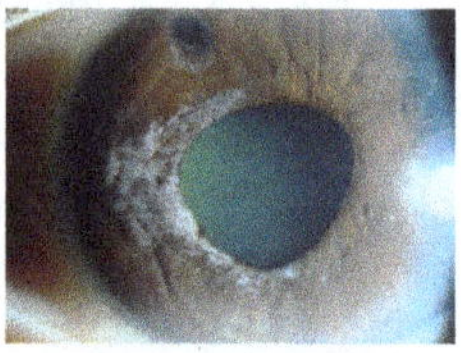
5. **Conjunctival injection** and **hazy oedematous cornea** due to the high intraocular pressure and ocular inflammation.	**Fig. 4.7** 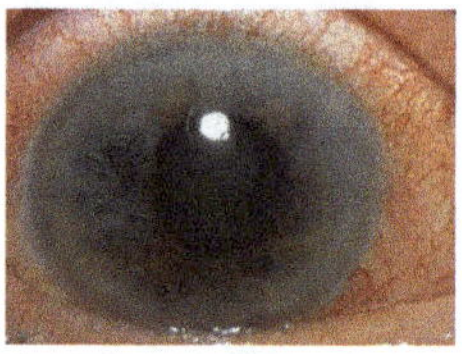

What is the Immediate Treatment for APAC?

APAC is an ocular emergency that requires urgent treatment to reduce intraocular pressure and relieve the pupil block. The key is prompt diagnosis and referral to the ophthalmologist.

The principles of management of APAC are highlighted in Table 4.5.

Table 4.5. Principles of Management of APAC

Principle	Management
1) Reduce IOP promptly	• Fast-acting topical IOP-lowering drugs, e.g. brimonidine, timolol • Topical steroids • Topical miotics • Systemic acetazolamide • Peripheral laser iridoplasty • AC paracentesis • Anderson's manoeuvre (corneal indentation with goniolens) • Lie supine

Principle	Management

2) Eliminate pupil block and non-pupil-block mechanisms	• Laser peripheral iridotomy
	• If the above measures fail, consider:
	  • Surgical iridectomy
	  • Urgent cataract extraction

3) Assess and treat the fellow eye	• Prophylactic laser peripheral iridotomy • Other treatments based on mechanisms
4) Monitoring for progression into chronic angle closure glaucoma (CACG)	• Anterior segment imaging (ASOCT) • Visual fields • Optic nerve head imaging

Take Home Messages

- All patients with suspected glaucoma should have a thorough assessment of the anterior chamber to rule out angle closure disease.
- The management of angle closure depends on the mechanism of angle closure, stage of disease and adequacy of preceding treatment.
- Acute angle closure is an ocular emergency. It requires prompt diagnosis and early treatment.

4.3 Primary Open Angle Glaucoma

Learning Objectives

- Learn the definition of primary open-angle glaucoma and the investigations required to make an accurate diagnosis.
- Identify the characteristic visual field defects associated with glaucoma.
- Definition of congenital glaucoma and its management principles.

What is Primary Open Angle Glaucoma (POAG)?

POAG is a subtype of glaucoma characterised by open angles on gonioscopy. It is commonly, but not always, associated with raised IOP.

1. Raised IOP does NOT equate to POAG.
   a. Ocular hypertension (OHT) is characterised by open angles, raised IOP and absence of glaucoma nerve damage and secondary causes of raised IOP.
2. Normal tension glaucoma (NTG), a subset of POAG, is not associated with raised IOP.

In POAG, the anterior chamber angles are open for at least 270° on gonioscopy without any evidence of ITC (iridotrabecular contact). Clinically, there must not be any secondary cause of trabecular outflow obstruction (Fig. 4.8)

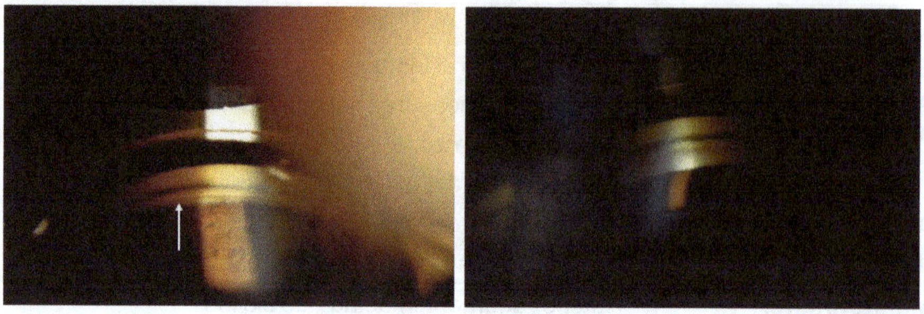

Fig. 4.8. Photographs showing gonioscopic comparison of open angle (Left) and angle closure (Right). In POAG, the angle structures can be visualised, especially the posterior trabecular meshwork on gonioscopy (brown pigmented band indicated by white arrow). There is the absence of new vessels, PAS, pigmentation and blood in Schlemm's canal (signifying raised episcleral venous pressure). In contrast, the image on the right shows angle closure — none of the normal anterior chamber angle structures can be seen.

What are Risk Factors of POAG?

Risk factors for POAG can be divided into major and minor factors. (Table 4.6.)

Table 4.6. Risk Factors for POAG

Major	Minor
• Afro-Caribbean race • Family history of POAG (2–3x increased risk) • Increased intraocular pressure • Increased age	• Myopia • Hypertension • Diabetes

What are Symptoms of POAG?

Patients with POAG are most commonly asymptomatic.

Peripheral vision is typically affected first; hence, in the early stages, most patients are still seeing well as central vision is still preserved. With time, there is a gradual loss of peripheral vision resulting in "tunnel vision". People who are symptomatic with blurred vision typically have advanced disease involving central vision.

Sometimes, patients can have headaches or eye pain when the intraocular pressure builds up or when the cornea begins to decompensate.

What is Normal Tension Glaucoma?

Normal Tension Glaucoma (NTG) is a subset of POAG where glaucomatous optic neuropathy occurs despite having normal IOP.

Although IOP remains one of the main modifiable risk factors, other risk factors at play include poor blood flow to the optic nerve (due to underlying conditions such as migraine, Raynaud's disease, low blood pressure, ischaemic vascular disorders), obstructive sleep apnoea and genetics (family history of glaucoma).

The visual defects in NTG patients tend to be more focal and closer to fixation, compared to those seen in POAG.

What are Optic Nerves Changes Characteristic of Glaucoma?

- **Characteristic "hard" signs:**
  - Gradual thinning of neurosensory rim starting at the inferior and superior quadrants first (Fig. 4.9)
  - Vertical cup-disc ratio > 0.6
  - Vertical cup-disc ratio asymmetry between eyes > 0.2 (Fig. 4.10)
  - Optic disc drance haemorrhage (Fig. 4.11)
  - Retinal nerve fibre layer defect (Fig. 4.12)
  - Acquired pit of the optic nerve
  - Focal notching of the neuro-retinal rim
  - Overhanging optic disc vessels crossing the neuro-retinal rim

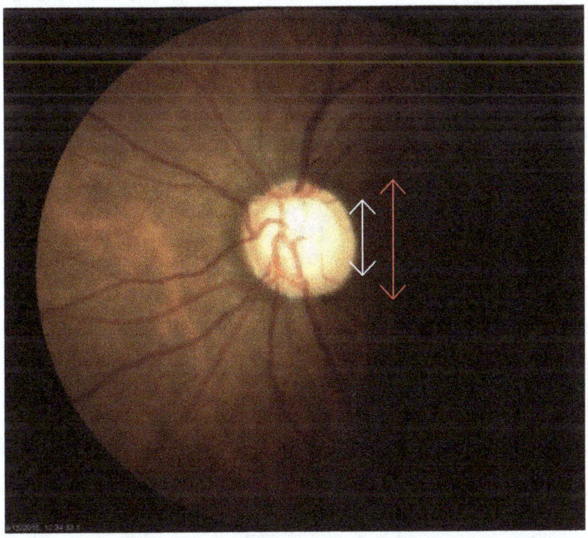

Fig. 4.9. Photograph showing an **increased vertical cup-disc ratio** (white arrow = cup height, red arrow = disc height.

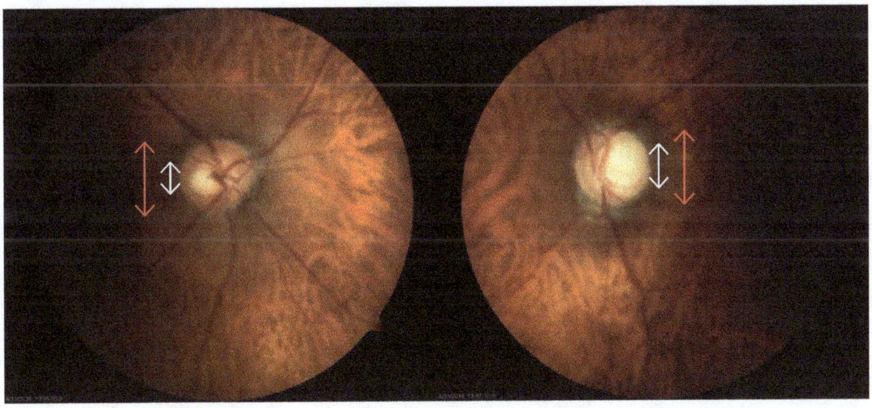

Fig. 4.10. The right and left eyes of the same patient showing **vertical cup-disc ratio asymmetry** of more than 0.2 (note: the right image shows the left eye).

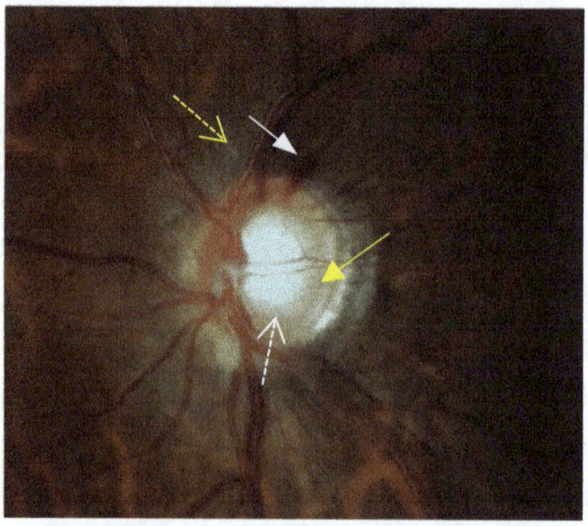

Fig. 4.11. Photograph showing optic disc **drance haemorrhage** (white arrow), thin inferior neuroretinal rim (yellow arrow), bayonetting of vessels (dotted white arrow) and nasalisation of vessels (dotted yellow arrow).

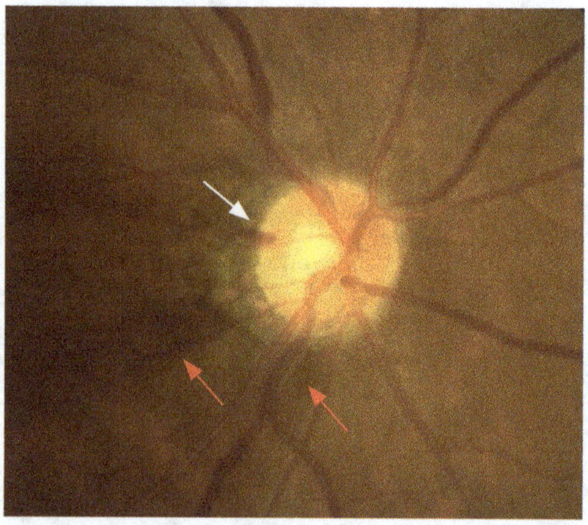

Fig. 4.12. Photograph showing a **wedge inferior retinal nerve fibre defect (red arrows)** and a **drance haemorrhage** of the optic nerve (white arrow).

- Minor changes
  - 360° of peripapillary atrophy (thinning of retina or RPE around the optic nerve)
  - Bayonetting of the blood vessels crossing the optic nerve (Fig. 4.11)
  - Nasalisation of optic nerve blood vessels (Fig 4.11)

What are Typical Visual Field Defect Patterns on Automated Perimetry?

- Visual defects associated with glaucoma can be classified into early and late. It can also be classified based on anatomy.

Table 4.7. Classification of Visual Field Loss According to the Stage of Glaucoma

Early Visual Field Loss	Late Visual Field Loss
Nasal step (Fig. 4.13) Seidel's scotoma (where paracentral scotoma reaches blindspot) Bjerrum scotoma (Fig. 4.13) (where the visual field defects extend in an arcuate manner to involve nasal field)	Arcuate visual field loss Altitudinal field loss Constricted visual fields with "tunnel vision"

- In glaucoma, it is important to note that the visual field defects should correspond to the structural abnormality.
  - e.g. A vertical cup-disc ratio of 0.9 can be expected to have a constricted visual field and vice versa. Similarly, an inferior neuroretinal rim notch is associated with a superior visual field defect.

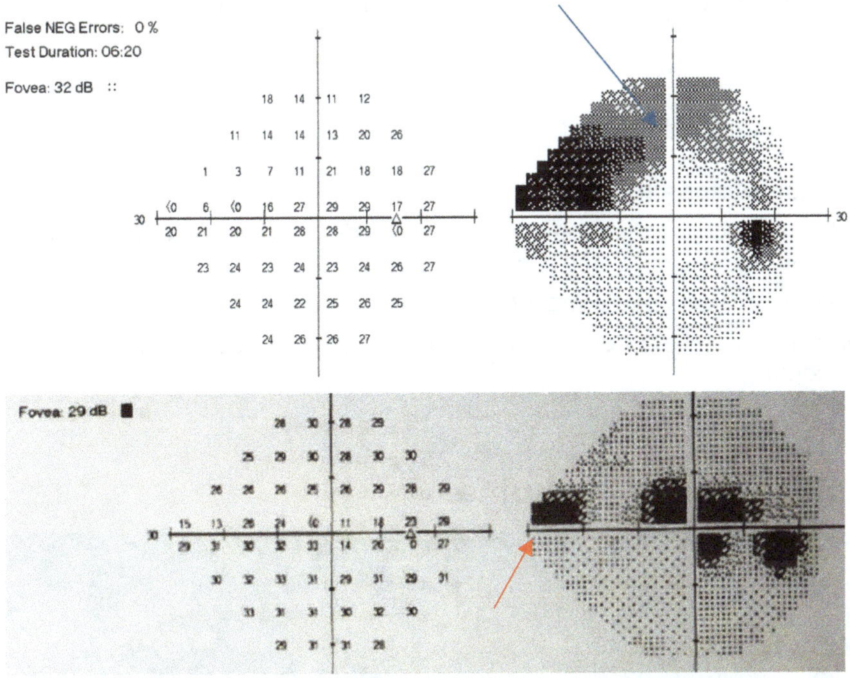

Fig. 4.13. Static automated visual field test showing nasal step (bottom, red arrow), and Bjerrum's scotoma (top, blue arrow) of the right eyes of different patients.

What is Ocular Hypertension?

This is a condition characterised by

1) Raised intraocular pressure
2) No evidence of glaucomatous optic neuropathy — this distinguishes OHT from POAG

The Ocular Hypertension Treatment Study (OHTS) looked at the risk factors associated with the progression of OHT to POAG.

- Risk factors for progression include increased cup-disc ratio, older age, thinner central cornea thickness, higher baseline IOP and higher pattern standard deviation on visual field testing
- Study found that reducing IOP in patients with OHT reduced the risk of developing POAG by about 50% over a 5-year period

Clinical Case Study

A 2-month-old baby was referred to the ophthalmologist after the paediatrician notices that there were bilateral cloudy corneas and the baby's eyes appeared "bigger than usual".

What are the Differentials?

- Congenital glaucoma (most important diagnosis to consider)
- Sclerocornea
- Peter's anomaly
- Muchopolysacharidosis

Take Home Messages

- POAG is associated with an increased cup-disc ratio with characteristic optic nerve appearance and corresponding visual field defect.
- Raised IOP is one of the main risk factors for POAG.
- Apart from a raised cup-disc ratio, there are other optic nerve features of glaucoma.

4.4 Secondary Glaucoma

Learning Objectives

- Identify the different types and mechanisms of secondary glaucoma.
- Outline the main principles of management specific to the aetiology of secondary glaucoma.

What are the Types of Secondary Glaucoma?

1. **Open angle**
   - Causes can be divided into pre-trabecular meshwork (TM), trabecular meshwork and post-trabecular meshwork
     - Pre-TM: Iridocorneal Endothelial (ICE) syndrome (Fig. 4.14), epithelial downgrowth, tumours, aphakia
     - TM: Hyphaema, inflammatory (uveitis, tumours), NVG, pigments (Fig. 4.16), PXF (Fig. 4.15), steroids, iatrogenic (silicone oil)
     - Post-TM: Carotid-cavernous fistula, Sturge–Weber syndrome

2. **Angle closure**

   Causes can be divided into push and pull mechanisms:

   - Push: lens-induced, lens subluxation, ciliary body cysts/tumours, iatrogenic (SO or scleral buckle), aqueous misdirection/drugs (topiramate, sulfonamide, anti-cholinergics)
   - Pull: AAU, NVG (in the presence of peripheral anterior synechiae), ICE, aniridia

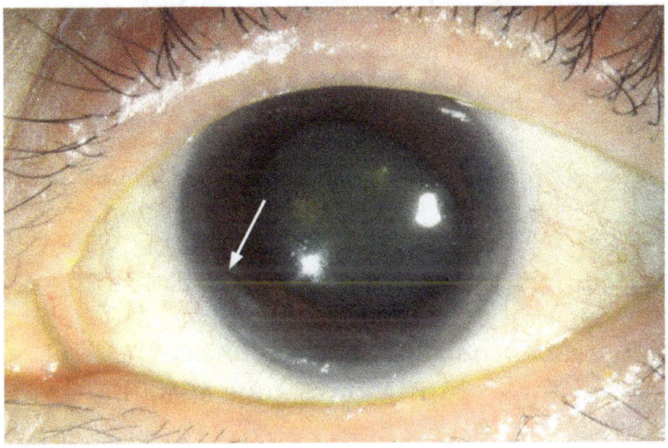

Fig. 4.14. Showing high peripheral anterior synechiae (white arrow) characteristic of ICE syndrome.

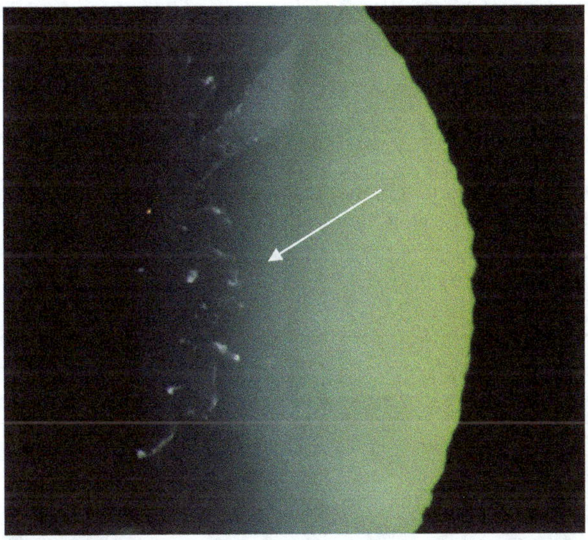

Fig. 4.15. Showing hoarfrost ring (white arrow) characteristic of pseudoexfoliation syndrome.

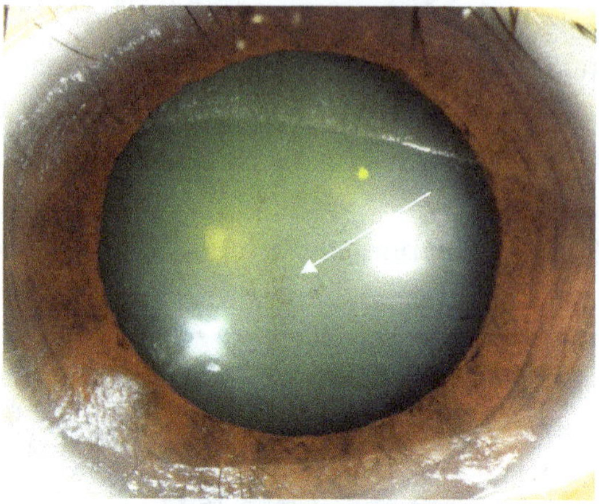

Fig. 4.16. Showing pigments (white arrow) on the anterior lens capsule in a patient with pigment dispersion syndrome.

What is Traumatic Glaucoma?

- Subtype of secondary glaucoma following significant ocular trauma, resulting in either open or closed angle obstruction of aqueous outflow from the eye

What are the Mechanisms of Traumatic Glaucoma?

Mechanisms of traumatic glaucoma can be classified according to the angle status.

Table 4.8. Classification of Mechanisms of Traumatic Glaucoma According to Angle Status

Open Angle	Angle Closure
• Angle recession glaucoma (Fig. 4.17) • Steroid-induced glaucoma • Hyphaema (risk of re-bleeding is highest around 3–5 days after injury; higher risk if hyphaema is more than 1/3 of AC depth, sickle cell disease, or on anti-coagulation drugs) (Fig. 4.18) • Ghost cell glaucoma	• Subluxed lens • Dense cataracts • Peripheral anterior synechiae (PAS)

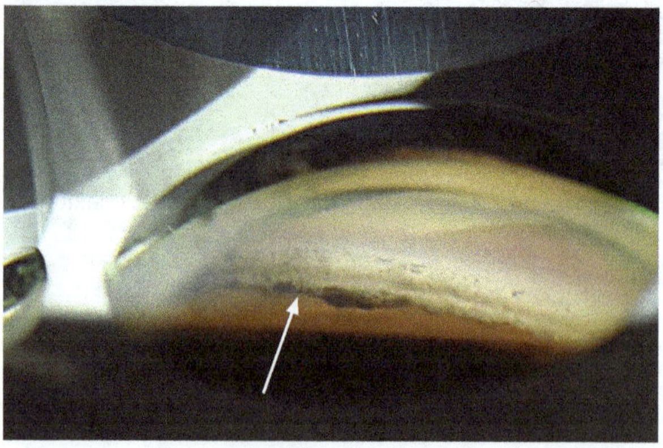

Fig. 4.17. Photograph showing a **prominent ciliary body** (white arrow) in angle recession syndrome after trauma.

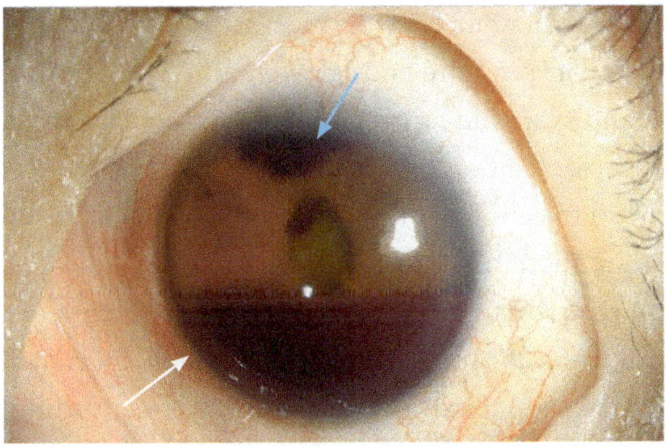

Fig. 4.18. Photograph showing **gross hyphaema** (white arrow) from **superior haemorrhage** (blue arrow).

What are the Causes of Neovascular Glaucoma (NVG)?

1. Most common causes of NVG (Fig. 4.19) are:
    - Proliferative diabetic retinopathy
    - Ischaemic central retinal vein occlusion
    - Ocular ischaemic syndrome
2. Less common causes include:
    - Chronic retinal detachment
    - Chronic uveitis (e.g. Vogt-Koyanagi-Harada Disease (VKH), Behçet's disease)
    - Ocular tumours (e.g. choroidal melanoma, retinoblastoma)
    - Carotid-cavernous fistula

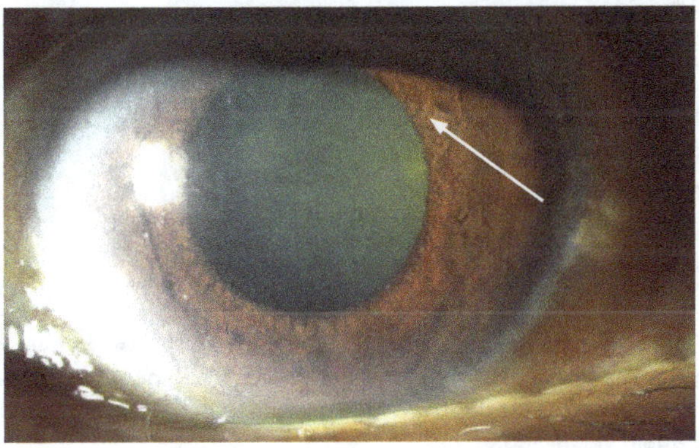

Fig. 4.19. Photograph showing florid iris neovascularisation (white arrow) in a patient with NVG. Iris neovascularisation is usually most prominent around the pupillary border.

How is NVG Treated?

1) NVG is a difficult condition to treat and the visual prognosis is usually guarded.
2) Management depends on the underlying cause, visual prognosis and patient symptoms.

3) Principles of management include:
   (a) Reduce intraocular pressure and relieve pain
      (i) Topical and systemic drugs to lower intraocular pressure
      (ii) Topical cycloplegics
      (iii) Intravitreal injection of anti-vascular endothelial growth factor
   (b) Determine the cause and reduce ischaemic drive
      (i) Perform panretinal laser photocoagulation if no media opacity
   (c) Subsequent intraocular pressure control depends on visual prognosis
      (i) Good visual prognosis: glaucoma surgery — including glaucoma shunt surgery
      (ii) Poor visual prognosis:
         1. Painful: trans-scleral cyclophotocoagulation
            a. If blind, consider evisceration
         2. Painless: conservative
            a. Topical IOP-lowering medications
            b. Topical cycloplegics

Clinical Case Study

A 30-year-old African American female with a history of sarcoidosis presented with right eye redness and blurring of vision for 1 week. Examination showed anterior chamber cells and granulomatous keratic precipitates (Fig. 4.20). Her intraocular pressure was 35 mmHg in the right eye.

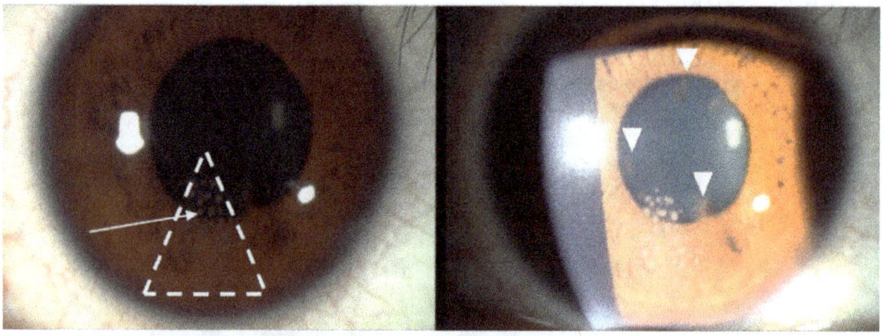

Fig. 4.20. (Left) Shows granulomatous keratic precipitates (white arrow) on inferior corneal endothelium forming the Arlt's triangle (dotted triangle). (Right) Shows the same eye with posterior synechiae, which is adhesion between the iris and anterior lens surface (arrowheads). The keratic precipitates are once again visualised.

What are the Mechanisms of Raised IOP in a Patient with Uveitis?

Mechanisms of raised IOP can be classified according to open or closed angle. (Table 4.9)

Table 4.9. Showing the Various Mechanisms of Raised IOP in Uveitis, Classified According to the Angle Status

Open Angle	Angle Closure
• Angle failure due to chronic and recurrent inflammation • Steroid-induced • Neovascularisation	• Peripheral anterior synechiae • Extensive posterior synechiae causing seclusio pupillae

What are the Causes of Hypertensive Uveitis?

The causes of hypertensive uveitis can be categorised according to infective versus non-infective causes. (Table 4.10)

Table 4.10. Classification of Causes of Hypertensive Uveitis

Infective	Non-infective
• Viral: CMV, HSV, VZV, rubella • Bacterial: bacterial endophthalmitis, syphilis, toxoplasmosis	• Matsuo-Schwartz from retinal detachment • Sarcoidosis

Clinical Case Study

A 79-year-old man with pre-existing poor vision in the right eye was punched in the same eye during a domestic dispute. He presented with right eye pain, redness, nausea and vomiting 2 days after the incident. On examination, you find the following (Fig. 4.21):

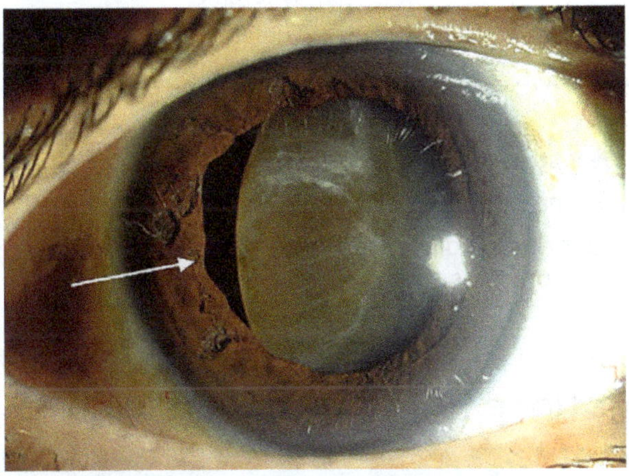

Fig. 4.21. Photograph of the patient's right eye showing infero-temporal subluxation of a cataractous lens. The zonular fibres are not well visualised, and the iris margins are irregular nasally (white arrow), suggesting possible sphincter rupture.

What has Happened to the Right Eye of this patient?

He has a dense cataract, which has also subluxed inferiorly.

What are the Types of Lens-induced Glaucoma?

Lens-induced glaucoma can be classified according to the angle status (Table 4.11.)

Table 4.11. Classification of the Types of Lens-induced Glaucoma According to the Angle Status

Angle Closure	Open Angle
• Subluxed lens • Dense cataract causing **phacomorphic** glaucoma	• **Phacoanaphylactic:** breached lens capsule with the resulting leak of lens material inciting AC inflammation • **Phacolytic:** intact anterior lens capsule through which lens material leaks, causing AC inflammation

What are Some Risk Factors for Lens Subluxation?

Risk factors for lens subluxation can be classified into congenital versus acquired factors. (Table 4.12.)

Table 4.12. Classification of the Causes of Lens Subluxation

Congenital	Acquired
• Ectopia lentis • Connective tissue disease: Marfan, Ehlers-Danlos • Metabolic disorders: Homocystinuria	• Ocular trauma • Dense brunescent cataract • Myopia • Pseudoexfoliation/pigment dispersion syndrome • Tumours (e.g. retinoblastoma, ciliary body melanoma)

Take Home Messages

- Secondary glaucoma can be subdivided into open angle and angle closure.
- Neovascular glaucoma is a difficult condition to treat and management depends on aetiology, visual prognosis and symptoms.

4.5 Investigations Related to Glaucoma

Learning Objectives

- Familiarise with the common investigations performed for glaucoma patients.
- Learn how to interpret static automated perimetry in a systematic approach.

What are the Investigations Commonly Performed for Glaucoma patients?

1. Structural tests
   a. Anterior segment
      i. Anterior segment optical coherence tomography
      ii. Ultrasound biomicroscopy
      iii. Photo-gonioscopy
   b. Posterior segment
      i. Stereodisc photographs
      ii. Optical coherence tomography of the retinal nerve fibre layer and ganglion cell — inner plexiform layer
      iii. Confocal laser scanning ophthalmoscopy (less commonly used)
2. Functional tests
   a. Static automated perimetry

What are the Ways to Evaluate Anterior Chamber Angles?

The evaluation of the anterior chamber angles is important in determining the pathogenesis of glaucoma — open or closed angle. There are various modes including:

i) Slit-lamp gonioscopy

(1) Gold standard

(2) Performed in dark conditions at the slit lamp and using a gonioscope

(3) Light from the anterior chamber undergoes total internal reflection and so a contact lens is required to overcome this principle

(a) The goniolens has a similar refractive index as the cornea and alters the cornea–air interface to overcome the critical angle that prevents total internal refraction of light from the angles

(4) Gonioscope lenses can be direct or indirect

(a) Direct gonioscope allows direct visualisation of the angle and is usually used during angle surgery (e.g. goniotomy)

(b) Indirect gonioscope uses mirrors to overcome total internal reflection (Fig. 4.22). It can be divided into indentational and non-indentational.

(i) Indentation describes the process of applying gentle pressure on the cornea with a gonioscope to differentiate between appositional and synechial closure

(ii) In appositional closure, contact between the peripheral iris and trabecular meshwork is dynamic and can be broken by indentation of the cornea

(iii) In synechial closure, this contact cannot be broken despite pressure on the cornea. This is due to permanent adhesions, known as peripheral anterior synechiae, between the peripheral iris and cornea.

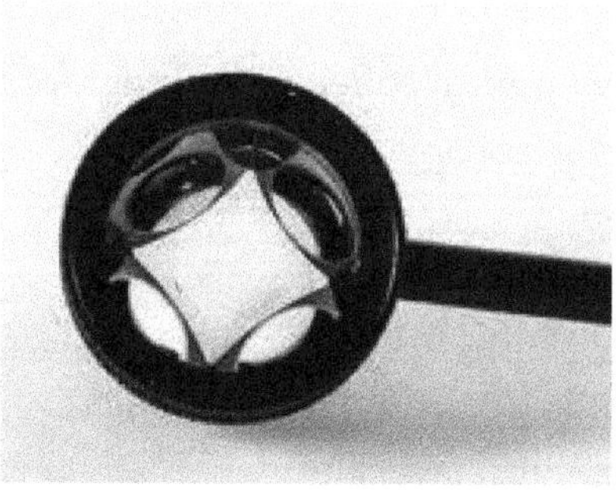

Fig. 4.22. Showing a picture of a 4-mirror goniolens used for indentational gonioscopy.

ii) Anterior segment optical coherence tomography (AS-OCT)

(1) Provides high-resolution cross-sectional images of the anterior segment of the eye (Fig. 4.23)

(2) Provides qualitative and quantitative assessment of the anterior chamber angles, mechanism of angle closure, lens position and even cornea pathology

iii) Ultrasound biomicroscopy (UBM)

(1) Uses 35–100 MHz frequency transducer, which provides a resolution of up to 25 μm

(2) It has better tissue penetration compared to AS-OCT, and allows evaluation of structures behind the iris (e.g. ciliary body, pars plana, zonules)

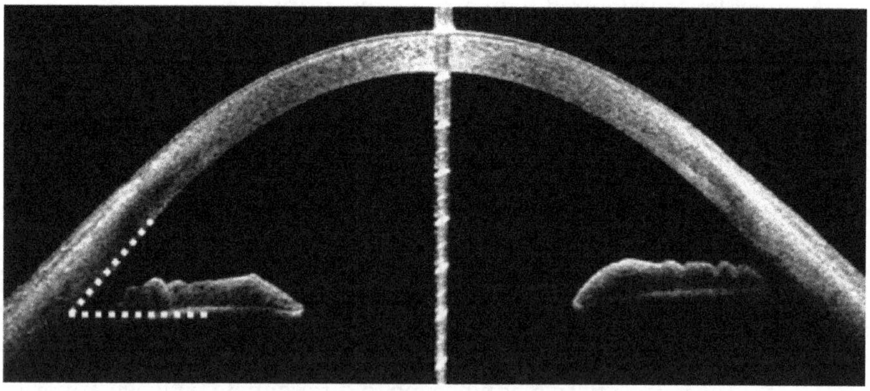

Fig. 4.23A. AS-OCT image showing open angle (white dotted lines).

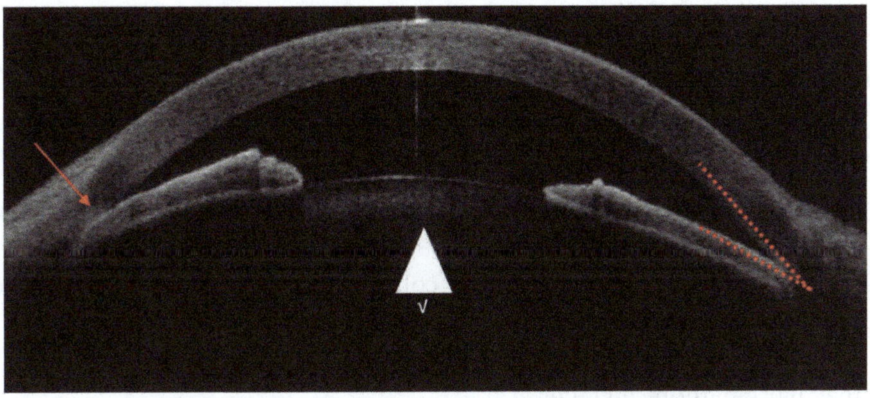

Fig. 4.23B. AS-OCT image showing narrow angles (red dotted lines) with closure in one quadrant (red arrow). The anterior lens vault from the cataract is also seen (white arrowhead).

Table 4.13. Summarising the Advantages and Disadvantages of Various Anterior Chamber Angle Imaging Modalities

	Advantages	Disadvantages
Gonioscopy	• Low cost • Less equipment required • Colour visualisation of the angles (e.g. tumours, FB, NVA) • Can indent to differentiate appositional vs. synechial angle closure	• Poor reproducibility • Not quantifiable • Operator dependent • Cannot visualise behind the iris
AS-OCT	• Non-contact • Fast • Reproducible • Latest Swept-Source OCT allows 360° assessment of the angles • Quantifiable parameters	• Cannot visualise behind the iris • Expensive
UBM	• Can visualise structures behind the iris (including ciliary body, lens zonules)	• Operator dependent • Only in supine position • Time-consuming • Expensive

Why is Structural Imaging of the Optic Nerve Head Important and How is it Done?

Histologic and imaging studies have shown that structural changes to the optic nerve head or retinal nerve fibre layer precedes functional changes — up to 40% of retinal ganglion cell loss may have occurred before any detectable visual field loss appears.

Common imaging modalities used in the clinical setting:

1. Stereodisc photographs
    - The earliest form of optic nerve imaging
2. Optical coherence tomography (e.g. Cirrus® OCT-RNFL)
    - Uses low coherence laser interferometry to acquire high-resolution cross-sectional images of the eye
    - Current spectral domain OCT can collect up to 55,000 A-scans per second with a resolution of 5 μm
    - Measures parameters of the optic nerve head, retinal nerve fibre layer and the macular ganglion cell layer

Table 4.14. Summarising the Advantages and Disadvantages of Various Optic Nerve Head Structural Imaging Modalities

	Advantages	Disadvantages
Stereodisc (Fig. 4.24)	• Affordable • Colour images can show disc haemorrhages or disc pallor • Not affected by a change in technology upgrades	• Cannot detect small changes in optic nerve head, making monitoring difficult • Only 2-dimensional: only certain structural defects (e.g. cup-disc ratio and disc size) are seen
OCT (Fig. 4.25)	• Non-contact • Fast • Highly reproducible • Guided progression analysis to detect structural progression using retinal nerve fibre layer thickness	• Expensive • Floor effect: for advanced disease, OCT measurements level off and do not fall below 50–70 μm • Media opacity can affect signal quality • Normative database does not include eyes with high myopia

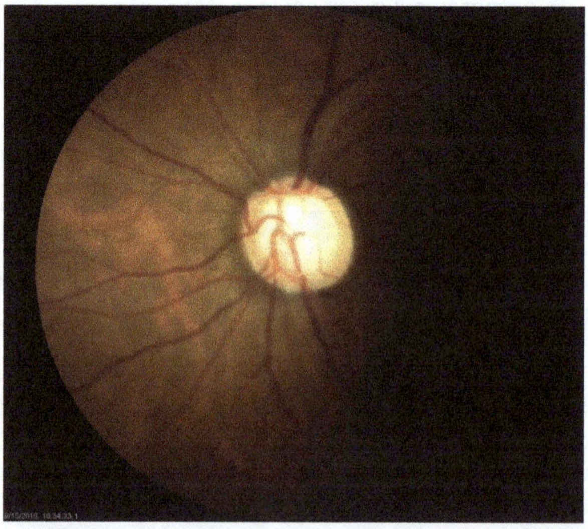

Fig. 4.24. Disc photograph showing increased cup-disc ratio. Colour disc photographs are useful as an objective documentation of disc appearance as a baseline.

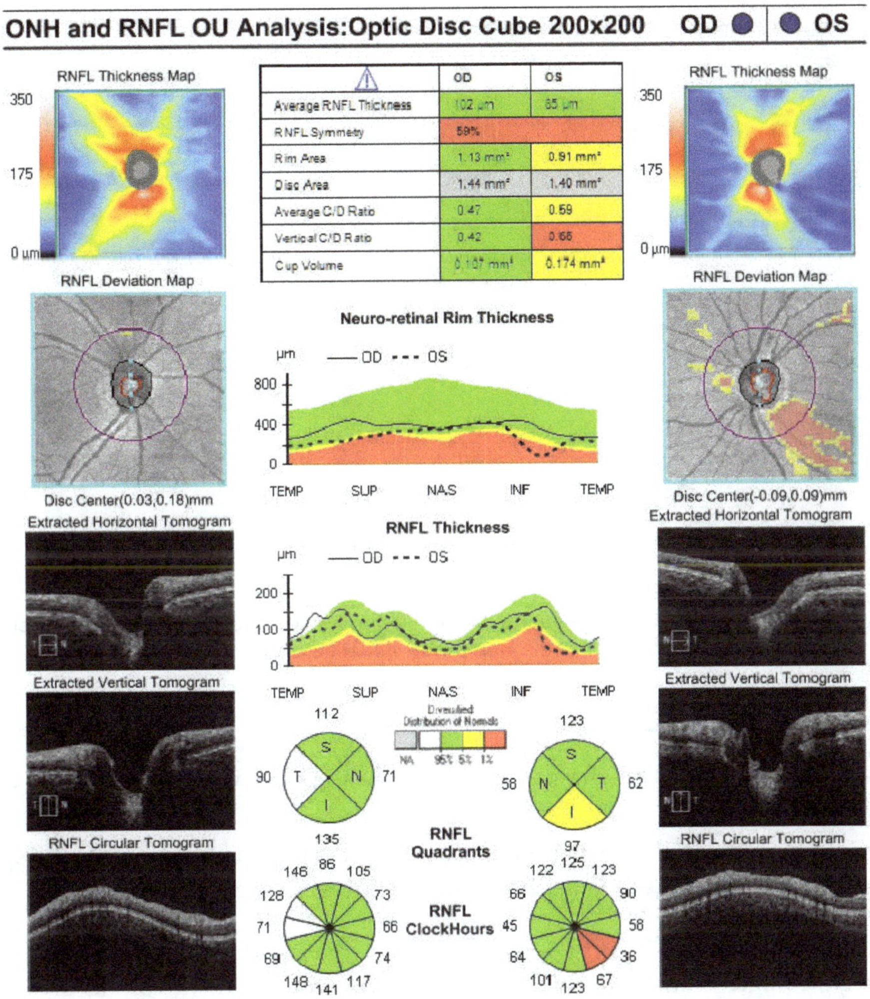

Fig. 4.25. Image showing a typical OCT printout, demonstrating inferior retinal nerve fiber layer (RNFL) thinning in the left eye.

Clinical Case Study

A 50-year-old Chinese female with a family history of glaucoma wants to check her risk of glaucoma. The following test (Fig. 4.26) was performed in the clinic:

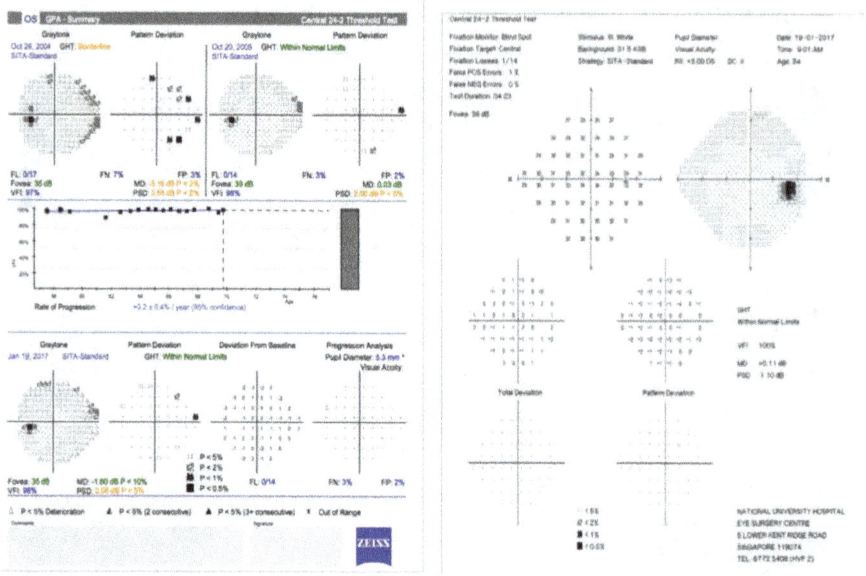

Fig. 4.26. Left image showing the **Glaucoma Progression Analysis (GPA)** summary of the left eye. Right image shows a typical printout of the **Humphrey visual field** test.

What is the Test Being Shown Below?

- Static automated perimetry testing the central 24° of fixation using the SITA standard algorithm
- Perimetry refers to the measurement of one's visual field — defined as the space that one eye can see while maintaining fixation at a single target

What Testing Strategies are Available?

Testing strategies can be divided into suprathreshold, full threshold and SITA (Table 4.15).

Table 4.15. Showing the Characteristics of Various Testing Strategies

Suprathreshold	Full Threshold	SITA
• Rapid screening test • Light stimulus is very intense and is the same across the whole visual field • Output is categorical — "Yes" or "No" only	• Retinal sensitivity is tested at each point using bracketing method • Time-consuming but provides point-by-point qualitative data • Duration of test can be shortened using artificial intelligence such as the Swedish Interactive Threshold Algorithm (SITA)	• Based on Bayesian probability and estimates the retinal sensitivity at each point • Uses real-time calculation to estimate adjacent threshold values based on the patient's individual response • Preferred by clinicians due to the shorter test duration without affecting diagnostic performance

How to Interpret the Static Automated Perimetry Results (Fig. 4.27)

1. Determine the boundary of visual field testing (common: central 24, 30 or 10 degrees) and the reliability of the test (see below)
2. Check the test strategies used and whether they are consistent with previous tests, especially when monitoring for progression
3. Raw values plots provide the raw threshold values of each point for the individual patient
4. Total deviation plots refer to the deviation of each individual test point compared to the age-matched normal controls
5. Pattern deviation plots adjust for generalised reduction in retinal sensitivity (due to refractive errors or cataracts) and reveal the underlying localised visual field defects or scotomas
6. Global indices: These secondary summary values are derived from the raw data and provide the clinician with an overall impression of the results
   - Glaucoma Hemifield Test (GHT): compares 5 zones in the superior and corresponding 5 zones in the inferior hemifield. The extent of asymmetry is

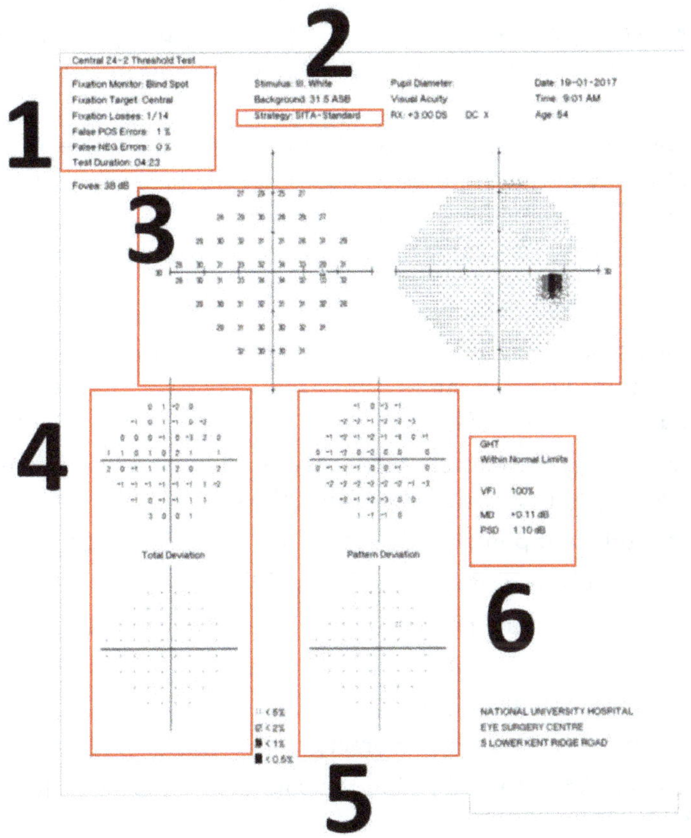

Fig. 4.27. A printout of a **Humphrey 24-2 visual field** of a normal patient's right eye.

used as an indicator for glaucoma. The possible results are: within normal limits, outside normal limits and borderline.

- Visual field index (VFI): Expresses visual field status as a percentage of a normal age-matched visual field
    i. Greater weight is given to points closer to fixation to adjust for differential ganglion cell density
    ii. Less affected by cataracts or after cataract surgery
    iii. Commonly used as a marker to track visual progression
- Mean deviation (MD): Average deviation of each point from age-matched normal controls. In general, more minus is bad (**M** for MD).
- Pattern standard deviation (PSD): Indicator of the variability of all the points within the visual fields. In general, more plus is bad (**P** for PSD).

How Do You Evaluate the Reliability of This Test?

- Static automated perimetry is a subjective test and has 3 main reliability indices
    - Fixation loss: a surrogate measure of how well the patient keeps fixation at a fixed target in primary gaze. In general, a fixation loss of less than 20% is acceptable.
    - False positive: a high value indicates a "trigger-happy" patient who responds even though he/she did not detect any light stimulation. A value of less than 30% is acceptable.
    - False negative: a high value suggests an "inattentive" patient who did not respond to a repeated stimulation, which he/she has responded to earlier in the test. A value of less than 30% is acceptable.
    - Other tests of reliability include the eyelid movement and eye movement tracker

How Can Static Perimetry be Monitored in a Patient with Glaucoma?

Serial visual fields can be monitored manually or using automated software. The latter can be broadly classified into:

- Event-based progression analysis
    - Glaucoma progression analysis (GPA) was the first event-based change analysis software to be put into widespread clinical use
    - Identifies significant point-wise progression based on statistical probabilities
    - Requires at least three sequential visual fields
    - Does not require as many fields to detect progression compared to trend-based analysis
- Trend-based progression analysis
    - For clinical practice, this is more practical
    - Allows the clinician to determine the rate of progression/deterioration in visual fields
        i. Provides extrapolated data based on trend analysis
        ii. Uses either the visual field index or mean deviation as the summary measure of the global retinal sensitivity

Take Home Messages

- Gonioscopy is still the gold standard for anterior chamber angle evaluation, but anterior segment optical coherence tomography and ultrasound biomicroscopy imaging are alternatives.
- Structural imaging of the optic nerve head provides an objective measurement for monitoring purposes.
- Static automated perimetry is a subjective test and the reliability indices need to be assessed prior to interpretation.

4.6 Management of Glaucoma and its Complications

Learning Objectives

- Learn the principles and indications for medical, laser and surgical therapy for glaucoma.
- Identify the potential side effects or complications associated with therapy.

What Do You Understand by Target Intraocular Pressure (IOP)?

Target IOP is the estimated IOP level on/below which functional and structural progression of glaucoma is less likely to happen. Target IOP needs to be individualised based on the age and life expectancy of the patient, presenting IOP and the severity of glaucoma.

How Can the Target IOP be Achieved?

This can be achieved using medications, laser therapy, and ultimately, surgery, should conservative options fail.

1. **Medical therapy:**
   - Most glaucoma medications aim to reduce aqueous humour production and/or increase outflow of aqueous through the trabecular meshwork or uveoscleral outflow pathways.
   - **Aqueous Suppressants:**
     - **A**lpha agonist (Brimonidine-Alphagan ®)
     - **B**eta-blocker (B1 non selective antagonist — Timolol; B1 selective — Betaxolol)
     - **C**arbonic anhydrase inhibitor, both topical and systemic — Acetazolamide (Azopt ®), Dorzolamide (Trusopt ®)
   - **Increase aqueous outflow**
     - i. Alpha-2 agonist (Brimonidine — Alphagan ®, Apraclonidine)
     - ii. Prostaglandin analogues (Latanoprost — Xalatan ®; Bimatoprost — Lumigan ®; Travoprost — Travatan ®; Tafluprost — Taflotan ®)
     - iii. Prostanoid E2 receptor agonist (Omidenepag isopropyl — Eybelis ®)
     - iv. Rho kinase inhibitors (Ripasudil — Glanatec ®; Netarsudi — Rhopressa ®)
     - v. Cholinergics (Pilocarpine)

- **Hyperosmotic agents**
  i. Mannitol
  ii. Glycerine
- Fixed combination drugs
  i. Usually in combination with a beta-blocker
  ii. Improve compliance to medications by rationalising daily regime

2. Lasers

- **Iris**
  - Laser peripheral iridotomy (Fig. 4.28)
    - One of the key treatments for angle closure
    - Relieves pupil block (most common mechanism for angle closure) and widens anterior chamber angle
    - Pupil block results from relative resistance between the lens and pupillary margin, leading to a differential pressure between the posterior and anterior chamber
    - Classic iris bombe configuration: Forward bowing of the iris results in contact between the trabecular meshwork and peripheral iris. This occlusion of the anterior chamber angles prevents aqueous drainage and results in a build-up of intraocular pressure.
    - Laser iridotomy neutralises the differential pressure gradient anterior and posterior to the iris, resulting in iris flattening
  - Laser peripheral iridoplasty (Fig. 4.28)
    - Treats plateau iris syndrome
    - Can be used to temporarily reduce IOP in acute angle closure

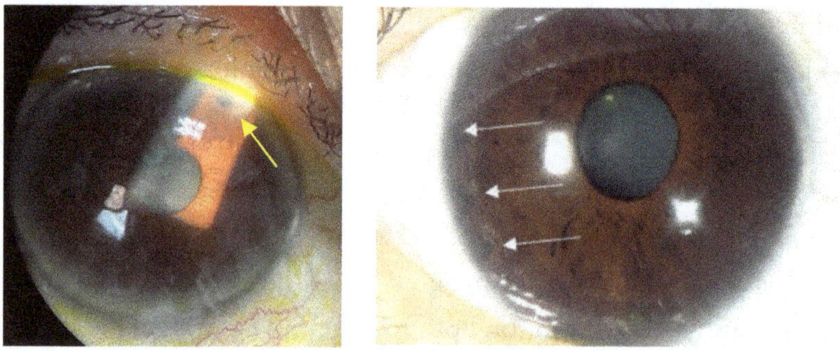

(a) (b)

Fig. 4.28. (A) Peripheral laser iridotomy (yellow arrow). (B) Iridoplasty scars (white arrows).

- **Trabecular meshwork**
  i. Selective laser trabeculoplasty
    - Increases aqueous outflow through the trabecular meshwork due to both mechanical and biochemical mediators
    - Effective for POAG, OHT and pigmentary glaucoma

        - May be used following failed medical therapy, as an adjunct to medical therapy or as primary treatment (if appropriate)
        - It is also suitable for the following patient groups:
            - Unfit for surgery
            - Not keen for surgery
            - Pregnancy
        - Effect may be temporary
    - **Ciliary body**
        - Cyclophotocoagulation
            - Reduces aqueous production by reducing ciliary body volume
            - Can be delivered transscleral (transscleral cyclophotocoagulation, TCP) or endoscopically (endoscopic cyclophotocoagulation, ECP)
            - Typically reserved for refractory glaucoma with poor visual prognosis
            - Risk of phthisis bulbi and sympathetic ophthalmia
            - Micropulse mode (micropulse transscleral cyclophotocoagulation, MPTCP) is increasingly popular (Fig. 4.29)
                - More gentle to the ciliary body compared to traditional TCP
                - Can be repeated multiple times if necessary
                - Lower risk of phthisis bulbi

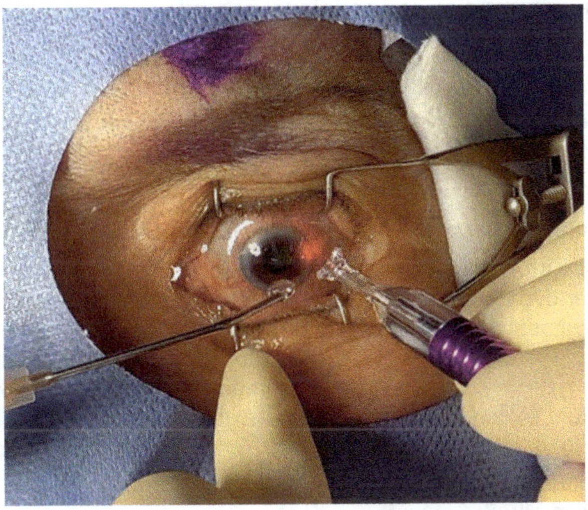

Fig. 4.29. Patient undergoing micropulse transscleral cyclophotocoagulation.

3. **Surgery**
    - Surgical interventions for glaucoma aim to improve aqueous drainage by maximising innate outflow facility or create an alternative outflow path. These interventions range from cataract extraction to minimally invasive glaucoma surgery (MIGS) or more invasive options such as trabeculectomy and glaucoma drainage implants (GDI).

- Glaucoma Filtration Surgery (Trabeculectomy) and GDI were the most commonly performed glaucoma surgeries in the past and were indicated when the patient demonstrated functional or structural deterioration and the inability to achieve target IOP despite maximum tolerable medical therapy.
  - However, in recent years, MIGS has been increasingly popular and is typically performed in patients with mild to moderate glaucoma or OHT.

- **Phacoemulsification**
  - Indicated for angle closure eyes in which the "bulky" lens (usually also has significant cataract) contributes to angle narrowing
  - Removal of the cataract and replacement with a thinner intraocular lens improves the trabecular meshwork drainage of aqueous and lowers IOP
  - Can be combined with goniosynechialysis to release early peripheral anterior synechiae
  - In eyes with mild glaucoma, phacoemulsification can be augmented with MIGS to increase aqueous outflow to the Schlemm canal, subconjunctival space or suprachoroidal space
- **Minimally Invasive Glaucoma Surgery (MIGS)**
  - Describes a group of procedures that have been shown to help reduce medication burden, lower IOP, have a better safety profile and are less invasive in nature, compared to trabeculectomies or GDI
  - Typically performed in patients with mild to moderate glaucoma, or OHT. May be performed as a standalone procedure or combined with cataract surgery.
  - Can be broadly classified into 3 categories: Trabecular meshwork Subconjunctival and Suprachoroidal. (Table 4.16)

Table 4.16. Summary of Various MIGS Procedures

Trabecular Meshwork	Subconjunctival	Suprachoroidal
Trabecular bypass stents: – iStent trabecular bypass stents (Fig. 4.30) (Glaukos, Laguna Hills, CA, USA) – Hydrus microstent (Alcon, Geneva, Switzerland) (Fig. 4.31) **Ab interno Schlemm's canal dilation/ trabecular excision MIGS:** – iTrack Advance Microcatheter (Ellex, Adelaide, Australia) – Kahook dual blade (New World Medical, Rancho Cucamonga, CA, USA) – Trabectome (Tustin, CA, USA) – Gonioscopy-assisted transluminal trabeculectomy (GATT)	Preserflo microshunt (Santen Pharmaceutical Co., Lte, Japan) (Fig. 4.32) Xen gel implant (Allergan, Irvine, CA, USA)	MINIject glaucoma drainage device (iStar Medical SA, Wavre, Belgium) CyPass Micro-Stent (Alcon, Fort Worth, Texas)

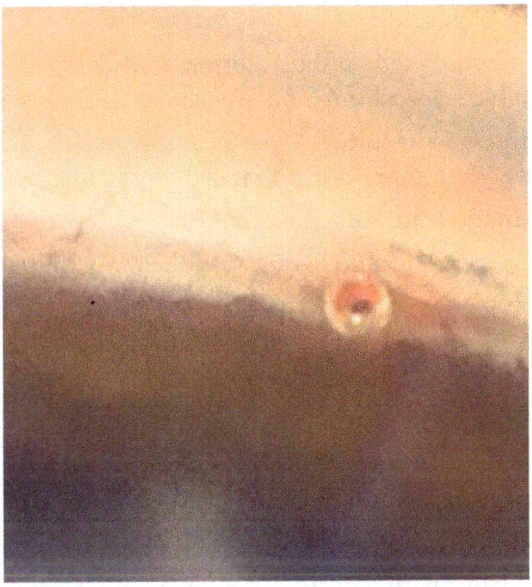

Fig. 4.30. Showing a picture of an iStent implant lodged at the angles of a patient's eye.

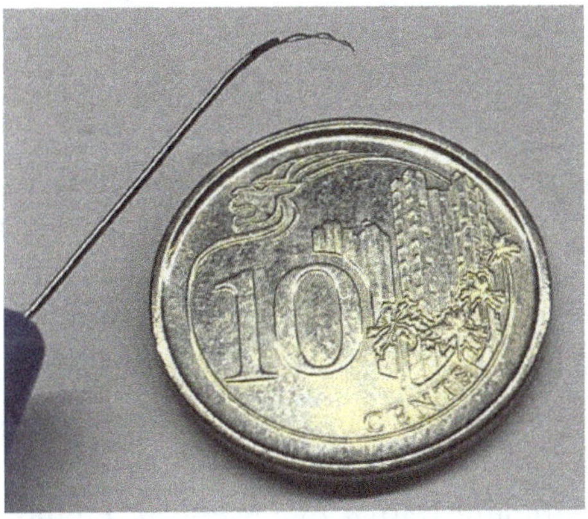

Fig. 4.31. Showing the size of a Hydrus implant, relative to a 10-cent coin.

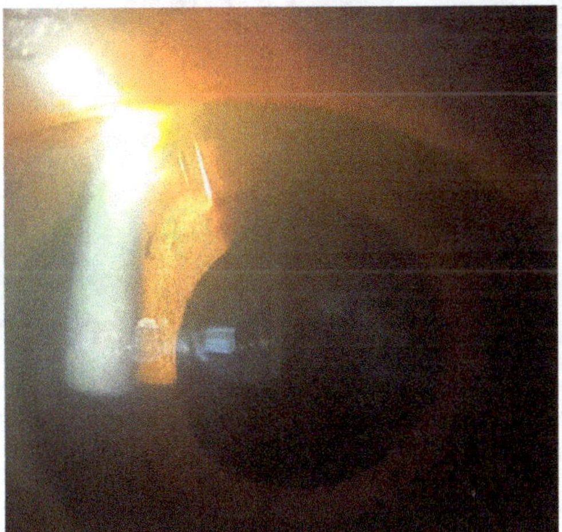

Fig. 4.32. Showing a Preserflo implant in the anterior chamber of a patient's eye.

- **Trabeculectomy (Fig. 4.33)**
  - i. A guarded fistula between the anterior chamber and the subconjunctival space through a sclerostomy and a partial thickness scleral flap
  - ii. Still one of the most commonly performed first-line surgical interventions for patients with moderate to advanced glaucoma.
- **Glaucoma Drainage Implants**
  - i. Reserved for eyes at high risk of trabeculectomy failure or previous failed trabeculectomy
  - ii. Involves the use of a silicone tube shunting aqueous from the anterior chamber to the post-equatorial subconjunctival space
  - iii. The conjunctiva at the equator has less fibroblasts and is less exposed to the external environment, making it less likely to scar down
  - iv. Classified into valved and non-valved implants
    - Valved implant
      - Built-in valve within the tube regulates aqueous flow and could prevent post-operative hypotony
      - For example, Ahmed glaucoma implant (New World Medical, Rancho Cucamonga, CA, USA) (Fig. 4.34)
    - Non-valved implant
      - The lack of any flow regulator means these implants require supplemental constriction of the tube calibre, using restorable sutures or reduction of tube lumen size using stenting sutures. These sutures can be removed subsequently when conjunctival healing around the base plate is deemed adequate, with a formed bleb around the plate.
      - Risk of hypotony is higher for this group of implants
      - For example, Baerveldt implant (Johnson and Johnson Vision, Irvine, CA, USA), Paul Glaucoma Implant (AOI, Singapore) (Fig. 4.35), Molteno implant (Nova Eye Medical, Fremont CA, USA), Ahmed ClearPath (New World Medical, Rancho Cucamonga, CA, USA)

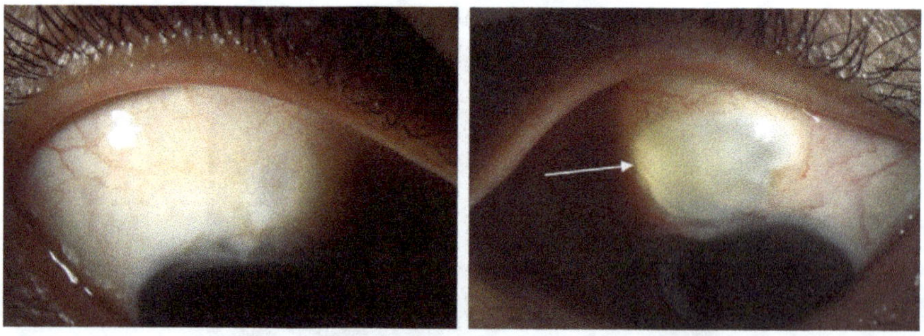

Fig. 4.33. Left image shows a diffuse and healthy trabeculectomy bleb. Right image shows a cystic, thin and avascular bleb (white arrow); this bleb is more prone to complications and failure.

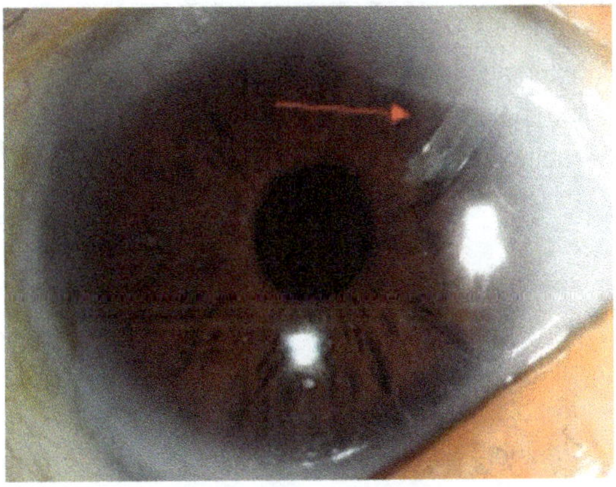

Fig. 4.34. Well-placed Ahmed tube (red arrow).

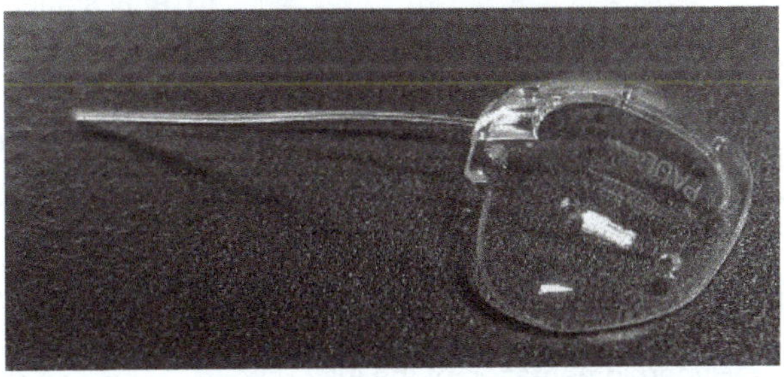

Fig. 4.35. Paul Glaucoma Implant (Image Credits: AOI).

What are the Potential Side Effects of IOP-lowering Medications?

IOP-lowering medications may have both ocular and systemic side effects (Table 4.17).

Table 4.17. Summarises the Ocular and Systemic Side Effects of IOP Lowering Medications

	Ocular	Systemic
Beta-blockers	• Reduced corneal sensation • Punctate keratitis	• Bronchospasm • Bradycardia • Lowered blood pressure • CNS depression, mood changes • Lethargy • Decreased libido • Masks hypoglycaemic effect in diabetics • May aggravate myasthenia gravis

	Ocular	Systemic
Alpha-agonists	• Conjunctival hyperaemia • Allergic conjunctivitis • Reactivation of HSV keratitis	• Central nervous system depression in children (crosses the immature blood-brain barrier) • In adults, may cause fatigue, hypotension, dizziness, dry mouth, depression

Carbonic anhydrase inhibitor (CAI)	• With topical CAI:
	  • Stinging sensation (esp. with dorzolamide)
	  • Transient blurred vision
	  • Reduced endothelial pump function
		• More common with systemic CAI:
		  • Allergy/anaphylaxis
		  • Stevens-Johnson syndrome
		  • Metabolic acidosis
		  • Hypokalaemia
		  • Renal stones
		  • Reduced appetite and metallic taste
		  • Tingling sensation on fingertips and toes

Prostaglandin analogue	• Conjunctival hyperaemia • Allergic conjunctivitis • Eyelash hypertrichosis • Hyperpigmentation of the iris and periocular tissue • Prostaglandin associated periorbitopathy syndrome (PAPs): Periorbital fat atrophy, deepening of the upper eyelid sulcus, tight eyelids, upper lid ptosis (Fig. 4.36) • Cystoid macular oedema • Pro-inflammatory and breaks down blood-aqueous barrier (relative contraindication for uveitis) • Reactivation of herpetic keratitis	• Minimal

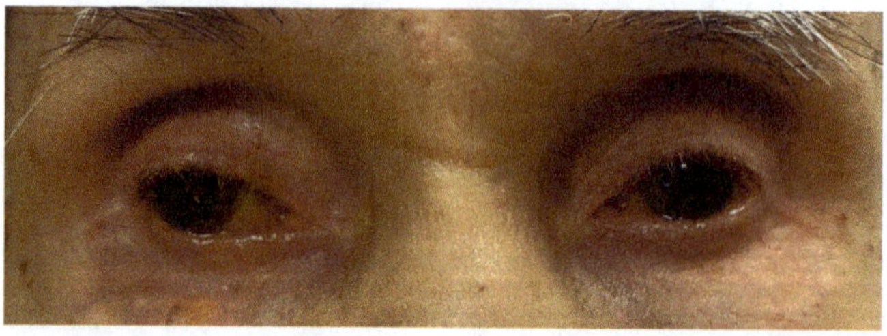

Fig. 4.36. This is a patient who had bilateral prostaglandin-associated periorbitopathy following the use of one of the prostaglandin analogues.

What are the Complications Associated with Laser Iridotomy?

- Photopsia
  - Due to light entering the eye through the iridotomy site
  - More common if the iridotomy site is near the upper eyelid resting position
- Corneal decompensation
  - Associated with the loss of endothelial cell loss
  - Higher risk if there is a chronic or acute rise in intraocular pressure
- Hyphaema
  - Risk of hyphaema can be reduced by performing sequential argon-YAG laser
  - Argon laser has photocoagulation properties and helps to coagulate blood vessels on the iris as the iris thins out
  - YAG laser aids to widen the iridotomy
- Intraocular pressure spike
- Malignant glaucoma
- Post-laser inflammation
- Localised lens damage and cataract progression

What are the Risks and Complications of Trabeculectomy?

- Intraoperative
  - Suprachoroidal haemorrhage
  - Scleral perforation
  - Hyphaema
  - Conjunctival buttonhole
- Early post-operative
  - High IOP:
    1. Shallow AC: Suprachoroidal haemorrhage, pupil block, aqueous misdirection
    2. Deep AC: Blocked sclerostomy, tight sutures, retained viscoelastics
  - Low IOP:
    1. Raised Bleb: Overfiltration
    2. Flat bleb: Conjunctival wound leak
  - Hyphaema
  - Endophthalmitis
  - Wipe-out
    1. Loss of remaining vision in patients with advanced visual field loss
- Late post-operative
  - High IOP due to subconjunctival fibrosis
  - Chronic hypotony
    1. From bleb leak
    2. From cystic avascular bleb

- Blebitis and endophthalmitis
- Cataract progression

What are Risk Factors for Trabeculectomy Failure?

The risk factors for trabeculectomy failure can be divided into patient and ocular factors (Table 4.18).

Table 4.18. Summarises the Risk Factors for Trabeculectomy Failure

Patient Factors	Ocular Factors
• Young patient • Asian, African Americans • Prone to scarring (e.g. keloid formation)	• Secondary glaucoma • Chronic use of IOP-lowering eye drops • Previous failed trabeculectomy

What are the Complications Associated with Glaucoma Drainage Implants?

The complications can be divided into:

- Intraoperative
  - Suprachoroidal haemorrhage
  - Conjunctiva button-hole
  - Hyphaema
  - Scleral perforation
  - Damage to ocular muscles
- Early post-operative
  - High IOP:
    i. Shallow AC: malignant glaucoma, suprachoroidal haemorrhage
    ii. Deep AC: Blocked tube, retained viscoelastic
  - Low IOP
    i. Overfiltration, wound leak
  - Hyphaema
    i. Usually self-limiting
    ii. Blood can block the tube, causing raised intraocular pressure
- Endophthalmitis
- Late post-operative
  - Cornea decompensation
    i. Due to tube-cornea touch, persistent iritis, anterior chamber fluctuation
  - Hypertensive phase
    i. Due to conjunctiva healing and fibrosis
    ii. Happens between 2–6 weeks after surgery
  - Conjunctiva erosion and exposure of tube/plate, with risk of endophthalmitis

- Diplopia
- Bleb encapsulation resulting in surgical failure
- Cataract progression

What are the Symptoms and Signs of Blebitis/Bleb-related Endophthalmitis? How Do You Manage Them?

Blebitis and/or bleb-related endophthalmitis are ocular emergencies because they can progress rapidly and lead to blindness. The symptoms and signs are summarised in Table 4.19.

Table 4.19. Symptoms and Signs of Blebitis and Endophthalmitis

Symptoms	Signs

• Red and painful eye
• Reduced vision
	• Swollen periocular tissue
	• Corneal oedema
	• Anterior chamber inflammation, including hypopyon
	• Leaking bleb
	  ▪ Bleb may be thin, avascular and cystic
	  ▪ Bleb contents are opaque and filled with fibrin/pus
	• Conjunctiva surrounding the bleb is congested (Fig. 4.37)
	• If endophthalmitis is present
	  ▪ Presence of relative afferent pupillary defect
	  ▪ Loss of red reflex
	  ▪ Presence of vitritis
	  ▪ Hypopyon

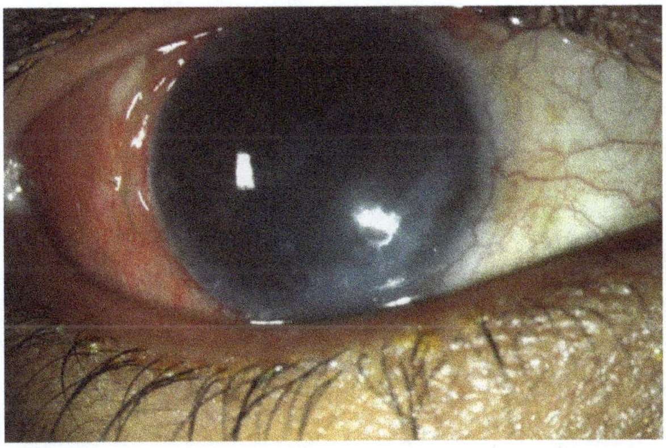

Fig. 4.37. Photograph showing **sectoral conjunctival injection** and **hyperaemia**, and opacification related to blebitis in this patient. Note the corneal oedema and consequent loss of iris details.

What are the Risk Factors for Blebitis/Bleb-related Endophthalmitis?

The risk factors for blebitis/bleb-related endophthalmitis can be classified into systemic and ocular factors. (Table 4.20.)

Table 4.20. Risk Factors for Blebitis and Bleb-related Endophthalmitis

Systemic	Ocular
• Immunocompromised (e.g. renal transplant, elderly, diabetes mellitus)	• Poor ocular surface • Lid disorders (e.g. Meibomian gland dysfunction, blepharitis, trichiasis) • Use of anti-metabolites during trabeculectomy • Repeated bleb needling with anti-metabolites

How do you Manage Blebitis or Bleb-related Endophthalmitis?

This requires admission and close monitoring of the patient.

Principles of management include:

- Microbiological diagnosis
  - Conjunctival swab around the bleb
  - Vitreous tap if endophthalmitis suspected and inject intravitreal antibiotics in the same setting
- Identify risk factors and treat (e.g. optimise diabetes control, treat blepharitis)
- Anti-microbial therapy
  - Empirical treatment with broad spectrum topical antibiotics
  - If endophthalmitis is suspected, treat with intravitreal antibiotics and systemic antibiotics
  - Subsequent anti-microbial regime depends on organism sensitivity
- Repair of bleb
  - Once active infection is treated, the trabeculectomy bleb at risk needs to be addressed
  - Bleb exploration and repair may be required
  - If not possible, compromised bleb needs to be excised and a separate filtration surgery at another site performed

Take Home Messages

- The target intraocular pressure can be achieved by either increasing aqueous outflow or reducing aqueous production. This can be achieved by medical, laser and/or surgical therapy.
- Laser iridotomy is indicated for angle closure to increase the anterior chamber angle width.
- The indication for surgical intervention is the presence of functional or structural deterioration and the inability to achieve target IOP despite maximum tolerable medical therapy.

References

1. American Academy of Ophthalmology — *Glaucoma.*
2. Shibal Bhartiya — *Manual of Glaucoma.*
3. Tarek M Shaarawy — *Glaucoma.*
4. Asia Pacific Glaucoma Guidelines — *4th Edition.*

Chapter 5

UVEITIS

Chan Hwei Wuen, Dawn Lim Ka-Ann

5.1 Classification

Learning Objectives

- Understanding the definition and classification of uveitis.
- Understanding the descriptors and terminologies used in uveitis.

Classification of Uveitis

Uveitis is defined as inflammation of the uveal tract. The uveal tract comprises the iris, ciliary body and choroid. Various classifications and grading systems for uveitis are available.

- Anatomical
- Clinical
- Aetiological
- Pathological

Definitions

Anterior Uveitis

- Iritis: Inflammation confined to the anterior chamber
- Iridocyclitis: Inflammation involving the ciliary body is termed as cyclitis. In iridocyclitis, cells are also seen in the retrolental (behind the crystalline lens) space.
- Keratouveitis: Inflammation involving the cornea and uveal tract
- Sclerouveitis: Inflammation involving the sclera and uveal tract

Intermediate Uveitis

- Inflammation primarily involving the middle portion of the eye, namely, the posterior ciliary body and pars plana
- Inflammatory cells are seen in the vitreous

Posterior Uveitis

- Inflammatory cells may be seen diffusely in the vitreous cavity, over the foci of active inflammation, on the posterior vitreous face or they can be absent (e.g. in immunodeficient patients)
- Inflammation can also affect the blood vessels, resulting in vasculitis

Panuveitis

- Diffuse inflammation involving the anterior and posterior segment

Anatomical Classification

The Standardisation of Uveitis Nomenclature (SUN) Working Group (2005) amended the anatomical classification that is commonly used today.

Table 5.1. The SUN Working Group Anatomical Classification of Uveitis

Type	Primary Site of Inflammation	Includes
Anterior uveitis	Anterior chamber	Anterior chamber
Intermediate uveitis	Vitreous	Vitreous
Posterior uveitis	Retina or choroid	Retina or choroid
Panuveitis	Anterior chamber, vitreous, and retina or choroid	Anterior chamber, vitreous, and retina or choroid

The SUN working group also provided descriptors of uveitis based on the following features:

Table 5.2. The SUN Working Group Descriptors of Uveitis

Category	Descriptor	Comment
Onset	Sudden insidious	
Duration	Limited	<3 months' duration
	Persistent	≥3 months' duration
Course	Acute	Episode characterised by sudden onset and limited duration
	Recurrent	Repeated episodes separated by periods of inactivity without treatment ≥3 months duration
	Chronic	Persistent uveitis with relapse in <3 months after discontinuing treatment

Clinical Classification

The clinical classification is formalised by the International Uveitis Study Group (IUGS):

Table 5.3. The IUSG Clinical Classification of Uveitis

Group	Subgroup
Infectious	Bacterial Viral Fungal Parasitic Others
Non-infectious	Known systemic association No known systemic association
Masquerade	Neoplastic (e.g. lymphoma, leukaemia) Non-neoplastic (e.g. TB)

Aetiological Classification

The aetiological classification expands on the cause of the disease and the treatment options. Nevertheless, often in uveitis, the true underlying aetiology is not known.

Pathological Classification

The pathological classification separates granulomatous from non-granulomatous uveitis. Granulomatous uveitis is characterised by large "mutton-fat" keratic precipitates (KPs) formed by macrophages and iris nodules, which include Busacca (located within the iris stroma) and Koeppe (located at the pupillary border) nodules.

Take Home Messages

- Uveitis encompasses a complex set of inflammatory pathologies in the eye.
- Understanding the classification of uveitis will aid in establishing the underlying aetiology and subsequent management.

5.2 Clinical Assessment and Investigations

Clinical Assessment

Learning Objectives

- Learning the approach to assessing a patient with uveitis.
- Learning when to investigate a patient with uveitis.
- Learning the roles of investigation in aiding the management of a patient with uveitis.

A thorough ophthalmic history and systematic review followed by detailed examination is paramount in all patients with uveitis.

In certain cases, systemic examination and co-management with an internal physician may be required.

Table 5.4. Ophthalmic History

Symptoms	Dependent on which segment of the uveal tract is inflamed • Anterior: redness, pain, photophobia, blurring of vision • Intermediate: blurring of vision, floaters, photopsia, photophobia • Posterior: typically painless blurring of vision, floaters, scotoma
Past ocular history	Previous similar episode: ask if any investigations were performed, results of investigations, any treatment? Previous history of ocular trauma or surgery (think of sympathetic ophthalmia)
Past medical history	• Systemic inflammatory disorders (e.g. sarcoidosis, Behçet's disease) • HLA-B27 associated spondyloarthropathies, rheumatoid arthritis • Chronic infection (e.g. TB, syphilis, HSV) • Immunocompromised status (e.g. malignancy, post-transplant, intravenous drug user)
Family history	Family history of uveitis or systemic inflammatory disorders
Drug history	Systemic immunosuppression and medications
Occupational history	

Table 5.5. Ophthalmic Examination

Visual function	Presenting visual acuity Relative afferent pupillary defect (RAPD), colour vision
Signs of uveitis (anterior) on slit-lamp examination	Conjunctiva • Perilimbal (Fig. 5.1) or diffuse injection Cornea • Keratic precipitates (Fig. 5.2) Anterior chamber: • Cells • Flare (proteinaceous influx) • Fibrin (Fig. 5.3) • Hypopyon Iris • Nodules • Anterior or posterior synechiae • Atrophy • Heterochromia Intraocular pressure • Hypotony • Secondary glaucoma — open or closed angle
Signs of uveitis (posterior) on slit-lamp examination with condensing lens (e.g. 90D for better evaluation of vitreous cells, 78D for better assessment of macular details)	Vitreous • Cells (single or clumped), snowballs • Tractional bands Pars plana • Snowbanking Retina • Unifocal or multifocal retinitis (fluffy white lesions which may progress to necrosis, atrophy which may lead to retinal detachment in the presence of atrophic retinal holes) • Cystoid macular oedema • Serous retinal detachment • Epiretinal membrane • Vasculitis Choroid • Unifocal or multifocal choroiditis (blurred yellowish lesions deep to the retina)

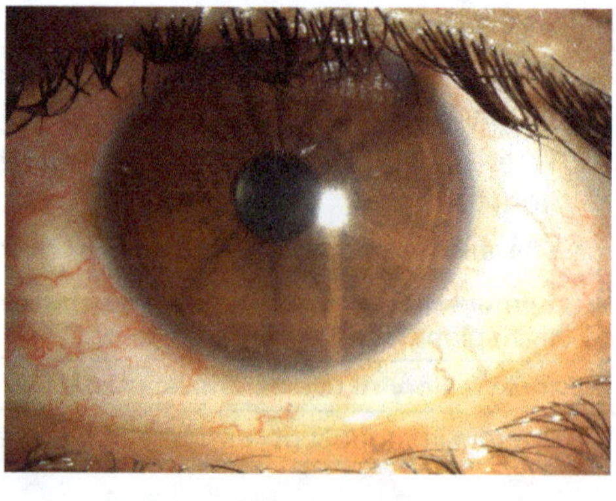

Fig. 5.1. Perilimbal injection.

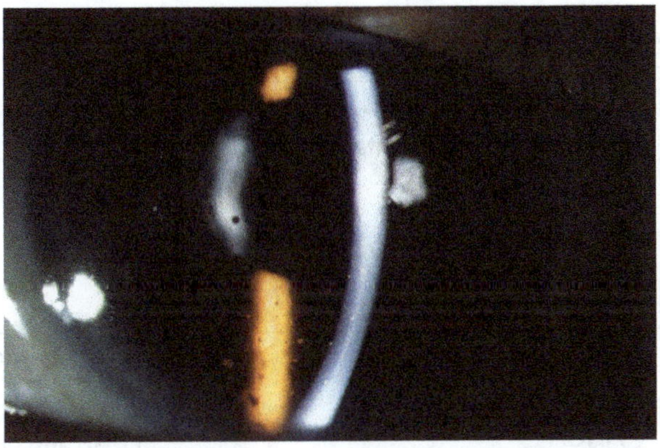

Fig. 5.2. Mutton-fat keratic precipitate in granulomatous uveitis.

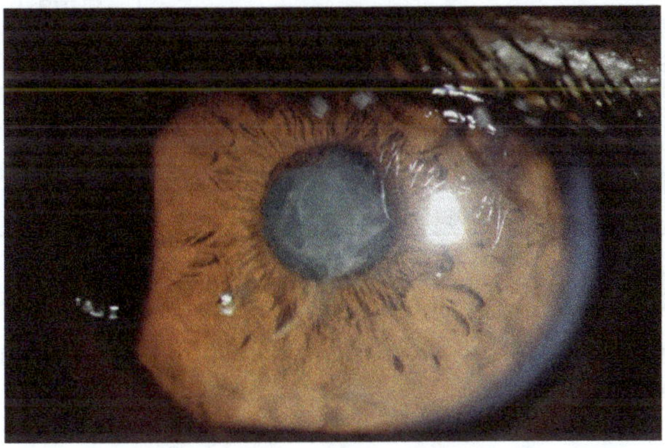

Fig. 5.3. Fibrin overlying the pupil.

Clinical Investigations

The objectives of performing investigations in uveitis patients are:

- Confirmation of diagnosis — often the underlying aetiology is unknown, but it is always important to rule out infective causes.
- Aid in management — for monitoring of disease activity, efficacy of treatment and associated side effect(s).

Baseline investigations are required in patients who have bilateral uveitis on presentation or recurrent disease. Special investigations are ordered on a case-by-case basis.

When there is a suspicion of possible infective aetiology, or any associated underlying connective tissue disease or oncological condition, such cases should be co-managed with the relevant specialists prior to initiating any treatment.

Patients who require immunosuppression therapy may need to be co-managed with the rheumatologist.

Table 5.6. Clinical Investigations

	Investigation	Possible Aetiology(ies)
Baseline	• Full blood count (FBC) • Erythrocyte sedimentation rate (ESR) • Syphilis serology • Mantoux, T-Spot.TB or TB quantiferon • Chest X-ray • Urinalysis	
Special (systemic)	• ANA, anti ds-DNA • Serum ACE, CT Thorax • ANCA • HLA-B27 • Toxoplasma serology	• Vasculitis work-up • Sarcoidosis • Granulomatosis with polyangiitis • HLA-B27 associated disease • Toxoplasmosis
Special (ocular)	• FFA and ICG • Endothelial cell count • Aqueous tap and PCR • Vitreous biopsy	• Posterior uveitis • Hypertensive uveitis

Management

Uveitis is a challenging condition to treat and the aim is to abolish the underlying inflammation, which could result from various infectious and non-infectious aetiologies.

The Basic Therapeutic Principles Are:

- To treat specific infectious causes, such as ocular tuberculosis, syphilis, viral retinitis (e.g. acute retinal necrosis or CMV retinitis, toxoplasmosis, endophthalmitis)
- To treat non-infectious uveitis with corticosteroids (systemic or topical)
- To consider the use of immunomodulatory agents if the patient has suffered steroid-induced complications, when steroids are not tolerated or contraindicated, in the presence of frequent flare-ups on tapering steroids, or if the underlying uveitis is associated with an ocular or systemic condition for which immunomodulatory agents are clinically indicated (e.g. Behçet's disease, granulomatosis with polyangiitis)

Treatment Modalities

Steroids

These are available in various formulations

Topical steroids, e.g. prednisolone acetate 1%, are typically indicated for anterior chamber inflammation

Periocular or intravitreal steroids, e.g. triamcinolone (periocular or intravitreal), OZURDEX® (dexamethasone intravitreal implant), can be considered in cases of intermediate uveitis with significant inflammation and cystoid macular oedema. Systemic steroids are used either as an adjunct to treatment for specific aetiologies or as a primary treatment, for bilateral or severe intermediate or posterior uveitis.

Cycloplegics

For example, atropine 1% or the less potent homatropine 1% eyedrop. This acts to stabilise the blood aqueous barrier and to break existing posterior synechiae. Adding a mydriatic such as phenylephrine 2.5% or 10% can act synergistically with a cycloplegic to break the posterior synechiae.

Immunomodulatory Agents

For example, azathioprine, methotrexate, mycophenolate mofetil, tacrolimus, infliximab, and adalimumab have been used in uveitis. (Details of these agents are beyond the scope of this chapter.)

Complications

Anterior Segment Complications

Iris

Posterior synechiae that is extensive could lead to seclusio pupillae (Fig. 5.4) and increase the risk of secondary angle closure from pupil block. Early administration of cycloplegics and mydriatics play a role in breaking existing posterior synechiae.

Iris atrophy can be a diagnostic feature of herpetic uveitis. Sector iris atrophy is seen in zoster-related uveitis.

The following pictures demonstrate the effects of cycloplegics and mydriatics in an uveitic eye with seclusio pupillae (Fig. 5.5).

Surgical iridectomy may sometimes be indicated in eyes that have failed to respond to pharmacological measures and where the intraocular pressures remain elevated in the presence of maximal tolerated medical treatment.

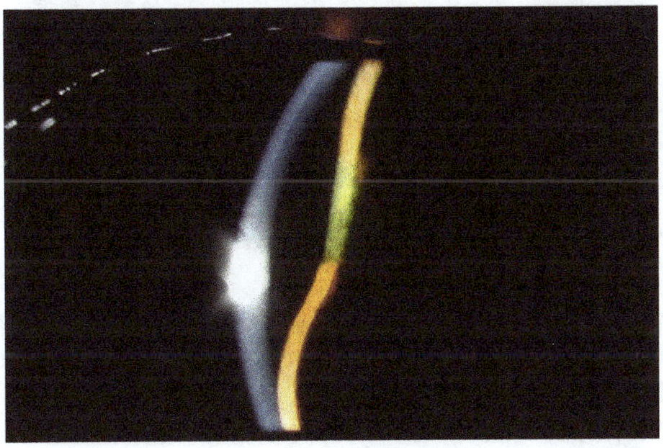

Fig. 5.4. Secondary angle closure with pupil block from seclusio pupillae.

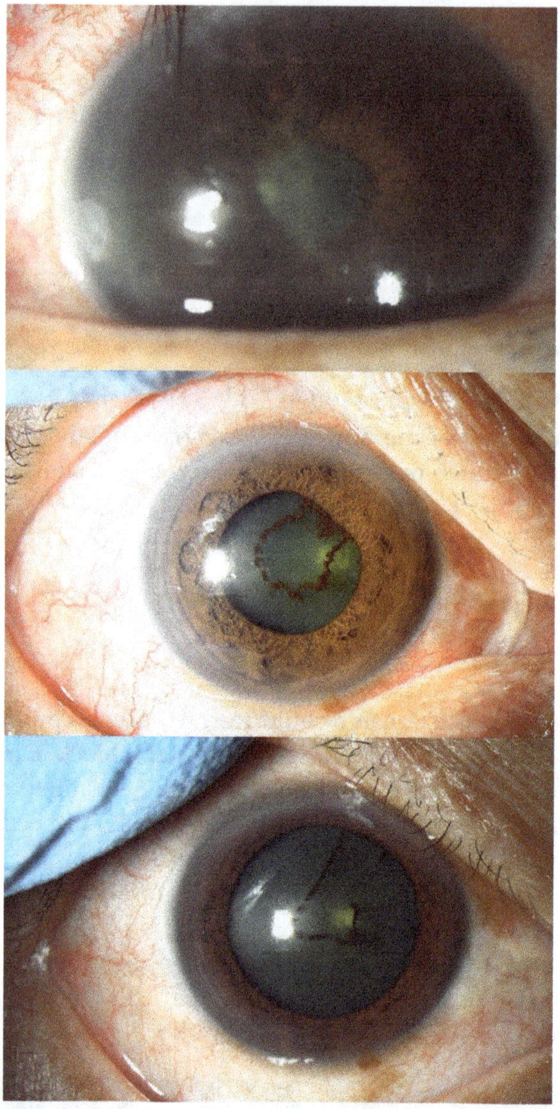

Fig. 5.5. (From top to bottom) The effects of cycloplegics and mydriatics in an uveitic eye with seclusio pupillae.

Intraocular Pressure (IOP)

Low IOP may result from ciliary body shutdown in active or uncontrolled ocular inflammation.

Factors that result in elevated IOP include peripheral anterior synechiae formation, which results in secondary angle closure, or from various causes of secondary open angle mechanisms, such as steroid therapy, trabeculitis or accumulation of inflammatory material and debris in the trabecular meshwork.

Anterior Chamber

Inflammatory ciliochoroidal effusion (e.g. in Vogt-Koyanagi-Harada disease) can give rise to shallow anterior chambers, which usually improve with systemic steroids or immunotherapy.

Lens

Cataract may develop due to a combination of factors, which include inflammation (recurrent or chronic) or the long-term use of steroids.

Posterior Segment Complications

Macula

Anterior and posterior segment inflammation or chronic inflammation can lead to cystoid macular oedema, exudative macular detachment and choroidal neovascular membrane.

Optic Nerve

Optic disc inflammation can occur isolated or concurrently with other signs of anterior and posterior uveitis. Sometimes, isolated optic disc swelling may be observed in cases of posterior scleritis. Sarcoid granulomas can infiltrate the optic disc and give the appearance of a disc swelling (Fig. 5.6 and Fig. 5.7).

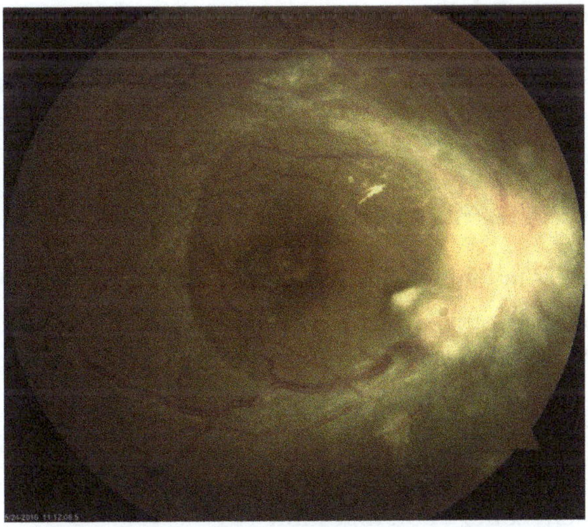

Fig. 5.6. Optic disc infiltrated with sarcoid granulomas.

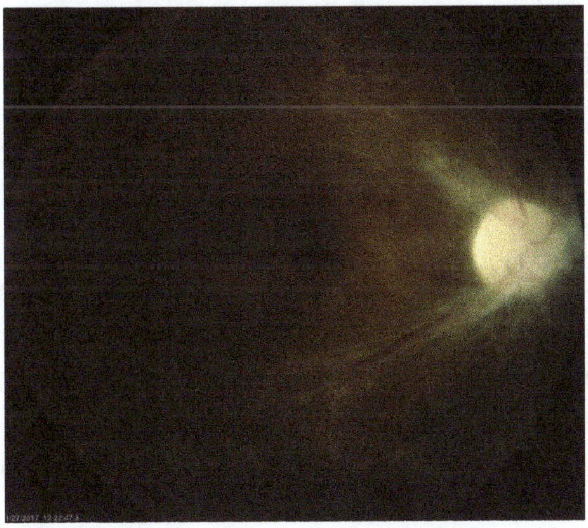

Fig. 5.7. Resolution of optic disc granulomas with treatment.

Retina

Retinitis and vasculitis can sometimes lead to occlusive vasculitis, and consequently vascular occlusion, with its attendant problems such as neovascularisation.

Exudative retinal detachment may also occur in some instances of uveitis.

Take Home Messages

- A systematic approach to assessing a patient with uveitis is paramount and this includes a detailed history and thorough ocular examination.
- The initial assessment will then guide the clinician on the necessary investigations.
- Investigations will aid the management of a patient with uveitis.
- Certain uveitis cases may require co-management with internal physicians, such as rheumatologists and infectious disease specialists.

5.3 Toxoplasmosis

Learning Objectives

- Understanding the clinical manifestation of congenital and acquired toxoplasmosis.
- Understanding the management of ocular toxoplasmosis.

- *Toxoplasma gondii* is an obligate intracellular parasite
- Transmission of the protozoa varies demographically — consumption of raw or undercooked meat in more developed countries versus drinking untreated water in under-developed countries
- Cats are the definitive hosts, whereas humans and livestock are intermediate hosts
- The oocysts excreted in cat faeces become encysted (bradyzoite) or actively proliferating (tachyzoite) upon ingestion
- Congenital toxoplasmosis from vertical transmission is more severe if contracted early in the pregnancy

Clinical Presentation

Patients with toxoplasmosis can have either of the following presentations:

- Bilateral poor vision with strabismus — congenital toxoplasmosis typically causes bilateral retinochoroiditis affecting the macula, resulting in poor vision and strabismus
- Acute onset blurring of vision with floaters — acquired toxoplasmosis is often asymptomatic and can affect both eyes in 40% of cases. It is imperative to maintain a low index of suspicion for immunocompromised status in bilateral, simultaneously active cases with large and/or multiple lesions.

Table 5.7. Clinical Presentation of Ocular Toxoplasmosis

Ophthalmic	Systemic
Symptoms • Blurring of vision • Floaters **Signs** • Vitritis with retinitis (classic "headlight in a fog" appearance) — retinitis is white and fluffy in appearance and may be adjacent to a previous toxoplasmosis scar (Figs. 5.8, 5.9), satellite lesions adjacent to the scar are also commonly seen • Others: scleritis, neuroretinitis, serous retinal detachment, punctate outer retinal toxoplasmosis (PORT) **Complications** • Cataract • Glaucoma • Choroidal neovascularisation	**Congenital** • Hydrocephalus • Cerebral calcification • Hepatosplenomegaly • Retinochoroiditis **Acquired** • Fever • Lymphadenopathy • NB: If immunocompromised, there is a risk of a life-threatening disease, e.g. encephalitis, intracerebral cysts, hepatitis, myocarditis

Patients with a history of ocular toxoplasmosis presenting with new onset blurring vision or floaters, whether in the affected or fellow eye, warrant an urgent ophthalmology referral.

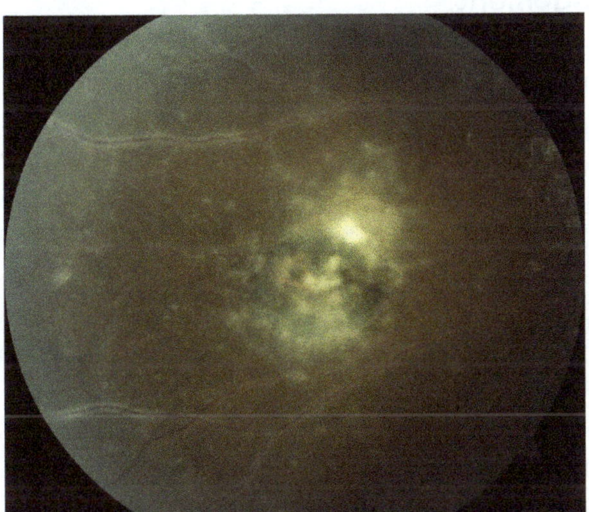

Fig. 5.8. Active retinochoroiditis with vasculitis adjacent to an old toxoplasmosis scar.

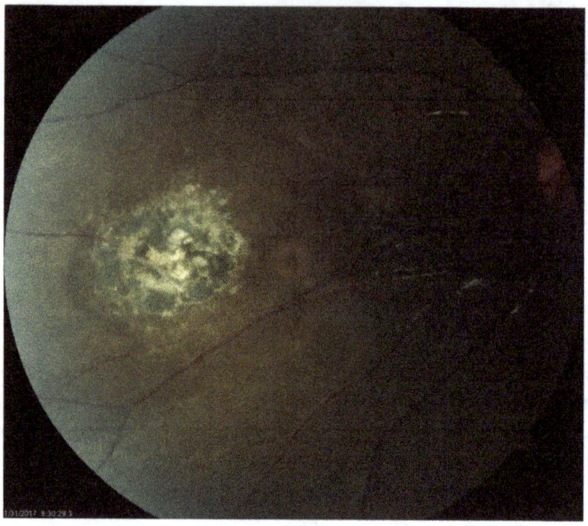

Fig. 5.9. Toxoplasmosis scar.

Clinical Investigation

Ocular toxoplasmosis is a clinical diagnosis. However, it is important to exclude other causes of retinitis, in which case PCR of intraocular fluid is useful. *Toxoplasma* serology is useful but should be interpreted with care, as anti-toxoplasma IgG are positive in many adults. The presence of IgM antibodies suggests acquired infection.

Clinical Management

Indications for treatment:

- Lesion(s) involving the optic disc, macula or papillomacular bundle
- Lesion(s) threatening major vessels
- Lesion(s) larger than 1 disc diameter in size
- Marked vitritis
- Immunocompromised patients

Various treatment regimens are available:

- Prednisolone + sulphadiazine + pyrimethamine + folinic acid (this is the classic "triple therapy" with folinic acid supplementation)
- Prednisolone + sulphadiazine + pyrimethamine + clindamycin + folinic acid ("quadruple therapy")
- Prednisolone + co-trimoxazole
- Prednisolone + clindamycin
- Prednisolone + atovaquone
- Prednisolone + azithromycin

Systemic steroids are typically commenced at least 24 hours after initiation of anti-toxoplasmosis therapy. Patients are co-managed with the infectious disease specialist. In the case of pregnant patients, the obstetrician should be involved in the management as well.

In immunocompetent patients, the disease is self-limiting; hence, treatment is only required for sight-threatening lesions. Recurrence is possible and patients should be informed.

All patients require regular follow-up until resolution of the disease, which is seen as complete scarring with the resolution of inflammation. Patients should be advised to seek medical attention should they develop blurring of vision or floaters upon discharge.

Take Home Messages

- Ocular toxoplasmosis is a potentially sight-threatening condition, e.g. in immunocompromised patients, or lesions involving the macula.
- Ocular toxoplasmosis is a clinical diagnosis; however, investigations are occasionally required to rule out other causes.
- Acute ocular toxoplasmosis is often co-managed by ophthalmologists and infectious disease specialists.
- Special attention must be paid to pregnant patients with acute ocular toxoplasmosis.

5.4 Cytomegalovirus Retinitis

Learning Objectives

- Understanding the clinical presentation of CMV retinitis.
- Understanding the management of CMV retinitis.

Cytomegalovirus (CMV) is a double-stranded DNA virus belonging to the Herpesviridae family. CMV retinitis can be seen in immunocompromised patients with malignancy (e.g. lymphoma or leukaemia, post-transplant patients, and retroviral-positive individuals).

CMV retinitis occurs in up to 40% of AIDS cases, typically when the CD4 count falls under 50/mm^3.

Clinical Presentation

Patients may be asymptomatic, particularly if the retinitis does not involve the macula. Screening is, therefore, important, especially when the CD4 count is low.

Severely immunocompromised patients are often unable to mount any immune response, hence the absence of ocular inflammation. On the contrary, marked immune response can be seen in immune reconstitution uveitis (IRU) upon recovery of the immune system, typically seen after initiation of highly active antiretroviral therapy (HAART).

Table 5.8. Ocular Presentation of CMV Retinitis

Symptoms	• Blurring of vision • Visual field loss • Floaters
Signs	Anterior • Anterior chamber inflammation — mild or typically absent Posterior • Vitritis — mild or typically absent Retinitis — 3 variants have been described • Classic or fulminant retinitis ▪ Classic "tomato and cheese" appearance with retinal haemorrhage and yellowish, fluffy retinitis often seen in the posterior pole from the optic disc (Fig. 5.10) along the arcade in the distribution of the retinal nerve fibre layer • Granular or indolent form ▪ Typically found in the peripheral retina ▪ Minimal or no haemorrhage or retinal oedema or vasculitis ▪ Active retinitis along the edge of the lesion • Perivascular form ▪ A variant of frosted branch angiitis — idiopathic retinal perivasculitis
Complications	• Retinal detachment (up to 30%) • Retinal atrophy • Optic nerve disease

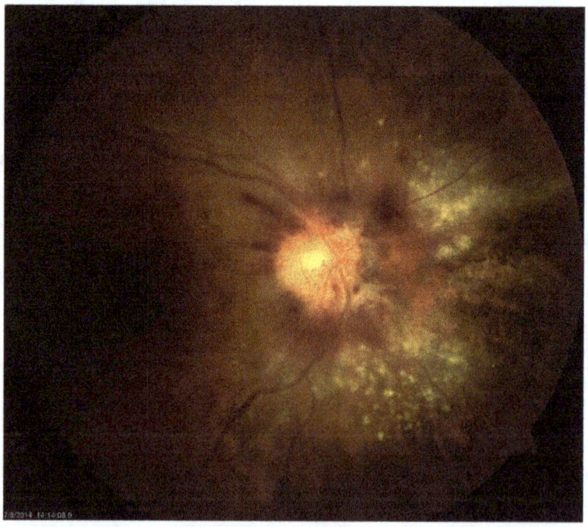

Fig. 5.10. CMV retinitis with optic disc involvement.

Clinical Investigations

CMV retinitis is a clinical diagnosis. Baseline blood investigations are performed for monitoring of treatment and side effects (e.g. agranulocytosis from ganciclovir).

Clinical Management

A multi-disciplinary approach is essential.

Treatment

- HAART for HIV patients, to sustain CD4 count above 50 mm^3
- Anti-CMV treatment: This involves an "induction" and "maintenance" regime. Combination therapy may be required depending on the disease severity.
  - Systemic: valganciclovir, ganciclovir, foscarnet, cidofovir
  - Intravitreal: ganciclovir, foscarnet
  - Intravitreal implant: ganciclovir

  Patients should be monitored for immune recovery uveitis and retinal detachment.

Take Home Messages

- CMV infection can be congenital or acquired.
- A high index of suspicion must be maintained in patients with AIDS having a CD4 count $<50/mm^3$ or other immunocompromised status, e.g. following a bone marrow or organ transplant.
- Immunocompromised patients may be completely asymptomatic.
- Referral to ophthalmology is paramount when there is a CD4 count $<50/mm^3$ or when there is any clinical suspicion.

5.5 Endogenous Endophthalmitis

Learning Objectives

- Understanding the clinical presentation of endophthalmitis.
- Understanding the management of endophthalmitis.

Endogenous endophthalmitis is an intraocular infection arising from haematogenous dissemination of bacterial or fungal organisms from a remote primary source, typically from liver abscesses or urinary tract infections. Although endogenous endophthalmitis is uncommon, it is a potentially blinding condition and should always be considered as a differential for acute, painful, red eye with blurring of vision.

Who is at Risk?

- Immunocompromised patients
- Predisposing conditions
  - Diabetes mellitus
  - Systemic malignancy
  - Sickle cell anaemia
  - AIDS
  - Extensive gastrointestinal surgery

- Potential sources of infection
  - Pneumonia
  - Urinary tract infection
  - Bacterial meningitis
  - Liver abscess

Table 5.9. Common Pathogens Causing Endogenous Endophthalmitis

Bacterial	Fungal
Gram-positive organisms • *Streptococcus* species (endocarditis) • *Staphylococcus aureus* (cutaneous infection) • Bacillus species (IVDU)	• *Candida albicans, Candida glabrata* • *Aspergillus fumigatus* • *Cryptococcus neoformans* • *Coccidioides immitis*
Gram-negative organisms • *Neisseria meningitides* • *Haemophilus influenza* • Enteric organisms (e.g. *Klebsiella* species, *Escherichia coli*)	

Clinical Presentation

Bacterial endophthalmitis tends to present acutely with pain, whereas fungal endophthalmitis tends to develop slowly and may be painless.

Table 5.10. Ocular Presentation of Endogenous Endophthalmitis

Symptoms	• Pain • Photophobia • Blurring of vision
Signs	• Severely reduced vision • Periorbital and eyelid oedema • Anterior chamber fibrin, hypopyon • Vitritis • Choroiditis (Fig. 5.11), retinitis ± necrosis
Complications	• Retinal detachment • Vitreous haemorrhage, suprachoroidal haemorrhage • Hypotony • Phthisis bulbi

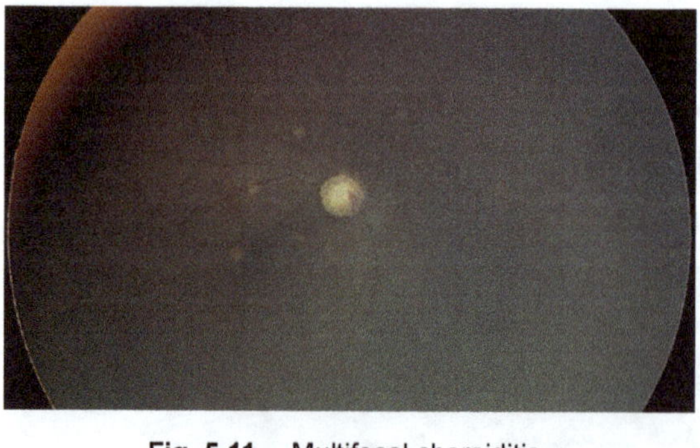

Fig. 5.11. Multifocal choroiditis.

Management

Confirmation of Diagnosis

- Blood culture
- Ocular culture: vitreous tap

Endogenous endophthalmitis is sight-threatening and rapid commencement of empirical anti-microbial treatment is crucial. If fungal endophthalmitis is suspected, concurrent anti-bacterial and antifungal treatment is initiated. Depending on the severity, a combination of systemic and intravitreal treatment may be required.

Prognosis is dependent on the organism and the immune status of the patient.

Take Home Messages

- Endogenous endophthalmitis is a serious, potentially blinding condition.
- It is commonly caused by haematogenous dissemination of bacterial or fungal organisms.
- The most common bacterial organism in the South East Asia region is *Klebsiella* spp.
- Patients with systemic infections secondary to the organisms listed, especially *Klebsiella* spp., must be referred to an ophthalmologist for screening.

5.6 Systemic Diseases Associated Uveitis

Learning Objective

Identify the systemic diseases associated with uveitis and its management.

Juvenile Idiopathic Arthritis (JIA)

Juvenile idiopathic arthritis (JIA)-associated uveitis is a challenging condition whereby both inflammation and treatment might result in problems that present themselves to the Ophthalmologist. Medical and surgical treatment options might have to be considered in the management of these problems. A multidisciplinary approach is often required in the management of JIA (International League of Associations for Rheumatology (ILAR) nomenclature), also known as juvenile rheumatoid arthritis.

American College of Rheumatology Criteria for Juvenile Rheumatoid Arthritis

JRA can be diagnosed if the age at onset is under 16 years; there is arthritis in 1 or more joints; disease duration is 6 weeks or greater; and other forms of juvenile arthritis (e.g. psoriatic and inflammatory bowel disease-associated arthritis) are excluded.

Disease type is defined by the type of disease present in the first 6 months.

- Systemic-onset JRA: daily (quotidian) fever spiking to more than 39°C (102.2°F) for 2 weeks or greater in association with arthritis of 1 or more joints.
- Pauciarticular JRA: arthritis in 4 or fewer joints in the first 6 months of disease.
- Polyarticular JRA: arthritis in 5 or more joints in the first 6 months of disease.

Risk Factors for Developing Uveitis

JIA-associated uveitis is usually described as chronic, bilateral, non-granulomatous anterior uveitis, with an insidious onset. As this is usually asymptomatic, screening for JIA-associated uveitis in at-risk patients is important. Majority of cases are diagnosed within 4 years from the onset of arthritis.

Risk factors for the development of uveitis

- Oligoarticular arthritis
- Young age at the onset of the disease
- Antinuclear antibodies (ANA) seropositivity
- Rheumatoid factor (RF) seronegativity
- Female gender

Complications of JIA-associated Uveitis

- Band-shaped keratopathy
- Cataract
- Glaucoma
- Hypotony
- Epiretinal membrane
- Macular oedema

Treatment Options

- Topical glucocorticoids and cycloplegics
- Immunosuppressants (e.g. methotrexate)
- Biological therapy

HLA-B27-associated Acute Anterior Uveitis

HLA-B27-associated acute anterior uveitis is relatively common.

It has been estimated that up to 20% of people carrying the HLA-B27 antigen have at least one of the several following associated conditions, which include:

- Ankylosing spondylitis
- Reactive arthritis (including Reiter's syndrome)
- Psoriatic arthritis
- Undifferentiated spondyloarthropathies
- Enteropathic arthropathy
- Inflammatory bowel disease

It is, therefore, important to take a detailed history and to conduct a directed systemic examination of these patients.

Classically, HLA-B27-associated acute anterior uveitis presents as a sudden onset, acute anterior uveitis in a young patient, typically male. It starts in one eye but is usually asymmetrically bilateral. The inflammation may be associated with a fibrinous reaction, hypopyon and the formation of posterior synechiae.

These patients typically respond readily to topical corticosteroid therapy.

Take Home Messages

- Juvenile idiopathic arthritis is associated with chronic uveitis and its complications in younger patients.
- HLA-B27-associated uveitis should be co-managed with a rheumatologist so that the systemic conditions can be addressed.

5.7 Scleritis and Episcleritis

Learning Objective

Identify and differentiate scleritis from episcleritis.

Differentiation between the two entities is important as the manifestations, prognosis and complications differ.

Episcleritis refers to inflammation confined to the superficial episcleral tissue, whereas scleritis refers to the inflammation of the sclera, which might involve other ocular structures, such as the adjacent cornea.

Episcleritis is non-vision threatening, usually idiopathic and can be self-limiting.

Aetiologies

The most common systemic associations of scleritis include rheumatoid arthritis, granulomatosis with polyangiitis, relapsing polychondritis and polyarteritis nodosa.

Infectious scleritis can be bacterial, viral, fungal or parasitic.

Surgically induced necrotising scleritis (SINS) can occur following a variety of procedures.

Investigations

In scleritis (Fig. 5.12 and Fig. 5.13), these have to be tailored to exclude infectious causes and systemic associations.

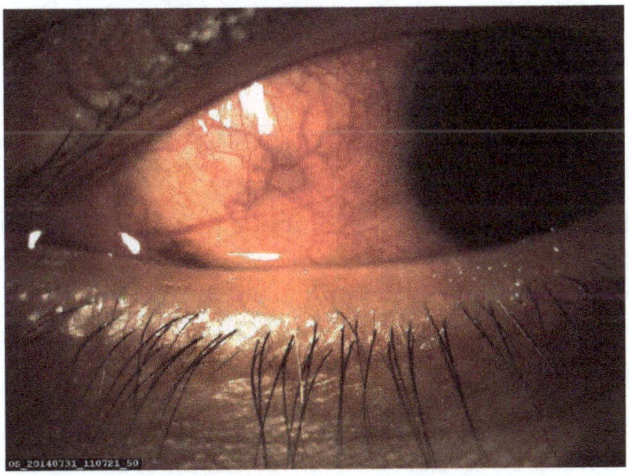

Fig. 5.12. Active scleritis.

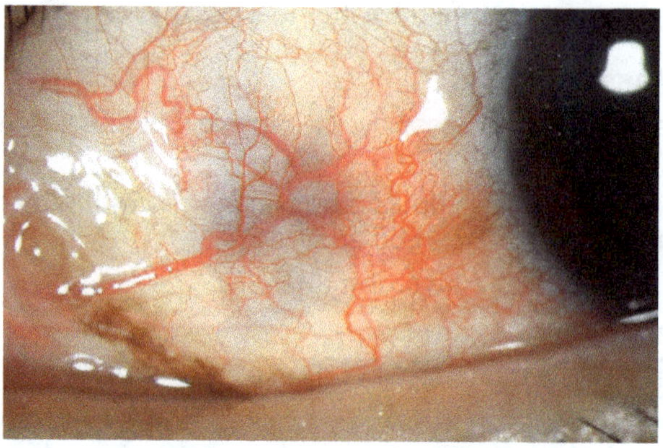

Fig. 5.13. Resolved scleritis with area of scleral thinning.

Treatment

Non-steroidal Anti-inflammatory Agents

Non-selective cox inhibitors, such as indomethacin or ibuprofen, can first be considered in the absence of any contraindications.

Gastrointestinal side effects and renal toxicity from the use of non-steroidal anti-inflammatory agents are some important considerations.

Corticosteroids

Steroids are commenced for those who do not respond to non-steroidal anti-inflammatory agents, posterior or necrotising disease. Systemic corticosteroids may be given orally or intravenously.

Steroid-sparing Agents

In the presence of contraindications or intolerance to steroids, or patients who relapse at doses of prednisolone >7.5 mg–10 mg per day, adjunctive immunosuppressive therapy should be considered. Options include methotrexate and azathioprine.

Take Home Message

Scleritis is associated with more ocular morbidity and should be investigated and managed with anti-inflammatory drugs.

References

1. Abu Samra K, Maghsoudlou A, Roohipoor R, *et al.* (2016) Current treatment modalities of JIA-associated uveitis and its complications: Literature review. *Ocul Immunol Inflamm* **24(4)**:431–439.
2. Denniston A, Murray PI (eds.) (2014) *Oxford Handbook of Ophthalmology. 3rd ed.* NY: Oxford University Press, pp. 410–413.
3. Brewer EJ Jr, Bass J, Baum J, *et al.* (1977) Current proposed revision of JRA criteria. JRA criteria subcommittee of the diagnostic and therapeutic criteria committee of the American rheumatism section of the arthritis foundation. *Arthritis Rheum* **20**(2 Suppl):195–199.

4. British Society for Paediatric and Adolescent Rheumatology, Royal College of Ophthalmology. (2006) Guidelines for Screening for Uveitis in Juvenile Idiopathic Arthritis.
5. Chang JH, McCluskey PJ, Wakefield D. (2005) Acute anterior uveitis and HLA-B27. *Surv Ophthalmol* **50(4)**:364–88.
6. Deschenes J, Murray PI, Rao NA, Nussenblatt RB. (2008) International Uveitis Study Group. International Uveitis Study Group (IUSG): Clinical classification of uveitis. *Ocul Immunol Inflamm* **16**:1–2.
7. Intraocular Inflammation and Uveitis, Section 9. Basic and Clinical Science Course, AAO, 2016.
8. Jabs DA, Nussenblatt RB, Rosenbaum JT. (2005) Standardisation of Uveitis Nomenclature (SUN) for reporting clinical data. *Am J Ophthalmol* **140:**509–16.
9. Okhravi N, Odufuwa B, McCluskey P, Lightman S. (2005) Scleritis. *Surv Ophthalmol* **50** :351–363.
10. Smith JR. (2002) HLA-B27-associated uveitis. *Ophthalmol Clin North Am* **15(3)**: 297–307.
11. Yang P, Liu X, Zhou H, *et al.* (2011) Vogt-Koyanagi-Harada disease presenting as acute angle closure glaucoma at onset. *Clin Exp Ophthalmol* **39**(7):639–47.

Chapter 6

VITREORETINAL DISORDERS

Yuen Yew Sen, Wong Meihua Wendy

6.1 Inherited Retinal Disorders

Learning Objectives

- Introduction to retinitis pigmentosa.
- Appreciate fundus changes in retinitis pigmentosa.
- Understand syndromes associated with retinitis pigmentosa.

Retinitis Pigmentosa

- Retinitis pigmentosa (RP) is a genetically heterogeneous group of disorders that primarily affects rod and cone photoreceptors.
- Hallmark symptoms include night blindness (nyctalopia) and loss of peripheral vision. Central vision may be affected in later stages of the disease, or if complications of macular oedema or epiretinal membrane develop.
- Most forms of RP are monogenic and may be transmitted in an autosomal dominant, autosomal recessive or X-linked recessive manner.

"Typical" findings in retinitis pigmentosa (Fig. 6.1)

- Bone spicule-like pigment changes
  - Can be generalised (affecting the entire retina) or sectoral (affect only a portion of the retina)
- Attenuated retinal vessels
- Waxy pallor of optic nerve

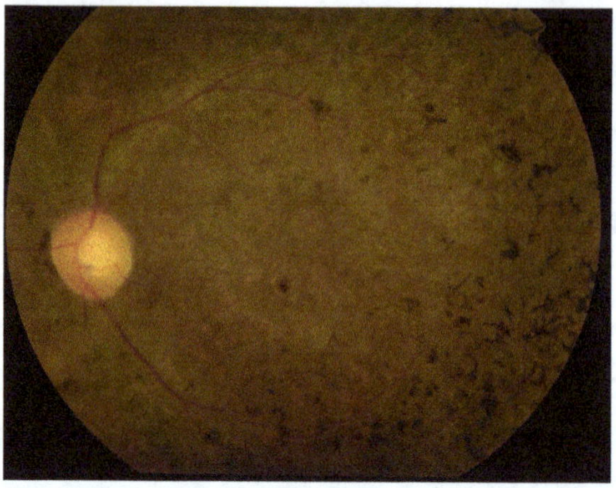

Fig. 6.1. Retinitis pigmentosa showing attenuated vessels and diffuse bone spicule-like pigmentation.

Other ocular findings in RP may include:

- Cataracts
- Cystoid macular oedema

Some forms of RP are associated with systemic disease

- Usher's syndrome: RP and deafness
- Lawrence-Moon-Bardet-Biedl syndrome: RP and polydactyly

At the time of printing, RP is generally managed conservatively, with efforts focused on maximising patients' vision with low vision aids and community support (e.g. Singapore Association of the Visually Handicapped). Research is ongoing, and therapeutic options such as gene therapy and retinal implants are being studied.

Take Home Message

Retinitis pigmentosa is a type of hereditary retinal disorder associated with constricted visual fields and nyctalopia.

6.2 Diabetic Retinopathy

Learning Objectives

- Classification of diabetic retinopathy.
- Understand mechanisms of vision loss due to diabetic retinopathy.
- Principles of management of diabetic retinopathy.

Concept of Ischaemic Drive

- Microvascular disease
- Reduction in oxygen supply to the retina

- Imbalance between demand for oxygen and supply for oxygen
- Production of growth factors for new blood vessels (including vascular endothelial growth factors (VEGF)

- New vessels grow in the retina and anterior chamber
- Vitreous haemorrhage or neovascular glaucoma

Diabetic Retinopathy

Diabetic retinopathy is a microvascular complication of diabetes mellitus throughout the body. Within the eye, diabetic changes are graded based on:

- Severity of the retinopathy
- Presence of diabetic macular oedema

International Clinical Diabetic Retinopathy Scale

Non proliferative diabetic retinopathy (NPDR)

- Mild NPDR
  - Microaneurysms only
- Moderate NPDR (Fig. 6.2)
  - More than just microaneurysms, but less severe than severe NPDR
- Severe NPDR
  - Defined as the "4-2-1" rule as any one of the following
    i. More than 20 intraretinal haemorrhages in each of the 4 quadrants
    ii. Definite venous beading in at least 2 quadrants
    iii. Prominent IRMA (intraretinal microvascular abnormalities) in at least 1 quadrant

Proliferative diabetic retinopathy (PDR)

- Presence of new vessels on the disc (NVD) (Fig. 6.3)
- Presence of new vessels elsewhere (NVE) (Figs. 6.4 and 6.5)
- Vitreous or preretinal haemorrhage

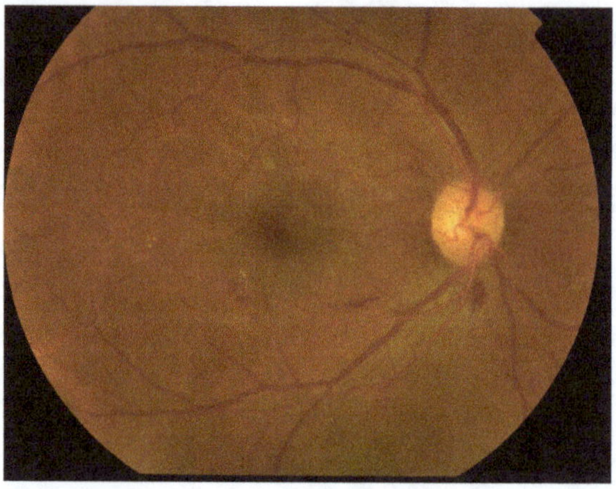

Fig. 6.2. Moderate nonproliferative diabetic retinopathy: Flame-shaped and blot haemorrhages are present. There are no new vessels.

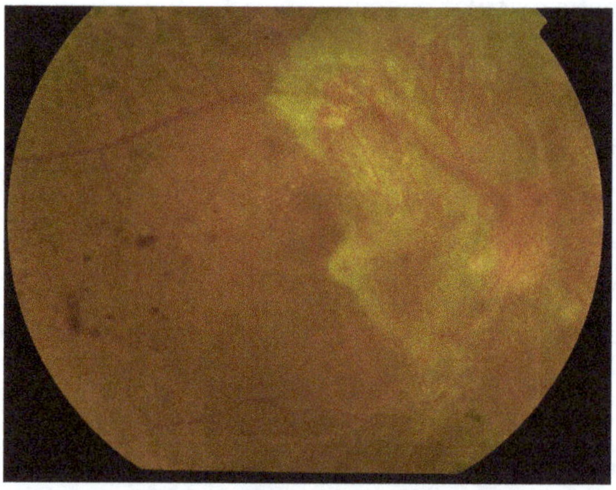

Fig. 6.3. Proliferative diabetic retinopathy with florid neovascularisation and fibrosis at the optic disc.

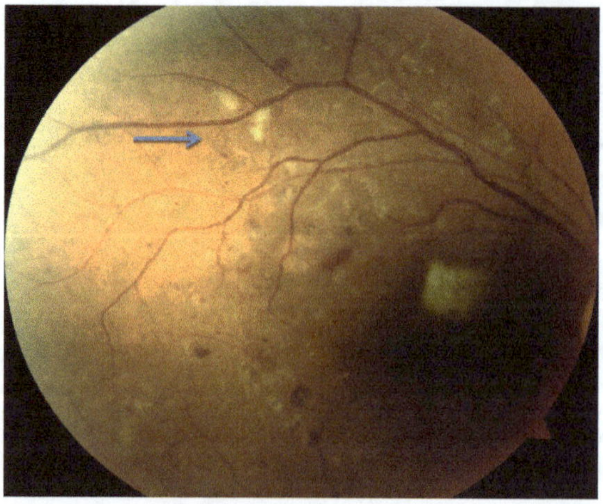

Fig. 6.4. Early new vessels seen.

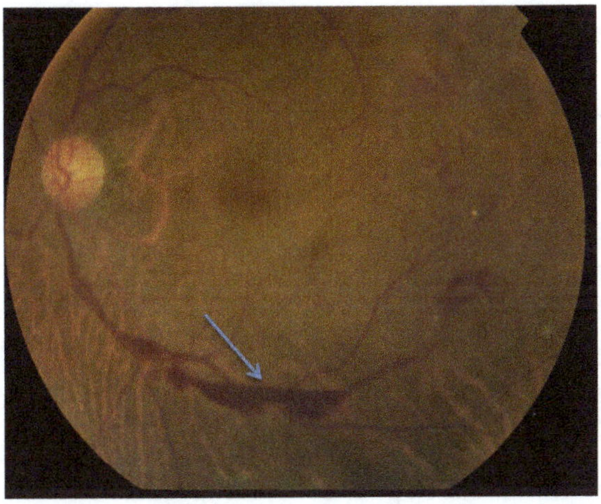

Fig. 6.5. Proliferative diabetic retinopathy: Subhyaloid haemorrhage seen indicating presence of bleeding from new vessels.

Clinically Significant Macular Oedema (CSME) (Fig. 6.6)

One of the following:

- Thickening within 500 μm of the fovea
- Hard exudates within 500 μm of the fovea with associated retinal thickening
- Area of retinal thickening of 1 disc area in size, any part of which is within 1 disc diameter of the fovea

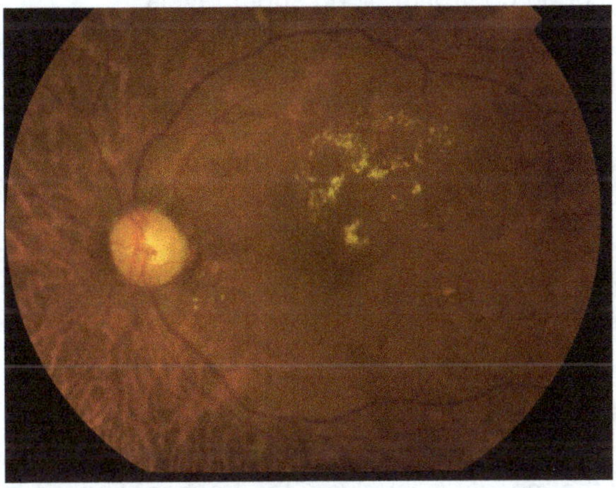

Fig. 6.6. Clinically significant macular oedema: Microaneurysms seen with surrounding hard exudates.

Patients with type 1 diabetes should commence screening 5 years after diagnosis, then at least annually thereafter. Patients with type 2 diabetes should be screened upon diagnosis, then at least annually thereafter.

Diagnosis and Classification

When examining the fundus, the severity of the diabetic retinopathy is graded (no apparent retinopathy, mild/moderate/severe NPDR or PDR), as well as the presence or absence of CSME.

Diabetic retinal disease can cause blurring of vision via a few mechanisms:

- Macular oedema from CSME
- Vitreous haemorrhage
- Tractional retinal detachment
- Neovascular glaucoma

Treatment

Systemic treatment involves the optimisation of glycaemic control. Tight control of blood sugar slows the progression of diabetic retinopathy. However, an important point to note is that rapid normalisation of the HbA1c after a period of prolonged poor diabetic control may paradoxically cause worsening of the macula oedema (Diabetes Control and Complications Trial).

With regard to the ocular management, treatment options depend on the severity of the diabetic retinopathy as well as the presence/absence of CSME.

Background retinopathy treatment
(ETDRS classification: Early Treatment of Diabetic Retinopathy Study)

Non proliferative diabetic retinopathy (NPDR)

Mild and moderate diabetic retinopathy is usually managed conservatively, aside from encouraging good control of blood sugar levels.

Severe NPDR can also be observed. However, most doctors would initiate treatment via pan-retinal photocoagulation (PRP; Fig. 6.7) by this stage to prevent visual loss.

Proliferative diabetic retinopathy (PDR)

PDR is managed with PRP.

- PRP involves the application of laser burns in the retinal periphery to reduce the oxygen demand of the retina, therefore reducing the imbalance between poor oxygen supply from diseased retinal vessels and the high demand from the photoreceptors in the retina

Tractional retinal detachment (TRD)

- TRD develops when new vessels that grow in PDR start to contract and pull on the retina. If the macula is involved, the tractional bands may cause vision to drop
- Once the macula is involved by the TRD, surgery is usually indicated

Clinically Significant Macular Oedema (CSME) treatment options

- Focal/Grid laser to leaking microaneurysms in the macula
  - Decreases risk of vision loss from macula oedema by 50% (ETDRS study)
- Intravitreal anti-vascular endothelial growth factor (Anti-VEGF)
  - Macular optical coherence tomography scans can be used to classify diabetic macular oedema as centre-involved or non-centre-involved. Treatment

with intravitreal anti-VEGF is indicated if there is centre-involved DME that impairs vision
- Intravitreal corticosteroid injection
  - This is an alternative pharmacological treatment to anti-VEGF agents

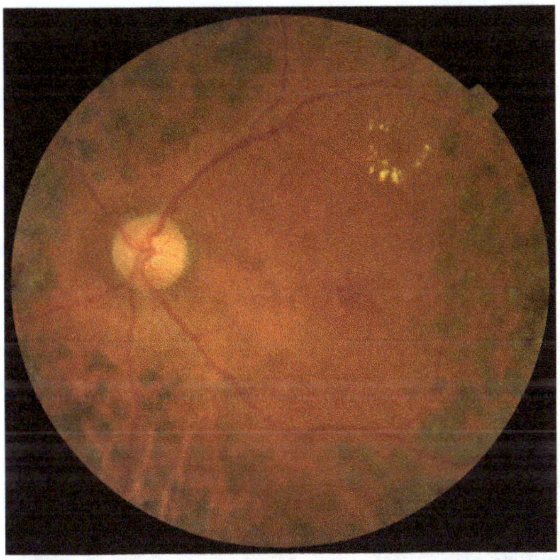

Fig. 6.7. Pan-retinal photocoagulation laser scars are seen in the peripheral.

Take Home Messages
- Patients with diabetes should undergo regular eye screenings.
- Vision loss may arise from diabetic macular oedema or complications of proliferative diabetic retinopathy.
- Management of vision-threatening diabetic retinopathy requires both systemic and ocular treatment.

6.3 Retinal Vein Occlusions

Learning Objectives
- Branch retinal vein occlusions (BRVO) vs. Central retinal vein occlusions (CRVO).
- Understand mechanisms of vision loss in retinal vein occlusions.
- Role of systemic illness in retinal vein occlusions.
- Principles of management of retinal vein occlusions.

The retinal veins allow blood to be drained from the retina and can be occluded at 2 sites:
- At or posterior to the lamina cribrosa (where the central retinal vein leaves the eyeball)
- At an arteriovenous crossing on the retina (where the vein shares a common adventitial sheath with a retinal artery)

Occlusion at the level of the lamina cribrosa obstructs the central retinal vein and results in a central retinal vein occlusion (CRVO; Fig. 6.8), whereas an obstruction at an arteriovenous crossing results in only a branch of the retinal veins being occluded (BRVO; Fig. 6.9). Venous occlusion results in backflow of blood, leading to the fundoscopic findings of multiple blot and flame-shaped haemorrhages. Cotton wool spots, representing small infarcts of the nerve fibre layer, may also be present.

Fundoscopic findings in a retinal vein occlusion

Acute presentation

- Flame-shaped and blot haemorrhages in the distribution of a retinal vein (BRVO) or in all four quadrants of the eye (CRVO)
- Cotton wool spots
- Dilated tortuous retinal veins
- Disc swelling

Chronic findings

- Sclerosed vein
- Opticiliary shunt
- Segmental/diffuse disc pallor
- Neovascularisation of the iris

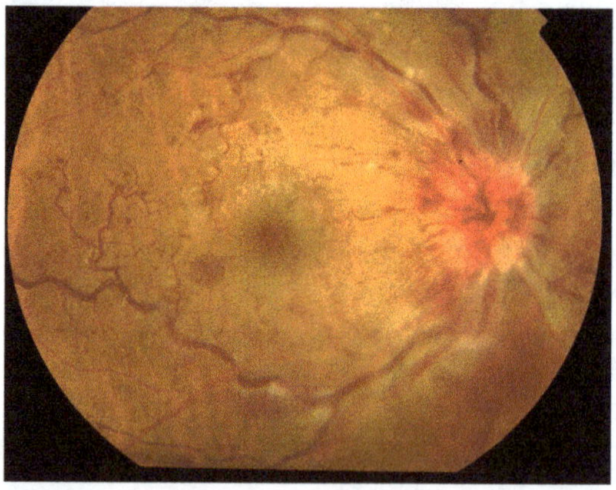

Fig. 6.8. Central retinal vein occlusion (disc swelling, dilated tortuous veins, scattered flame and blot haemorrhages, and cotton wool spots).

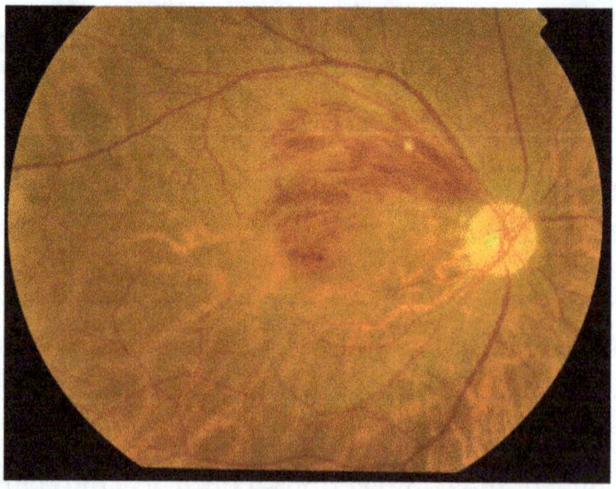

Fig. 6.9. Branch retinal vein occlusion (due to thickened atherosclerotic artery compressing on vein in the common shared adventitial sheath).

Vision Loss in Retinal Vein Occlusions

Vision loss can occur in a few ways:

- Macula involvement
  - Macular oedema
  - Macular ischaemia
- Neovascular glaucoma (usually due to an ischaemic central retinal venous occlusion, which leads to new vessel growth in the anterior segment, which, in turn, leads to raised intraocular pressure)
- Vitreous haemorrhage from new vessels on the disc (NVD) or elsewhere (NVE)

Role of Systemic Diseases in Retinal Venous Occlusions

The roles of systemic diseases differ slightly in BRVO versus a CRVO.

In a BRVO, venous occlusion usually occurs at an arteriovenous crossing. Atherosclerosis leads to thickening of the arterial wall. This, in turn, causes compression of the vein at the site of crossing (Fig. 6.10) and induces the BRVO.

The main risk factors for a BRVO are:

- Increasing age
- Systemic arterial hypertension
- History of smoking
- History of glaucoma

In CRVO, the main risk factors are slightly different:

- Systemic hypertension
- Open angle glaucoma
- Diabetes mellitus
- Hyperlipidaemia

Fig. 6.10. This image shows a typical arteriovenous crossing in the retina where the thinner arterial vessel crosses a larger, dilated retinal vein.

Retinal vein occlusion treatment

Management strategies can be broadly divided into

- Identifying and treating systemic risk factors
- Identifying and treating ocular complications

Ocular complications

Macular oedema

- The mainstay of treatment is the use of intravitreal anti-VEGF agents or intravitreal steroids
- In BRVOs, grid laser may be attempted. Grid laser is not useful in CRVO associated macular oedema.

Macular ischaemia

- Macular ischaemia is usually untreatable and has a grim prognosis for the patient's vision
- Low vision aids may be used for severe visual loss neovascular glaucoma
- A high threshold of suspicion must be maintained to identify and treat neovascular glaucoma early
- The mainstay in management is to reduce the ischaemic drive by performing laser photocoagulation to the ischaemic retina in the periphery
- Intravitreal anti-VEGF agents can also be used to reduce the high anti-VEGF levels and hopefully regress the new vessels that have appeared
- Anti-glaucoma eye drops are also started to reduce the intraocular pressure

Take Home Messages

- Vision loss from retinal vein occlusion can occur from macula involvement, neovascular glaucoma and vitreous haemorrhage.
- For macular oedema due to retinal vein occlusion, the mainstay of treatment is the use of intravitreal anti-VEGF agents or intravitreal steroids.

6.4 Retinal Artery Occlusions

Learning Objectives

- Branch retinal artery occlusions vs. Central retinal artery occlusions.
- Understand mechanisms of vision loss in retinal artery occlusions.
- Role of systemic illness in retinal artery occlusions.
- Principles of management of retinal artery occlusions.

The central retinal artery supplies blood to the inner layers of the retina and can cause sudden visual loss if occluded (CRAO: Central retinal artery occlusion; Fig. 6.11). Some patients (approximately 20%) are fortunate enough to have a cilioretinal artery, which arises from the choroidal circulation. If a patient with a CRAO has a concomitant cilioretinal artery, blood flow to the macula may be preserved, and, therefore, central vision may survive.

Retinal artery occlusion can occur along its branches as well (BRAO: Branch retinal artery occlusion; Fig. 6.12), causing a sudden onset partial visual loss in the affected segment.

Fundoscopic findings in a retinal artery occlusion

Acute presentation

- Retinal whitening
- Cherry red spot
- The offending emboli may be seen (Cholesterol, also known as Hollenhorst plaques, platelet fibrin, calcific emboli)

Chronic findings

- Disc pallor

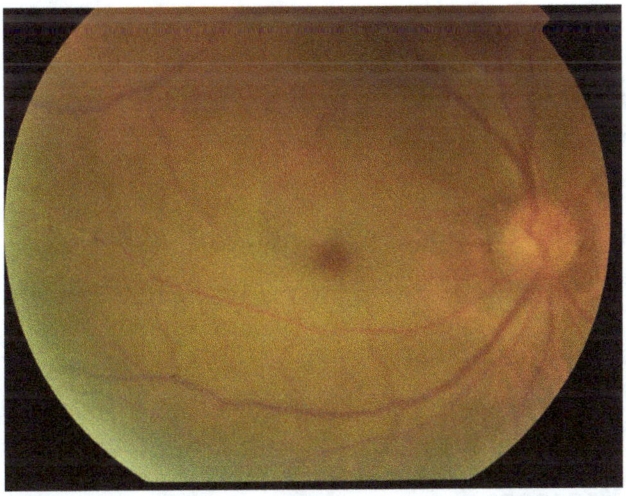

Fig. 6.11. Central retinal artery occlusion with a cherry red spot, diffuse oedema. This patient underwent an anterior chamber paracentesis and had the retinal artery emboli dislodged to the inferiotemporal branch of the retinal artery.

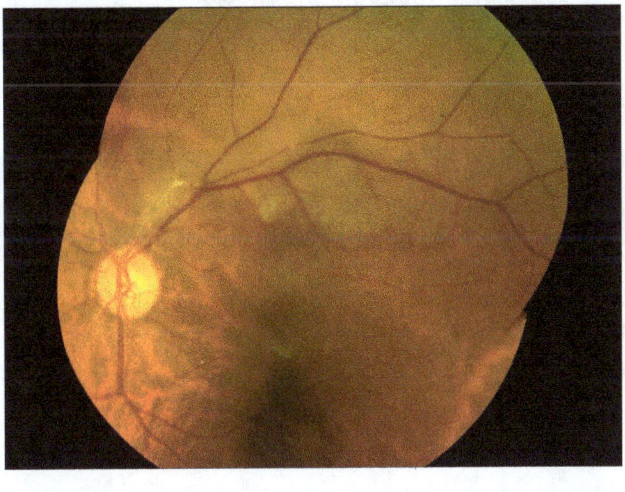

Fig. 6.12. Branch retinal artery occlusion with emboli seen in the retinal artery and retinal oedema in the area supplied by the blocked artery.

Role of Systemic Diseases in Retinal Artery Occlusions

Three main types of emboli have been described:

- Cholesterol emboli (Hollenhorst plaques) from the carotid arteries
- Platelet-fibrin emboli from atherosclerotic vessels
- Calcific emboli from abnormal cardiac valves

Generally, the underlying aetiology for retinal artery occlusion varies depending on the patient's age. Carotid artery atherosclerosis is the most common aetiology in older patients. In younger patients, the development of a retinal artery occlusion prompts a systemic evaluation for an underlying cause.

Potential causes may include:

i. Collagen vascular diseases (Giant cell arteritis, systemic lupus erythematosus)
ii. Prothrombotic conditions (Protein C/S deficiency, antithrombin III deficiency, oral contraceptives, pregnancy, cancer, haematological malignancies)
iii. Cardiac emboli

Retinal artery occlusion treatment

Management strategies can be broadly divided into:

- Identifying and treating systemic risk factors
- Acute management to dislodge the emboli to improve retinal circulation

Acute ocular intervention (aimed at dislodging clot)

- Digital ocular massage
- Carbogen inhalation
- Anterior chamber paracentesis
- Intravenous carbonic anhydrase inhibitor and other topical anti-glaucoma medications

Take Home Messages

- Retinal artery occlusion is an ocular emergency and should be identified promptly.
- The condition is associated with poor prognosis.

6.5 Hypertensive Retinopathy

Learning Objective

Classification of hypertensive retinopathy.

Hypertension has effects on the precapillary arterioles in the eye. Early stages of hypertensive changes may include:

- Diffuse/focal retinal arteriolar narrowing
- Arteriolar wall opacification (Silver/Copper wiring)
- Compression of the venules at the arteriovenous junction (AV nicking/nipping)

Traditionally, the Keith-Wagener-Barker classification has been used to characterise these changes.

Keith-Wagener-Barker classification

Grade 1

Mild generalised arteriolar narrowing/sclerosis

Grade 2

Generalised/focal arteriolar narrowing, silver/copper wiring, AV nicking/nipping (Fig. 6.10)

Grade 3

Haemorrhages (dot/blot/flame), microaneurysms, cotton wool spots, hard exudates (Fig. 6.13)

Grade 4 (Malignant hypertension)

Moderate changes + Disc swelling

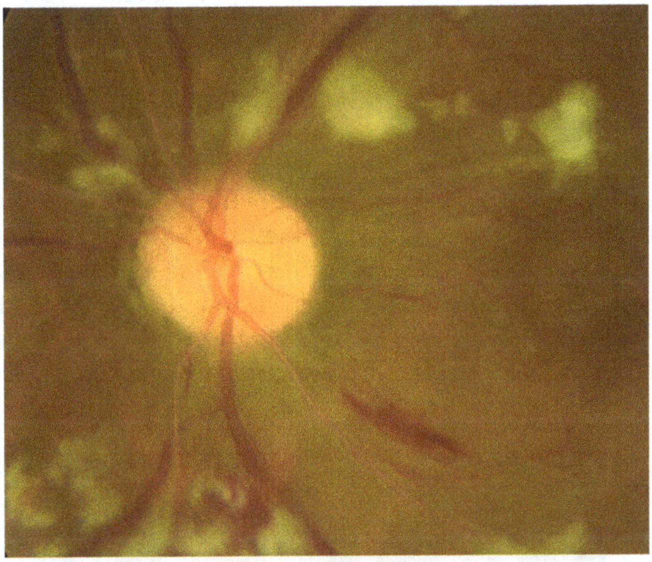

Fig. 6.13. Scattered cotton wool spots, with some flame haemorrhages seen.

Take Home Message

Hypertensive retinopathy can be classified based on the Keith-Wagener-Barker classification.

6.6 Age-related Macular Degeneration

Learning Objectives

- Difference between dry and wet age-related macular degeneration (AMD).
- Understand mechanisms of vision loss in AMD.
- Role of smoking in AMD.
- Principles of management of AMD.

Age-related macular degeneration (AMD) is a leading cause of central visual loss in persons above the age of 50. The hallmark finding in eyes with AMD is the presence of drusen in the macula.

Other findings may include:

i. Retinal pigment layer abnormalities (geographic atrophy)

ii. Haemorrhage

iii. Disciform scarring

Classically, AMD has been divided into "dry" and "wet" forms. The dry form is characterised by the presence of drusen in the macula, which are initially visually asymptomatic (Fig. 6.14). Later on, atrophic macular scarring may develop (geographic atrophy; Fig. 6.15). The progression to macular scarring is a chronic process and does not involve the formation of any abnormal choroidal neovascular membrane (CNVM).

In wet AMD, a CNVM forms at the macula. Histopathologically, the CNVM may lie above or below the retinal pigment epithelium (RPE). The actual formation of the CNVM is visually asymptomatic. However, these CNVM typically bleed (Fig. 6.16), causing a sudden drop in vision. Visual loss may manifest as mild metamorphopsia (due to the distortion in the photoreceptor layer from the oedema and bleeding) or may be more severe with the sudden loss of central vision (due to a thick layer of blood over the photoreceptors).

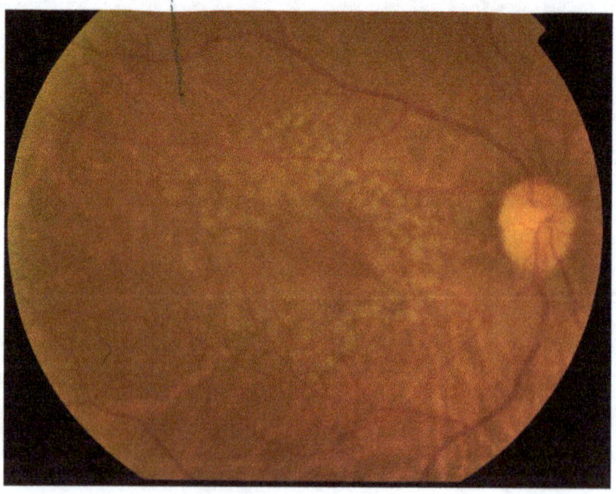

Fig. 6.14. Dry AMD with drusen seen around macula.

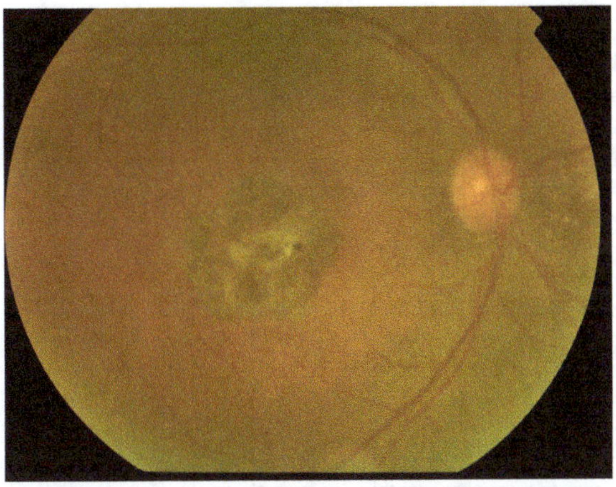

Fig. 6.15. Dry AMD with macula scar seen (also known as geographic atrophy).

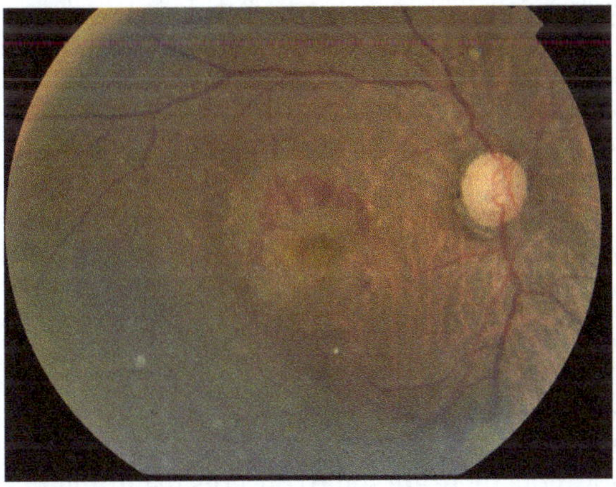

Fig. 6.16. Wet AMD: Haemorrhage noted in macula with surrounding drusen.

With regard to prevention, the main modifiable risk factor is smoking. Smoking cessation is an important aspect of managing all forms of AMD.

In addition, antioxidant supplementation in the form of the AREDS (age-related eye disease) vitamins have been shown to help in reducing the progression to advanced AMD in some patients. At 10 years, 44% of placebo patients compared to 34% of the patients receiving the AREDS supplementation developed advanced AMD (a 27% risk reduction).

However, this benefit was noted in only two groups of patients:

i. Individuals with intermediate AMD (extensive intermediate or at least 1 large drusen, or nonsubfoveal geographic atrophy)

ii. Individuals with advanced unilateral AMD (vision loss due to AMD in one eye)

Regular surveillance with an Amsler grid (Fig. 6.17) is important. Patients are instructed to close one eye and focus on the central dot in the Amsler grid and report to their doctor if they have a sudden distortion/disappearance of the lines on the Amsler grid

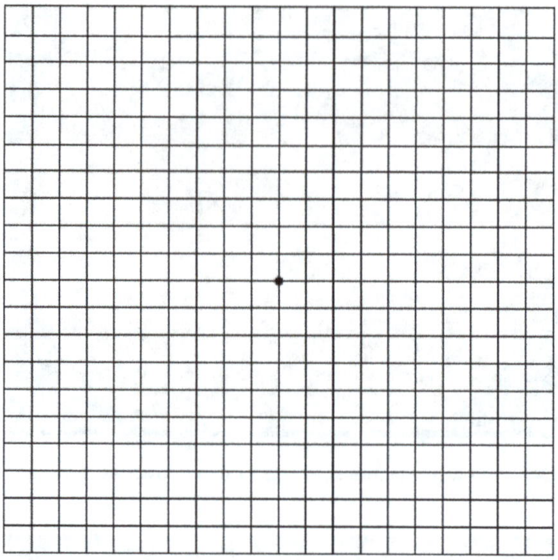

Fig. 6.17. Amsler grid.

Once the patient develops neovascular AMD, with haemorrhage and/or oedema in the macula, the mainstay of treatment is intravitreal injections of anti-vascular endothelial growth factors (anti-VEGF). Various anti-angiogenic agents are available:

- Bevacizumab (Avastin)
- Ranibizumab (Lucentis)
- Aflibercept (Eylea)
- Faricimab (Vabysmo)

These injections are generally safe but carry a small risk of endophthalmitis with each injection. In addition, there are some concerns regarding the use of anti-VEGF agents in patients with a recent history of stroke or heart attacks.

In some cases, laser therapy using Photodynamic Therapy (PDT) may be done. This involves the injection of a photosensitive drug into a peripheral vein, which is then activated by a laser with a specific wavelength in the retina circulation. The activated drug then creates free radicals, which then cause local damage in the abnormal retinal vasculature, where it is activated.

Take Home Messages

- Age-related macular degeneration can be classified into "dry" and "wet" forms.
- The underlying pathophysiology is related to choroidal neovascularisation.
- The mainstay of treatment for wet AMD is intravitreal injections of anti-vascular endothelial growth factors (anti-VEGF).

6.7 Retinal Tears/Retinal Detachments

Learning Objectives

- Understanding symptoms of a retinal tear.
- Development of a retinal detachment after a retinal tear.
- Role of early detection and prophylactic treatment of retinal tears.

Retinal tears are full thickness tears of the neurosensory retina. Typically, these tears are believed to occur due to traction from the vitreous body pulling on the retina. This tractional force is especially strong once a posterior vitreous detachment develops.

To understand a posterior vitreous detachment, one must first understand that the vitreous body has an outer cortex, which in the posterior part is known as the posterior vitreous cortex. This posterior vitreous cortex is adherent to the surface of the retina. With age, the gel in the vitreous body starts to degenerate and liquefy, causing a drop in the volume of the vitreous body. This leads to a contraction in the vitreous body and a subsequent detachment of its posterior cortex off the surface of the retina. This process is known as a posterior vitreous detachment (PVD).

When a PVD develops, patients typically experience floaters or photopsia. Patients with these symptoms should undergo a dilated fundus exam to exclude retinal tears.

Retinal tears provide an entry point for liquefied vitreous to enter the potential space between the neurosensory retina and the retinal pigment epithelium. As the liquefied vitreous enters this potential space, a neurosensory detachment occurs (retinal detachment), which can lead to visual field defects and, eventually, the loss of central vision when the macula is involved.

Once a retinal detachment occurs, surgery is typically required. Treatment options include a pneumatic retinopexy, vitrectomy or scleral buckle procedure.

However, if the patient is diagnosed early before the retinal tear has progressed to a retinal detachment (Fig. 6.18), prophylactic laser retinopexy (Fig. 6.19) can be

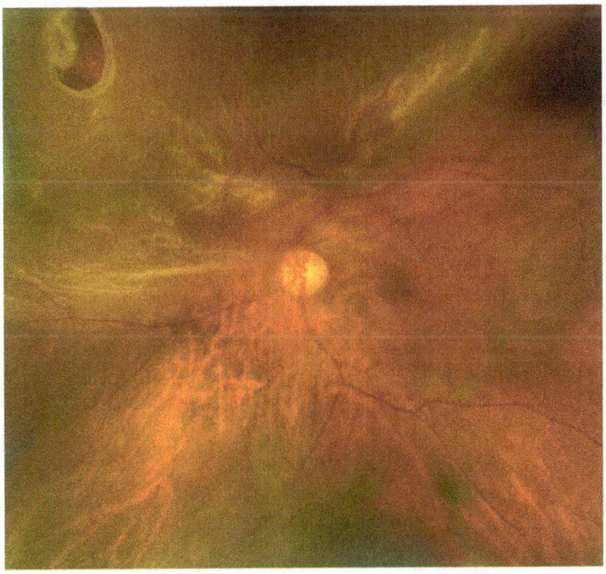

Fig. 6.18. Retinal detachment with horseshoe retinal tear seen superonasally.

done to surround the retinal tear with laser burns to seal the neurosensory retina to the retinal pigment epithelium. These laser scars then prevent further movement of the liquefied vitreous gel through the tear to reduce the risk of developing a retinal detachment.

There is no symptom that can distinguish which patient has a retinal tear or not. A dilated fundus exam is important to detect retinal tears or detachment.

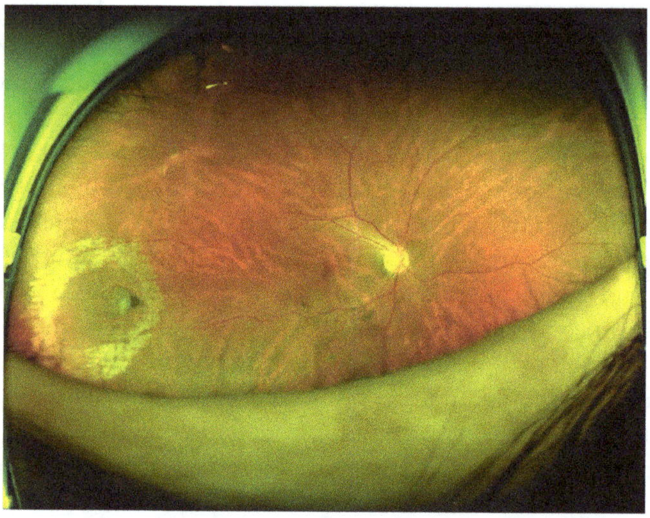

Fig. 6.19. Inferotemporal retinal tear surrounded by fresh laser retinopexy burns.

Take Home Message

Retinal detachment is an emergency, and surgical intervention is associated with high rates of success.

References

1. American Academy of Ophthalmology (Basic and Clinical Sciences Course).
2. Hayrey SS, Zimmerman MB. (2014) Branch retinal vein occlusion: Natural history of visual outcome. *JAMA Ophthalmol* **132(1)**:13–22.
3. *Kanski's Clinical Ophthalmology*.
4. The Diabetic Retinopathy Study Research Group. (1976) Preliminary report on effects of photocoagulation therapy. *Am J Ophthalmol* **81**:383–396.

Chapter 7

OCULOPLASTICS

Stephanie Ming Young, Blanche Xiaohong Lim, Maryanne Chew Romero, Gangadhara Sundar

7.1 Eyelid Disorders

Learning Objectives

- Be aware of common causes of eyelid lumps and bumps and be alert to malignant lesions.
- Know how to classify ptosis based on onset and cause and understand the mechanism of ptosis.
- Be familiar with common eyelid malpositions, including entropion and ectropion.
- Know how to evaluate a patient with eyelid injury and be familiar with the principles of management.

Lumps and Bumps

Due to the unique anatomic features of the eyelid, lesions on the eyelid may have distinct presentations compared with similar lesions elsewhere in the body. Clinical judgment is important for identifying benign eyelid lesions while recognising those with malignant potential that require biopsy.

Chalazion

- Chalazia typically appear as characteristically hard and usually painless (unless infected) lid nodules overlying the tarsus (Fig. 7.1)
- These growths occur due to obstruction of the orifices of the meibomian glands. Subsequently, the sebaceous contents of these glands are forced into the tarsus and surrounding soft tissues of the eyelid, leading to a chronic localised inflammatory response.

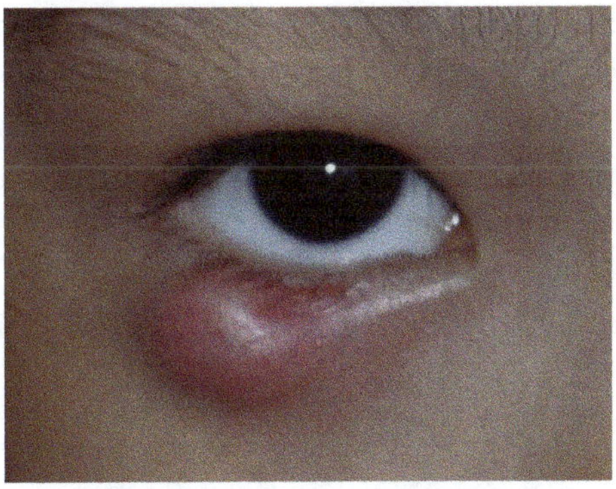

Fig. 7.1. A large lower lid chalazion with signs of inflammation.

- The classic histopathologic finding in chalazia is chronic lipogranulomatous inflammation
- Management: Most chalazia resolve by themselves within several days to weeks, but sometimes can take months to completely disappear. Medical therapy includes warm compresses, lid scrubs and antibiotic ointment. A large or persistent chalazion may require incision and curettage.

Hordeolum

- This is an acute focal infection (usually staphylococcal) involving either the glands of Zeis (external hordeola) or, less frequently, the meibomian glands (internal hordeola)
- Medical therapy for hordeola includes eyelid hygiene (lid scrubs), warm compresses and topical antibiotic ointment. If an external hordeolum is centred around a lash follicle, the lash can be pulled to enhance drainage. Systemic antibiotics may be indicated if the hordeola is complicated by preseptal cellulitis. Internal hordeola may occasionally evolve into chalazia, which may require surgical incision and curettage.

Benign and Premalignant Lesions

Embryologically, the skin and palpebral conjunctiva of the eyelid develop from the surface ectoderm, whereas the remaining structures originate from the mesoderm. Nearly all eyelid tumours arise from the epidermis, dermis, and adnexal structures. The adnexal structures include the sweat glands (glands of Moll), hair follicles, and sebaceous glands (Meibomian glands and glands of Zeis).

Table 7.1. Examples of Benign and Premalignant Eyelid Lesions Categorised According to their Layer of Origin

Layer	Lesions
Epidermis	Squamous cell papilloma, seborrhoeic keratosis, keratoacanthoma, actinic keratosis
Dermis	Nevus
Cystic lesions	Epidermal inclusion cyst, dermoid cyst
Sweat gland tumours	Hidrocystoma, syringoma
Hair follicle tumours	Pilomatrixoma, trichoepithelioma
Sebaceous gland tumours	Sebaceous adenoma

- Majority of tumours occurring on the eyelid are benign, and a number of these lesions may be difficult to distinguish from malignant tumours based on clinical examination alone
- Typically, benign lesions do not ulcerate, bleed, or cause loss of lashes or destruction of normal eyelid architecture
- Atypical lesions may be more difficult to identify accurately. Histopathologic confirmation is necessary to establish a definitive diagnosis in some cases.

Malignant Lesions

Skin cancer is one of the most common malignancies in the human body, with the eyelids being one of the frequent sites of involvement. There are geographic differences in the incidence of eyelid tumours as a result of skin type and sun exposure. In white populations, basal cell carcinoma (BCC) is the most frequent eyelid malignancy, followed by squamous cell carcinoma (SCC), sebaceous gland carcinoma (SGC), and melanoma. In more pigmented populations, appendageal tumours such as SGC make up a greater proportion.

Although each tumour has characteristic clinical features, there are certain signs that are suggestive of malignancy: loss of normal lid architecture, madarosis, tethering to deeper structures, and growth or change of a lesion's colour, border, or size.

Basal Cell Carcinoma

- Basal cell carcinoma (BCC) is one of the most common human malignancies
- Risk factors include ultraviolet (UV) light exposure, fair skin, immunosuppression, genetic disorders such as basal cell nevus syndrome (BCNS, Gorlin syndrome) and xeroderma pigmentosum
- BCC most commonly occurs on the lower eyelid, followed by the medial canthus, upper lid, and lateral canthus
- The following clinical presentations can occur:
    - Nodular: A pearly papule or nodule with surface telangiectasia and a rolled edge. It gradually enlarges to form a dome-shaped lesion, which may develop central ulceration
    - Superficial: A slow-growing, scaly, erythematous patch or plaque, which may resemble dermatitis
    - Morpheic (sclerosing): An indurated, poorly defined, white to pink, scar-like plaque. This appearance is also sometimes termed "infiltrative" BCC.
    - Pigmented (Fig. 7.2): BCC can have uniform or variegated brown, gray-blue, or black pigmentation and may mimic nevi or melanoma. This type is most common among pigmented races and is uncommon in whites.
- Metastasis is rare in BCC
- Excision with confirmation of 3–4 mm clear margins by histopathologic examination is the mainstay of treatment

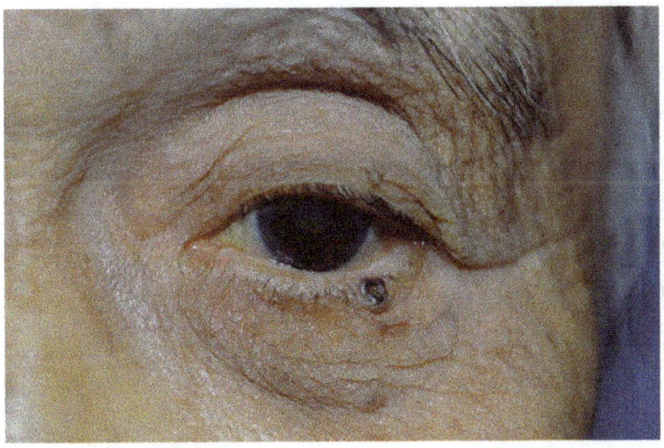

Fig. 7.2. Left lower lid pigmented BCC with rolled edges and an ulcerated crater in the centre.

Squamous Cell Carcinoma

- Squamous cell carcinoma (SCC) accounts for 5% to 10% of eyelid malignancies in whites but is rare in pigmented races
- Compared to BCC, it is a more aggressive tumour with a higher risk of perineural, nodal, and distant spread
- Risk factors include UVB radiation, pre-existing injured skin (e.g. ulcers, burns), immunosuppression, presence of precancerous lesions (e.g. actinic keratosis), genetic conditions (e.g. albinism, xeroderma pigmentosum)
- In the periocular area, they are most common on the lower lid, followed by the medial canthus, the upper lid, and the lateral canthus
- SCC has a wide range of clinical appearances
  - The majority are painless, scaling nodules or plaques with irregular rolled edges, fissuring and ulceration
  - Others can form cutaneous horns, papillomas, or large fungating masses
- SCC can be neurotrophic when perineural invasion facilitates tumour spread into the orbit and cranial cavity
- Regional and distant metastatic spread occurs in 2% to 10% of periocular SCC
- Periocular SCC should be excised with intraoperative margin control, with either a frozen section or Moh's micrographic surgery (MSS). A minimum 4 mm margin has been advised for SCC.

Sebaceous Gland Carcinoma

- Sebaceous gland carcinoma (SGC) can arise from the Meibomian glands, glands of Zeis, and sebaceous glands. They are most frequent in the eyelids because of the density of these glands. Other periocular sites include the eyebrow, caruncle, lacrimal gland and conjunctiva.
- Reported risk factors for SGC include advanced age, Asian or South Asian race, women and previous irradiation to the head and neck
- SGC (Fig. 7.3) may masquerade not only as various inflammatory conditions such as blepharoconjunctivitis or chalazion but also as premalignant lesions and other benign or malignant tumours
  - The nodular form of SGC presents as a discrete, hard, immobile nodule commonly located in the upper tarsal plate, having a yellowish appearance
  - The pagetoid variety of SGC occurs with intraepithelial infiltration of the lid margin and/or conjunctiva, causing diffuse thickening and loss of eyelashes, resembling chronic blepharoconjunctivitis
- Surgical excision, with 5 mm margins and margin control, is the recommended treatment. Orbital involvement usually necessitates exenteration, and nodal involvement is cleared with neck dissection. Adjunctive treatment (cryotherapy, radiotherapy and chemotherapy) may be used for advanced lesions or those with significant intraepithelial spread.

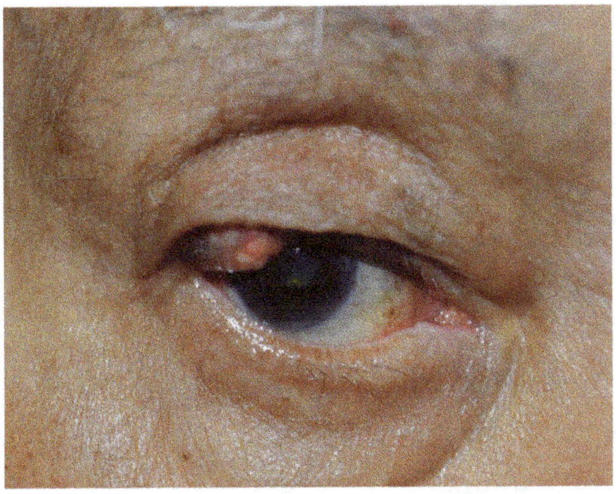

Fig. 7.3. Pigmented lesion on the right upper lid margin with yellowish deposits suspicious of lipid and overlying telangiectasia with loss of lashes. Incisional biopsy confirmed SGC.

Ptosis

"Ptosis" refers to the drooping or inferior displacement of any anatomical structure. "Blepharoptosis" (usually simply referred to as "ptosis") refers to the drooping or inferior displacement of the upper eyelid.

Ptosis can be classified by:

- Onset
  - Congenital
  - Acquired
- Cause
  - Myogenic
  - Aponeurotic
  - Neurogenic
  - Mechanical
  - Traumatic

Anatomy and Function

The upper eyelid retractors comprise the following:

- Levator muscle
  - Primary retractor of the upper eyelid
  - Supported at orbital aperture by Whitnall's ligament
  - Becomes collagenous aponeurosis that inserts on the tarsal plate
- Müller's muscle
  - Responsible for involuntary upper eyelid elevation

- Frontalis muscle
  - Lifts brows
  - Weak retractor of upper eyelids

Evaluation

History

Pertinent points to ask in any patient with ptosis include:

- Medical history
  - Medication history: anticoagulants
  - Previous eye or eyelid surgeries
  - Previous periorbital trauma
  - Onset and duration to distinguish congenital from acquired
  - Any variability in the degree of ptosis during the day to rule out myasthenia-related ptosis
  - Complaints of diplopia
  - Dysphonia, dyspnoea, dysphagia, proximal muscle weakness
  - Family history
  - How ptosis is affecting the patient's daily activities

Physical Examination

A complete examination of any patient with ptosis includes:

- Vertical interpalpebral fissure height
  - Widest point between the lower and upper eyelid
- Margin-reflex distance 1 (MRD-1)
  - Distance between the upper eyelid margin and corneal light reflex in primary position
- Upper eyelid crease position
  - A high crease and deep superior sulcus is suggestive of aponeurotic ptosis
  - An absent or poorly formed lid crease is suggestive of congenital ptosis
- Levator function
  - Measuring eyelid excursion from downgaze to upgaze with frontalis muscle function negated
- Position of ptotic eyelid in downgaze
  - Congenital ptosis: eyelid higher in downgaze than the contralateral side
  - Involutional ptosis: eyelid ptotic in all positions of gaze, usually worsens in downgaze
- Visual function and refractive error
  - Congenital or childhood ptosis: amblyopia occurs in approximately 20% of congenital ptosis
- Extraocular movements

- Extraocular muscle dysfunction associated with ptosis in various conditions
  - Oculomotor palsy
  - Ocular myasthenia gravis (MG)
  - Chronic progressive external ophthalmoplegia (CPEO)
- Pupils
  - Horner syndrome — miosis
  - CN 3 palsy — mydriasis
- Head position, chin elevation, brow position, brow action in attempted upgaze
- Tear film, lagophthalmos, Bell's reflex, corneal sensation
  - To identify factors that may predispose the patient to complications of ptosis repair, such as dryness and keratopathy
- Synkinesis
  - Marcus Gunn jaw-winking ptosis
  - Aberrant regeneration of 3rd or 7th CN palsy

Acquired Aponeurotic Ptosis

- Most common of all forms of ptosis
- Due to stretching or dehiscence of levator aponeurosis/Disinsertion of levator aponeurosis from the normal position
- Common causes
  - Senile changes of the levator aponeurosis and its insertion onto the tarsus
  - Frequent eye rubbing
  - Contact lens wear
  - Previous intraocular surgery
- Characteristics (Fig. 7.4)
  - High or absent eyelid crease
  - Deep superior sulcus
  - Levator function may vary but is usually fair to good
  - Ptosis may worsen in downgaze

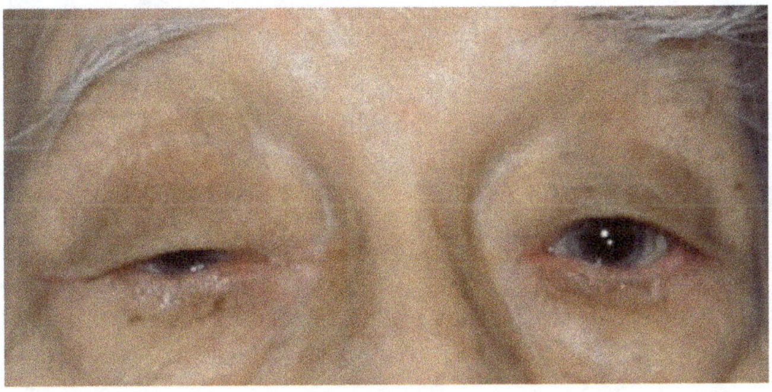

Fig. 7.4. Patient with right-sided aponeurotic ptosis causing obstruction of visual axis.

Congenital Myogenic Ptosis

- In most cases of congenital myogenic ptosis, the cause is idiopathic
  - Rarely, it may be associated with a genetic dysmorphic syndrome such as blepharophimosis syndrome
- Histologically, the levator muscles of patients with congenital ptosis are dystrophic. The levator muscle and aponeurotic tissues appear to be infiltrated with fat and fibrous tissue.
- Although not all patients with congenital ptosis need surgical intervention, patients need to be closely monitored for the possible development of amblyopia from visual deprivation or uncorrected astigmatism
- Characteristics (Fig. 7.5)
  - Decreased levator function, usually poor
  - Eyelid lag on downgaze
  - Lagophthalmos (sometimes)
  - Absent or poorly formed lid crease

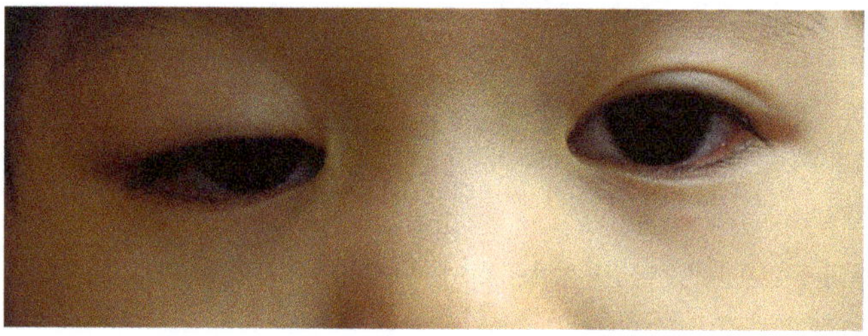

Fig. 7.5. Child with right congenital myogenic ptosis. Note the absent lid crease.

Myogenic Ptosis

- Other than congenital myogenic ptosis, causes of myogenic ptosis include CPEO (Fig. 7.6), myotonic dystrophy and oculopharyngeal muscular dystrophy
- **Myasthenia gravis** (MG) may be included in both the neurogenic and myogenic classifications. (See Chapter 9: Neuro-ophthalmology.)

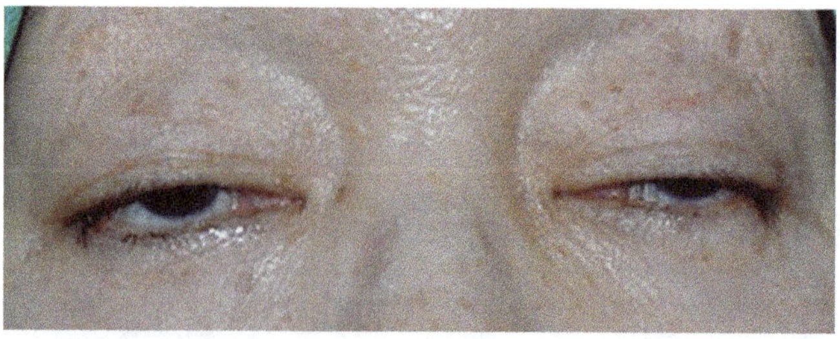

Fig. 7.6. Patient with myogenic ptosis with ophthalmoplegia secondary to CPEO.

Neurogenic Ptosis

- Causes
  - Dysfunction of the oculomotor nerve (aetiologies include vascular, ischaemic, demyelination, tumours and trauma)
  - Dysfunction of sympathetic innervation to Müller's muscle (Horner's syndrome)
  - Synkinetic ptosis, such as Marcus Gunn jaw-winking syndrome
- In cases of neurogenic ptosis due to dysfunction of the oculomotor nerve, there is innervational deficiency in the levator muscle function
  - There may be associated neurologic findings
  - Surgical correction of ptosis should be deferred until its cause has been thoroughly investigated and the condition has stabilised
  - The ocular misalignment must be addressed before ptosis correction
  - Levator function will remain defective despite the reestablishment of adequate eyelid height

Treatment of Ptosis

- Non-surgical treatment
  - Eyelid crutches attached to eyeglass frames
  - Taping of upper lid
- Surgical treatment
  - Usually done under local anaesthesia (except children)
  - Three broad categories:
    i. External/Transcutaneous/Anterior: Levator repair/resection
      - Skin incision
      - Tightening levator muscle to elevate eyelid
      - Reserved for fair to good levator function, although maximal levator resection can be attempted for poor levator function

    ii. Internal/Transconjunctival/Posterior: Conjunctivomullerectomy
      - No skin incision
      - Surgery on Müller's muscle from the conjunctival approach
      - Usually for mild (2 mm or less) ptosis with a positive phenylephrine test

    iii. Frontalis muscle suspension
      - Brow suspension
      - For patients with poor to absent levator function
      - Materials for brow suspension include autogenous or preserved fascia lata, silicon rods, monofilament nylon, braided polyester, etc.

Eyelid Malpositions

Entropion

Entropion is an eyelid malposition resulting in the inward turning of the eyelid margin (Fig. 7.7). This causes the myocutaneous border of the eyelid and lashes to be directed towards the globe, resulting in conjunctival irritation and corneal abrasion.

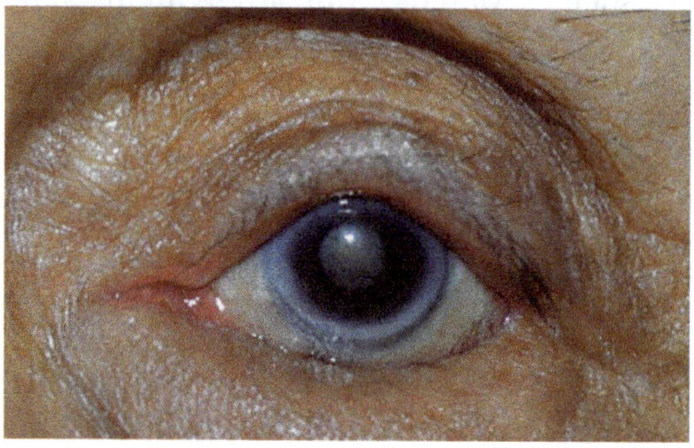

Fig. 7.7. Left lower lid involutional entropion. Note the inward rolling of the eyelid margin with lashes buried and touching the conjunctiva.

Classification

The pathophysiology depends on the type of entropion:

- Acute spastic
  - Following ocular inflammation/irritation
  - Sustained orbicularis contraction > inward rotation of eyelid margin
- Involutional
  - Weakness of inferior retractors
  - Horizontal lid laxity
  - Overriding of preseptal to pretarsal orbicularis oculi
  - Tarsal plate atrophy
- Cicatricial
  - Caused by vertical tarsoconjunctival contracture and internal rotation of the eyelid margin
    1. Autoimmune: ocular cicatricial pemphigoid (OCP)
    2. Inflammation: chronic meibomitis, Stevens-Johnson syndrome (SJS)
    3. Infection: trachoma, herpes zoster (HZ)
    4. Surgery, trauma

Management

Medical therapy may be warranted for patients who decline surgery and as a temporising manoeuvre in patients who may improve spontaneously

- Topical lubricants are helpful for protecting the ocular surface and may break the cycle in patients with spastic entropion due to dry eye syndrome
- Treatment of blepharitis may help alleviate spastic entropion

- Small amounts of botulinum toxin (BOTOX®) may be effective for spastic entropion by weakening the pretarsal orbicularis oculi muscle
- Treat underlying cause of cicatricial entropion, e.g. OCP and SJS

Multiple surgical procedures have been described for the management of entropion. The surgical correction must be directed at repair of the primary anatomic defects.

- For instance, in involutional entropion, both inferior retractor repair and horizontal lid shortening (e.g. lateral tarsal strip) are usually required to address inferior retractor weakness and horizontal lid laxity, respectively
- A less satisfactory and temporary procedure is the placement of full thickness Quickert-Rathbun type sutures to rotate the eyelid margin outwards (Fig. 7.8)

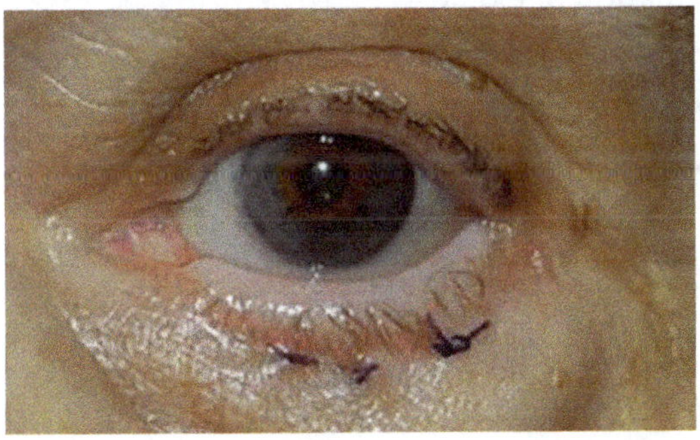

Fig. 7.8. Left lower lid entropion treated with Quickert sutures to rotate the eyelid margin outwards.

Ectropion

Ectropion is an eyelid malposition resulting in outward turning of the eyelid margin. This leads to lagophthalmos, inadequate corneal protection, discomfort, and, ultimately, epithelial and stromal injury. Tear drainage dysfunction results from poor apposition of the puncta to the globe. The causes are varied, and correction must be directed at the source of the pathologic process.

Classification

Ectropion can be classified by the cause:

- Involutional
  - Horizontal lid laxity + dehiscence of lower lid retractors
- Paralytic
  - Facial palsy (Fig. 7.9)
    - i. Loss of orbicularis tone results in outward displacement of the lower lid under the influence of gravity
    - ii. Paralytic ectropion is often associated with brow ptosis and secondary dermatochalasis
- Cicatricial
  - Loss of skin
    - i. Chemical/thermal burns
    - ii. Trauma (mechanical/surgical)

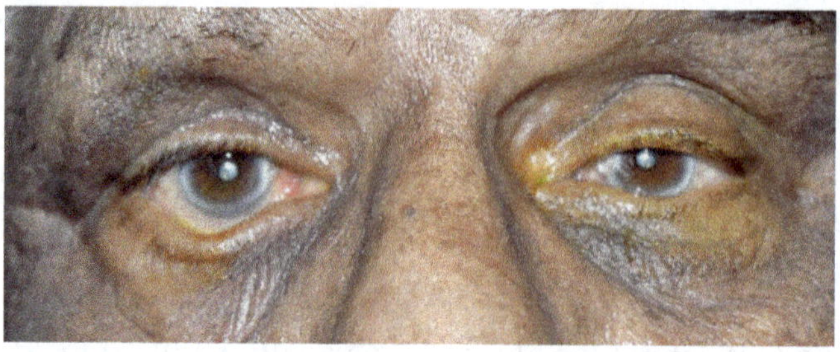

Fig. 7.9. Right lower lid paralytic ectropion secondary to lower motor neuron facial palsy. He had concurrent brow ptosis as well and had shaved his eyebrow to avoid the hairs from the eyebrow, causing irritation to his eye.

- Chronic inflammation of eyelid
  i. Rosacea
  ii. Atopic dermatitis
  iii. HZ infection
- Mechanical
  - Mass effect induced by bulk tumours of the eyelid

Management

Management is directed at the underlying cause

- In involutional ectropion, repair is directed at tightening the lax components of the eyelid structure. The most common and useful lid shortening procedure is the lateral tarsal strip procedure
- In paralytic ectropion secondary to facial nerve palsy, the goal in management is to protect the cornea. It is important to determine the likelihood of facial palsy recovery before offering more permanent surgical procedures. Surgical procedures for facial palsy are varied and include tarsorrhaphy, lateral tarsal strip, medial and lateral canthoplasty, mid-face lift, and direct brow lift

Eyelid Injuries

Head and facial injuries frequently involve the periocular area and can cause significant morbidity.

Initial Assessment

- When evaluating a patient who has sustained any type of trauma, life-threatening injuries should first be addressed or ruled out before assessing for ocular and adnexal trauma
- In the setting of trauma, the physician should not forget the basics of life support (airway, breathing, circulation) and systemic trauma assessments

History

- Evaluation should begin with a complete history
- This includes the medical, ocular, and surgical history and pointed questions about the injury

- The mechanism, timing and location of the injury should be recorded
- Tetanus status and any changes in the patient's vision or facial sensation should be noted
- The patient's allergies and last oral intake are important, and the patient should not be allowed to eat or drink until the evaluation and any surgical planning is complete

Examination

A full examination for any lid and adnexal trauma includes the following:

- Visual acuity
- Pupils
- Extraocular motility
- Eyelids
  - Any lacerations should be noted, including the location and depth
  - Fat protrusion through the eyelid is an indication of orbital septum penetration and requires ophthalmologic consultation before exploration and repair
- Canaliculi and lacrimal system
  - Eyelid lacerations medial to the puncta are assumed to involve the canaliculus (canaliculi) until proven otherwise (Fig. 7.10)
- Orbit (refer to Section 7.2: Orbital Trauma)

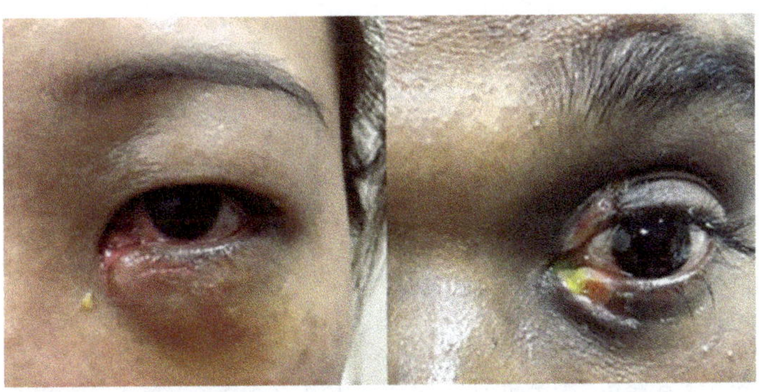

Fig. 7.10. Small lacerations in the medial aspect of the lower lid in different patients. Probing confirmed laceration of the lower canaliculus.

General Principles of Repair for Eyelid Lacerations

- Clean wound and remove the foreign body, if any
- Careful handling of tissues
- Careful alignment of anatomy
  - Lid margin, lash line, grey line, etc.
  - Lid margin lacerations usually repaired prior to extramarginal lacerations for better anatomical realignment
- Close in layers

- Timing
  - Ideally within 12–24 hours of injury, but can be delayed based on patient factors

Eyelid Margin Lacerations

- Carefully align lid margin with 6/0 silk suture to prevent notching
- Close tarsal plate with 6/0 Vicryl (partial thickness of tarsus)
- Additional margin silk sutures (Fig. 7.11)
  - Mucocutaneous junction (A)
  - Gray line (B)
  - Lash line (C)

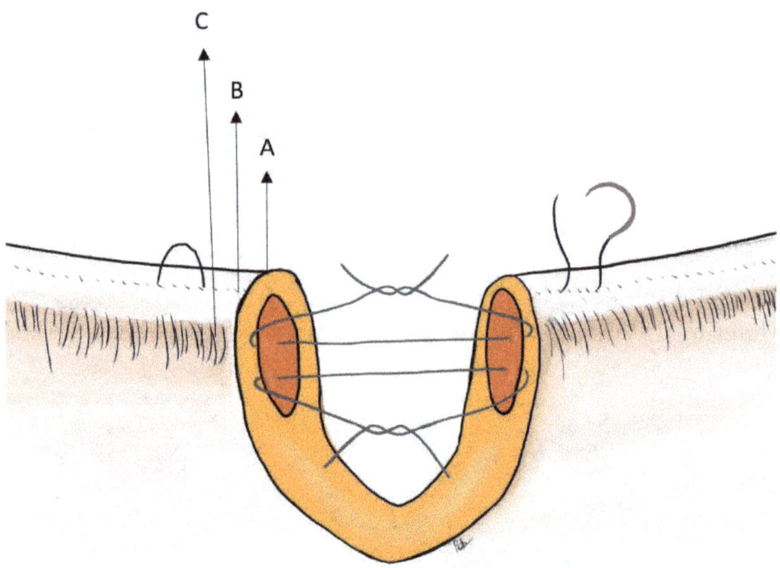

Fig. 7.11. Sutures placed at the tarsus and lid margin.

Take Home Messages

- Although most eyelid tumours are benign, some are clinically difficult to distinguish from malignant tumours and may require a biopsy.
- Common malignant tumours of the eyelid are basal cell carcinoma (BCC) and squamous cell carcinoma (SCC).
- Aponeurotic ptosis is the most common cause of adult-acquired ptosis, whereas the most common myogenic ptosis is congenital in origin.
- Entropion and ectropion are common malpositions of the eyelid and correction must be directed at the source of the pathologic process.
- General principles for the repair of eyelid lacerations include careful handling of tissues and proper alignment of the anatomy, especially for lid margin lacerations.

7.2 Orbital Disorders

Learning Objectives

- Know how to differentiate preseptal from orbital cellulitis and be familiar with their management.
- Be familiar with the signs and symptoms of thyroid eye disease (TED) and various sight-threatening complications.
- Understand the management principles of TED.
- Be aware of common orbital tumours and how they may present.
- Know how to assess a patient with trauma and what to look out for in a patient with suspected orbital fractures.

Orbital Cellulitis

Orbital cellulitis is one of the life-threatening ophthalmic conditions. It is considered on the same spectrum of disease with preseptal cellulitis; however, the distinction between these two conditions is important.

Orbital cellulitis is the infection of the ocular adnexal tissue posterior to the orbital septum, while preseptal cellulitis is an infection that only involves structures anterior to the septum, such as eyelid tissue. The septum is a layer of fascia extending superiorly from the orbital rim to the levator aponeurosis in the upper eyelid, as well as to the inferior border of the tarsus in the lower eyelid. In orbital cellulitis, the infection could spread posteriorly, causing cavernous sinus thrombosis as well as intracranial involvement, resulting in morbidity and mortality.

Chandler's Classification

It describes the level of involvement of cellulitis. Although this suggests a sequential progression, any infection may involve one or more stages and progress in either direction, so its usefulness is debated.

Stage 1: Preseptal cellulitis

Stage 2: Orbital cellulitis

Stage 3: Subperiosteal abscess

Stage 4: Orbital abscess

Stage 5: Cavernous sinus thrombosis

Aetiology

- Adjacent infection in the surrounding structures
  - Sinusitis
  - Eyelids (including hordeola)
  - Lacrimal sac
  - Dental infections

- External causes
  - Trauma
  - Surgery
- Endogenous causes (bacteraemia)
- Ophthalmic causes (e.g. endophthalmitis with extraocular extension)

Pathogens

The pathogens involved depend on the source and the patient's age

- *Staph. aureus* and streptococcal species (including *Pneumococcus*) are associated with eyelid and lacrimal sac infections
- Community-acquired MRSA is increasing in incidence in some regions and may penetrate small breaks in the skin
- In the past, *H. influenza* was a common organism in young children with dacryocystitis or haematogenous sources, but is rare in regions where HiB vaccination is available
- Sinus infections
  - In children under 9 years of age: commonly caused by a single aerobic non-spore-forming bacteria
  - In adolescents, and particularly adults: more likely to be polymicrobial and to include facultative anaerobes
- Penetrating trauma with organic foreign bodies may introduce fungi, especially *Aspergillus*

History

Preseptal Cellulitis

- Pain of the eyelid/periorbital tissues
- Eyelid redness and swelling

Orbital Cellulitis

- Symptoms of preseptal cellulitis, as well as:
- Blurring of vision
- Swelling and injection of conjunctiva
- Double vision
- Pain on eye movements
- Systemic symptoms, such as fever

Other Relevant History that Should Be Sought

- Symptoms of sinusitis (facial pain, post-nasal drip, etc.)
- Trauma
- Insect bites
- Immunocompromised status (uncontrolled diabetes, malignancies, etc.)

Examination

A full examination for periorbital cellulitis includes the following:

- Optic nerve function
  - Visual acuity
  - Colour vision (Ishihara, D-15 charting)
  - Pupils (RAPD)
  - Visual fields (by confrontation)
  - Examination of the optic disc (for disc swelling)
- Chemosis
- Ocular motility (looking for limitation)
- Proptosis
  - Using an exophthalmometer, if possible
  - If not available, this can be grossly observed from looking down from above the patient's head to observe protrusion of the corneal apex on the affected side
- Systemic evaluation, e.g. for fever and toxicity

Investigations

- Blood cultures before starting IV antibiotics
- Swab culture of purulent material (e.g. cutaneous wounds, nasal secretions, or conjunctival discharge)
- High-resolution computed tomography (CT) (Fig. 7.12) scanning is helpful to assess the severity of the infection and look for sinus disease and complications such as subperiosteal abscess and cavernous sinus thrombosis

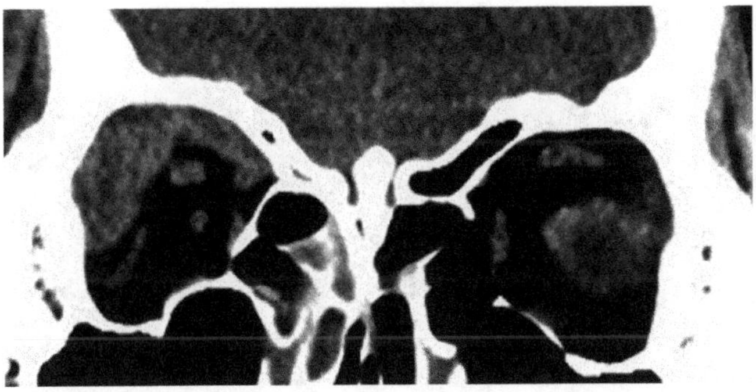

Fig. 7.12. Right superior subperiosteal abscesses in a patient with orbital cellulitis.

Management of Orbital Cellulitis

- Patients with orbital cellulitis should be admitted for treatment and close monitoring
- Systemic antibiotics should be instituted early and not be delayed while waiting for imaging studies

- Indications for surgery:
  - Progressive disease despite antibiotic use
  - Decrease in vision
  - Subperiosteal or orbital abscesses causing visual compromise, or large abscesses, especially in older patients >9 years
  - Invasive fungal disease (e.g. mucormycosis)
- Referral to an otolaryngologist if sinus disease is detected

Thyroid Eye Disease

Thyroid eye disease (TED), also known as thyroid-associated orbitopathy (TAO) or Graves orbitopathy (GO), is a tissue specific autoimmune orbito-facial inflammatory disorder. It is one of the most challenging syndromes to manage owing to its complex and poorly understood pathogenesis.

What is Thyroid Eye Disease and Why Does it Happen?

- Thyroid eye disease (TED) is an autoimmune disease. It is mainly associated with an over-active thyroid due to Graves' disease, although it does sometimes occur in people with an under-active or normally functioning thyroid.
- The eyes are particularly vulnerable to Graves' eye disease because the autoimmune attack often targets the eye muscles and connective tissue within the orbital socket. This likely occurs because the tissues within the orbit contain proteins that appear similar to the immune system as those of the thyroid gland.
- As a result of the autoimmune attack, the eye muscles and fatty tissue behind the eye become inflamed. This can cause the eyes to be pushed forward and the eyelids to be pulled upwards to some degree, giving rise to "staring" or "bulging" eyes. In the active state, the eyes feel painful and tight, and the eyes and eyelids often become swollen and red (Fig. 7.13).

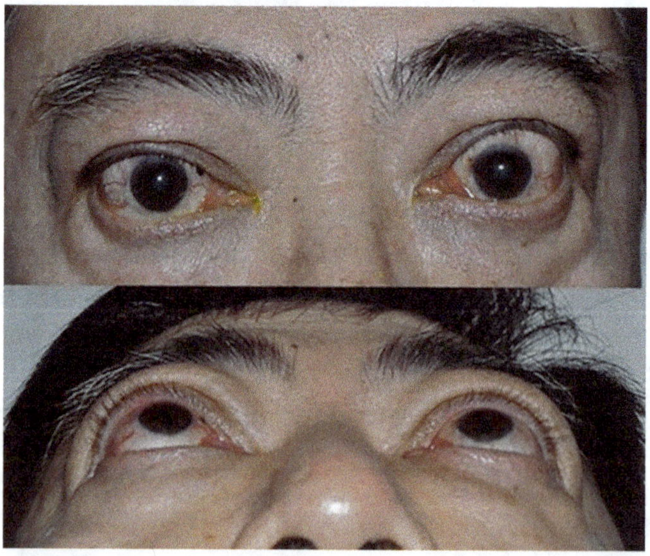

Fig. 7.13. Patient with active thyroid eye disease, characterised by swelling and redness of the upper and lower lids, conjunctival redness, swelling of the caruncle and orbital pain. This patient also has lid retraction and proptosis of both eyes.

- In the inactive or chronic phase, the extraocular muscles may become swollen and stiff, resulting in double vision. Rarely, TED can cause blindness from pressure on the optic nerve (compressive neuropathy) or exposure keratopathy.
- Apart from activity, TED is also classified based on severity (mild, moderate or severe)
    - In mild cases of TED, patients may only complain of sensitive and dry eyes, associated with increased tearing. Some mild cases may have associated lid signs, namely lid retraction and lid lag.
    - In moderate TED, the patient usually has worsening of soft tissue signs, with greater lid retraction and exophthalmos. The patient may also experience diplopia (double vision) outside 30° of the primary gaze.
    - In severe TED (Fig. 7.14), the patient may experience severe exposure keratopathy not amenable to conservative management, compressive optic neuropathy, or diplopia in primary gaze, or within 30° of primary gaze

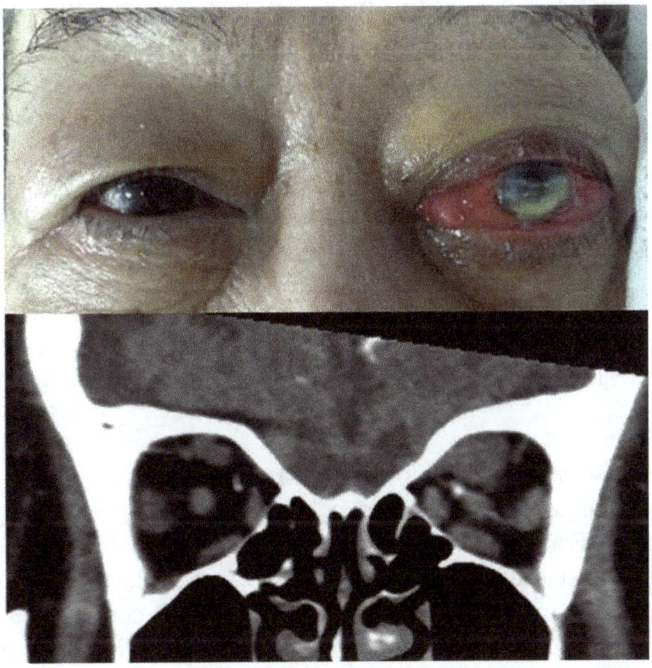

Fig. 7.14. Patient with severe active thyroid eye disease. This lady had an active flare of the disease with progressive proptosis resulting in exposure keratopathy and a resultant corneal ulcer. Corresponding computed tomography (CT) scan of the orbits shows enlargement and crowding of the extraocular muscles around the optic nerve in the left orbit.

What Can be Done for Thyroid Eye Disease?

- For all patients with TED, the following measures may prevent the disease progression:
    - Symptomatic treatment of dry eyes, including topical lubricants, sunglasses in bright sunlight or temporary punctal plugs
    - Give up smoking, both active and passive, in order to reduce the severity, duration of activity, degree of scarring, and risk of optic nerve involvement

  - Co-manage all patients with an endocrinologist, and ensure their thyroid disease is well-controlled at each visit
- Classifying the patient into active or inactive disease is very important from management point of view
  - Active disease requires immunosuppression, of which intravenous methylprednisolone is the treatment of choice
  - Steroid sparing immunosuppressant therapy, given in collaboration with the Rheumatology team, is considered for its steroid sparing effects, especially in cases of persistent inflammation
  - External beam radiotherapy, given by radiation oncologists, may also be considered in those patients who have contraindications or intolerance to various forms of corticosteroid/steroid sparing agents, but generally avoided both in the young and the elderly, as well as those with diabetes
- Surgical management for TED includes the following:
  - Orbital decompression and this may be done for several indications
    - i. Proptosis
    - ii. Persistent congestion after immunosuppression
    - iii. Compressive optic neuropathy
    - iv. As a staging procedure, in preparation for strabismus or eyelid surgery
  - Strabismus surgery: Surgery on the extraocular muscles is performed to correct the misalignment of the eyes
  - Eyelid surgery and these include surgery to correct
    - i. Upper or lower lid retraction
    - ii. Upper or lower blepharoplasty (to remove excess skin and fat)

Conclusion

Thyroid eye disease remains a major clinical and therapeutic challenge. It has been shown to have a negative impact on psychosocial functioning and quality of life, even in mild cases. Fortunately, there are continued advances in the understanding of pathogenesis and the risk-benefit profile of various medical and surgical interventions, making it a much more manageable disease compared to decades ago. The ultimate goal is early identification of TED, with effective halting and reversal of the active inflammatory process. The need for a patient-centred, multidisciplinary approach to these patients is important, to ensure careful and coordinated care.

Orbital Tumours

Orbital Tumours

- The orbit is the bony socket in which the eye is located. It consists of a floor, roof and walls on either side.
- It is possible for tumours to form in this space, between the eye and the bones
- These tumours range in seriousness, from benign lumps that can be observed to malignant tumours that require complex treatment regimens
- Tumours can be congenital or acquired

- They may involve other areas outside the orbit, including the sinuses or even the brain
- Orbital tumours may arise from any of the tissue types that are normally found in the orbit, including blood vessels, nervous tissue, bone and lymphoid tissue

Presentation

- A tumour in the orbit may initially cause fullness in the area around the eye or it may cause proptosis
- Patient may complain of double vision when the globe is moved significantly away from its normal position
- Certain tumours can also affect the nerves in the area and cause pain

Capillary Haemangioma

This is the most common tumour of the orbit in childhood. It is a vascular tumour, comprising a series of anastomosing small vascular channels. A range of presentations exists, from a small lesion away from the eye to a large lesion involving the eyelid and obstructing the visual axis of one of the eyes. The most concerning feature to the ophthalmologist is the proximity of involvement to the eye. Lesions of the eyelid can cause astigmatism (and possible resultant refractive amblyopia) from external pressure on the eye, as well as deprivational amblyopia if the visual axis is obstructed.

Presentation

- This tumour often presents in the first few weeks of life, with typical enlargement in size up to the age of 2 years with a subsequent reduction in size
- 70% of lesions tend to regress by 7 years of age

Clinical Appearance

- The tumour appears bright red when superficially located (earning the name "strawberry nevus") (Fig. 7.15)
- Deep tumours may cause a unilateral proptosis without any discolouration of the skin

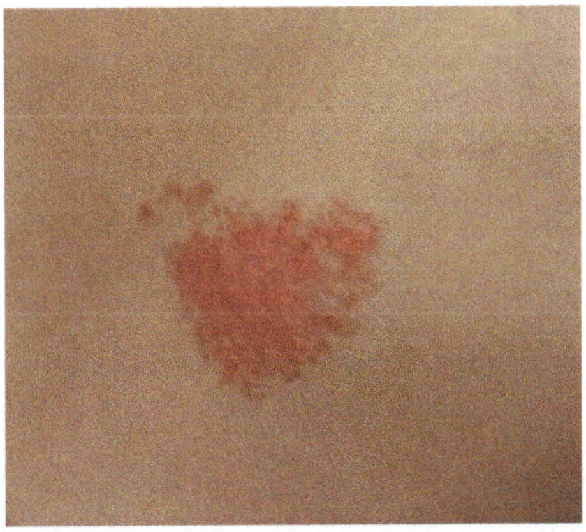

Fig. 7.15. Superficial capillary haemangioma (also known as strawberry nevus) appears as a raised, red, lumpy area of flesh anywhere on the body, including the head and neck.

Management

- Indications for treatment
  - Amblyopia due to astigmatism or obstruction of the visual axis
  - Optic nerve compression
  - Exposure keratopathy
- Treatment modalities
  - Beta-blockers
    i. Topical
    ii. Systemic: Propranolol is an effective medication and the mainstay of treatment for capillary haemangiomas
  - Steroids
    i. Local injection (only for superficial lesions)
    ii. Systemic
  - Surgical resection
    i. This is a last resort option as it is often difficult to remove the tumour while preserving normal anatomy
  - Laser treatments
    – can sometimes be used on superficial haemangiomas to prevent growth, diminish their size, or lighten their colour

Cavernous Haemangioma

Cavernous haemangioma is the old term for what is now classified as a venous malformation. It is a tumour that consists of a collection of vascular channels and is the most common benign orbital tumour in adults. It affects females more than males. Mean age of presentation is in the 4th to 5th decade of life. It often results in a tumour within the muscle cone that causes a unilateral axial proptosis. However, some cases are discovered incidentally on radiographic imaging studies.

History

- Duration of proptosis
- Diplopia
- Blurring of vision

Examination

- Visual acuity, intraocular pressure
- Ocular motility
- Exophthalmometry
- Complete ocular examination, looking for choroidal folds due to compression

Investigations

- CT scan of the orbits (Fig. 7.16) shows a well-circumscribed round lesion with contrast enhancement

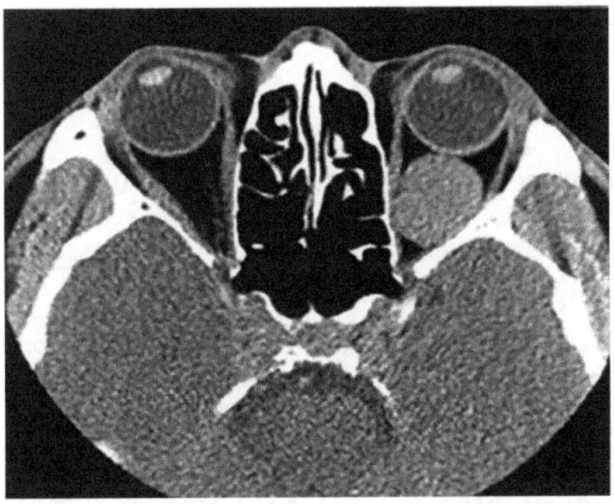

Fig. 7.16. CT showing a well-circumscribed intraconal mass in the left orbit. The mass was surgically excised and proven to be cavernous haemangioma.

Treatment Options

- Observation: for asymptomatic tumours not causing proptosis or disfigurement
- Surgical resection: for tumours causing proptosis, diplopia, disfigurement or optic nerve compression

Optic Nerve Glioma

Optic nerve glioma is a slow-growing tumour of neural tissue origin that typically affects young children. 30% of affected children have neurofibromatosis Type 1. The typical age of presentation is during the first decade of life.

Clinical Presentation

- Slow onset of visual loss
- Proptosis
- Fundoscopy shows optic disc swelling, then pallor
- Chiasmal and intracranial spread is possible

Investigations

- CT scanning shows a fusiform enlargement of the optic nerve
- MRI may be useful to evaluate any suspected intracranial involvement

Management

- Small tumours with minimal visual compromise can be observed
- Surgical excision is indicated if there is poor visual or very significant proptosis
- Radiotherapy may be considered for tumours with intracranial involvement, which are not suitable for resection

Optic Nerve Sheath Meningioma

Optic nerve sheath meningiomas (ONSM) arise from the meningoepithelial tissues around the optic nerve. They are typically slow-growing tumours, affecting middle-aged women most commonly.

Clinical Features

- Gradual impairment of vision
- Gradual proptosis
- May present with optociliary shunts and optic nerve atrophy

Investigations

- CT shows thickening and calcification of the optic nerve
- MRI studies with gadolinium contrast, as well as fat suppression, are ideal for evaluating ONSM. MRI will again demonstrate diffuse, tubular thickening of the optic nerve sheath encasing the optic nerve, often producing a characteristic "tram track" sign on axial cuts or a "doughnut" sign on coronal cuts. The tumour enhances with contrast infusion. MRI is particularly useful for delineating the extent of the tumour and for evaluating for intracranial extension.

Management

- Small tumours with minimal visual compromise can be observed
- Surgical excision is indicated if there is poor visual or very significant proptosis
- Radiotherapy may be considered for tumours with intracranial involvement, which are not suitable for resection

Orbital Metastases

Orbital metastases are not a common cause of proptosis and are less common as compared to choroidal metastases. However, the ophthalmologist may be the first doctor to detect the presence of a malignancy. The most common metastases in adults are from the breast, bronchus, prostate, skin, gastrointestinal tract and kidney.

Rhabdomyosarcoma

Rhabdomyosarcoma is the commonest primary orbital malignant tumour in children. It comprises poorly differentiated mesenchymal cells, which possess the potential to differentiate into striated muscle. It is an aggressive tumour that requires prompt recognition as it may masquerade as orbital cellulitis.

Clinical Features

- Typical presentation is during the first decade of life
- Rapid onset of unilateral proptosis that is progressive
- Swelling and redness of overlying skin
- Ptosis and strabismus may be present
- Skin is not warm to the touch, unlike orbital cellulitis
- May masquerade as an orbital inflammation or orbital cellulitis

Imaging Findings

- CT and MRI scanning usually shows an ill-defined mass
- There are often areas of bony destruction

Management

- An urgent workup is required for these patients

- Biopsy of the tissue is required for histological diagnosis
- Surgical debulking may improve staging and tumour response to treatment
- Radiotherapy and chemotherapy are options for tumours not amenable to surgery
- Exenteration is reserved for recurrent disease and carries significant morbidity

General Principles of Management for Orbital Tumours

Often, a multi-disciplinary team is required, including adult or paediatric oncologists, radiation oncologists, social workers, prosthetics specialists, geneticists and the ophthalmologist.

- Imaging with CT or MRI scan of the orbits and/or brain is required
  - CT is better than MRI for bone definition
  - MRI is better than CT for soft tissue definition
- Tissue diagnosis via biopsy or other tissue sampling method may be required
- This will be sent to a specialised laboratory to be analysed by a pathologist trained in ocular oncology
- Based on the tissue diagnosis and further ancillary tests, including tissue genetic or biochemical analysis, the ideal mode of therapy is decided after consideration of multiple factors, including:
  - The degree of systemic involvement
  - The aggressiveness of the tumour
  - The health of the patient
  - The wishes of the patient and family
  - The likely success rates of treatment

Orbital Trauma

Head and facial injuries frequently involve the periocular area and can cause significant morbidity.

Initial Assessment

- When evaluating a patient who has sustained any type of trauma, life-threatening injuries should first be addressed or ruled out before assessing for ocular and adnexal trauma
- In the setting of trauma, the physician should not forget the basics of life support (airway, breathing, circulation) and systemic trauma assessments

Orbital Fractures

Orbital wall fractures are commonly encountered in facial trauma. In more than 40% of all facial fractures, parts of the orbital rim and/or the internal orbit are injured, showing various fracture patterns.

- The very anatomy of the orbit makes it prone to fractures, and it is therefore involved in a majority of midfacial fractures. However, just as the bony orbit protects the globe normally, the bony orbit gives way at its weak points to protect the globe when traumatised. Hence, fractures are, in fact, a protective mechanism to the eye in times of trauma.

Typical Signs Pointing towards Orbital Fracture

- History of blunt trauma to face
- Periocular ecchymosis and oedema
- Enophthalmos (later sequelae)
- Infraorbital hypoaesthesia
- Ocular motility limitation; diplopia
- Hypoglobus
  - Severe orbital floor disruption
  - Roof fracture with superior orbital haematoma

Orbital Blow-out Fracture

- The orbital floor medial to the infraorbital groove and the lamina papyracea overlying the ethmoidal sinuses are relatively thin and may buckle and fracture when blunt force impacts the orbital soft tissue and bone margins, causing a sudden rise in hydraulic pressure and buckling of the thinner bone. This gives rise to orbital floor and medial wall blow-out fractures, respectively (Figs. 7.17 and 7.18).
- Orbital tissue herniating into the sinus through the resulting defect in the orbital floor may become entrapped, causing diplopia, and if the displacement of the bony fragment is large enough, enophthalmos may develop

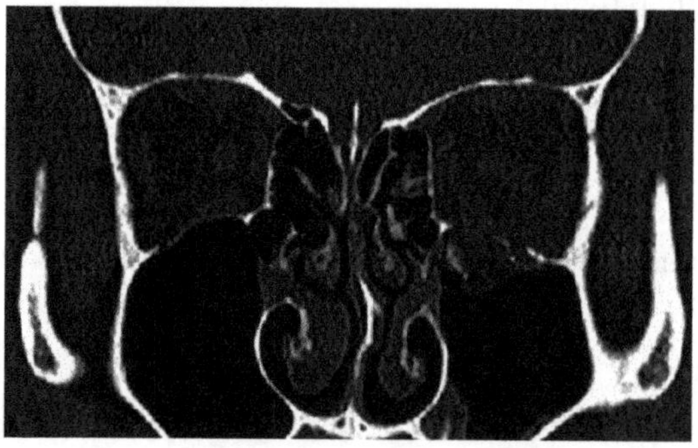

Fig. 7.17. Left orbital floor blow-out fracture, medial to infraorbital groove with mild herniation of orbital contents into the maxillary sinus. The inferior rectus is not entrapped.

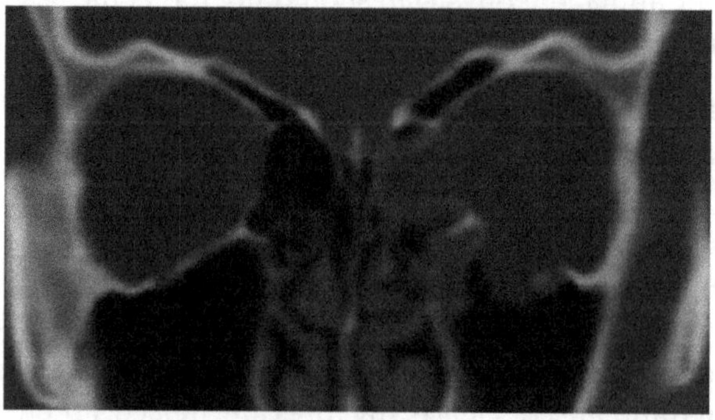

Fig. 7.18. Large blow-out fractures of the left orbital floor and medial wall, with herniation of the medial and inferior recti into the adjacent sinuses, along with the orbital contents.

- Two theories have been proposed — the "buckling" theory and "hydraulic" theory
  - In the former, blow-out fractures are believed to occur through force transmission from the more rigid infraorbital rim to the relatively weak orbital floor. Blunt trauma to the face causes the pressure wave to travel posteriorly, acutely compressing the bones of the orbit in the anterior-posterior direction. This increase in bony pressure causes the weakest point in the orbit to "buckle" and crack, with the bone fragment pushed inferiorly.
  - In the "hydraulic" theory, the eyeball, when struck directly by an object such as a fist or a baseball, is thrust posteriorly, transiently raising the pressure within the orbit. As the intraorbital pressure increases dramatically and suddenly, the floor of the orbit "blows out" inferiorly at the point of the greatest weakness. Hence, the hydraulic pressure from the globe is transmitted to the bony orbit, resulting in fracture of the thin medial orbital floor.

Trapdoor Fracture

- A "trapdoor" orbital fracture is an isolated orbital floor fracture, which occurs when a bony fragment, often hinged medially, is transiently displaced inferiorly, allowing herniation of orbital contents into the maxillary sinus, which are then entrapped as the bony fragment returns toward its initial position (Fig. 7.18)
- It is postulated that before puberty, a large portion of the orbital floor consists of immature bone and overlies a small maxillary sinus. Hence, the bony floor in children and adolescents is relatively pliable — even minimal force can result in a small fracture segment swinging down and snapping back, thereby incarcerating orbital tissue.
- Despite severe limitation of ocular motility, orbital oedema or sign of soft tissue injury is relatively minimal. Hence, it has also been termed "the white-eyed blow-out fracture" (Fig. 7.19). Such fractures are often associated with nausea and vomiting. An oculocardiac reflex can also occur, manifesting in bradycardia, especially on eliciting eye movements.

Take Home Messages

- Orbital cellulitis can be life-threatening, and treatment must be initiated promptly.
- Three questions to ask when assessing a patient with thyroid eye disease:
  - Is this thyroid eye disease?
  - Is it mild, moderate or severe?
  - Is it active or quiescent?
- Orbital tumours can arise from many structures, including blood vessels, nervous tissue, bone and lymphoid tissue.
- Principles of management of orbital tumours include assessing the extent of involvement, establishing a tissue diagnosis and starting specific treatment.
- The most common sites of orbital fractures are the medial part of the orbital floor and medial wall.
- Trapdoor fracture should be suspected in any child with blunt trauma.

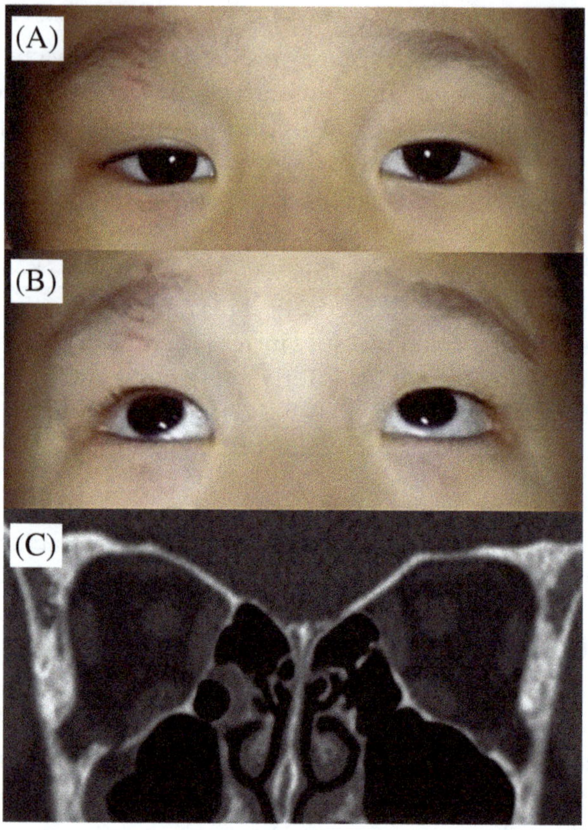

Fig. 7.19. (A) Five-year-old boy who fell and hit his right eye. On examination, the eye is white without much periorbital oedema and ecchymosis. (B) There is limitation of the right eye on upgaze, raising the clinical suspicion of a trapdoor fracture. (C) On imaging, the fracture may be easily missed as the bony fragment has "snapped back" into position, incarcerating some orbital soft tissue.

7.3 Lacrimal Disorders

Learning Objective

Be aware of symptoms and signs of nasolacrimal duct obstruction in adults and children.

Acquired Nasolacrimal Duct Obstruction

Tears play a critical role in providing nutrients and protection to the cornea, in creating a smooth surface for clarity and in conveying emotions. There are three phases in normal tear flow: 1) production — lacrimal secretion, release of mucin from goblet cells and lipid from Meibomian glands; 2) distribution through the eyelid blinking and the lacrimal pump; and 3) tear elimination through excretion and evaporation. Disorders in the lacrimal system may arise in any one of these three phases and require specific tests for confirmation and directed management dependent on the structures affected.

Obstruction of the drainage system can be congenital or acquired and may result in persistent epiphora and mucopurulent discharge.

What is the Anatomy of the Lacrimal Drainage System? (Fig. 7.20)

- The lacrimal system consists of:
  - **Puncta:** These are small openings of 0.2–0.3 mm diameter in the medial aspect of the upper and lower lid margin. Each punctum lies on the lacrimal papilla. The inferior punctum lies in apposition to the tear meniscus.
  - **Canaliculi:** Vertical canaliculi is 2 mm and horizontal canaliculi is 8 mm in length. They are 1 to 1.5 mm in diameter. Both the upper and lower canaliculi join to form the common canaliculus.
  - **Lacrimal Sac:** The common canaliculus then leads to the lacrimal sac. The lacrimal sac lies in the lacrimal sac fossa, which is bounded by the anterior and posterior lacrimal crests. The floor of the fossa comprises the maxillary bone anteriorly and the lacrimal bone posteriorly.
  - **Nasolacrimal duct:** The nasolacrimal duct lies within a bony canal, which is 12 mm long, 3–5 mm wide. It passes down posteriorly at a 15–30° angle to open in the inferior meatus within the nasal cavity.

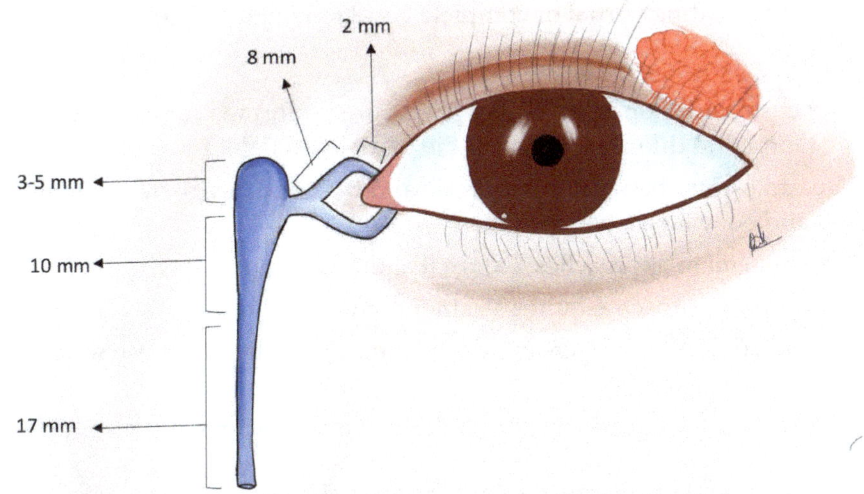

Fig. 7.20. Normal lacrimal drainage pathway.

Clinical Features

- Epiphora
- Ocular discharge
- Sometimes, lacrimal sac inflammation (dacryocystitis)

What is the Management of Nasolacrimal Duct Obstruction?

- In acute or chronic dacryocystitis (Fig. 7.21)
  - Topical and systemic antibiotics
  - Some surgeons believe in percutaneous drainage of lacrimal sac abscess
  - Dacryocystorhinostomy (DCR) is usually performed subsequently

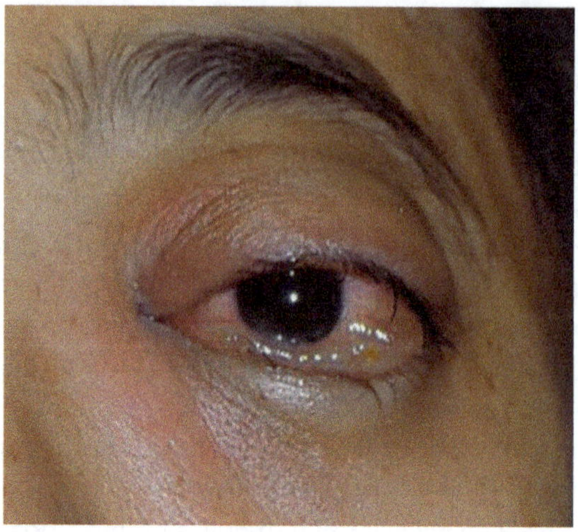

Fig. 7.21. Left acute dacryocystitis with erythema and swelling over the lacrimal sac region, chemosis, tearing and ocular discharge.

- More recently, endoscopic lacrimal ductal recanalisation (ELDR) has been gaining popularity in treating partial or complete nasolacrimal duct obstructions

What is a Dacryocystorhinostomy?

- A dacryocystorhinostomy (DCR) is a procedure performed for the treatment of tearing (epiphora) due to blockage of the nasolacrimal duct
- It creates an ostium between the tear sac and the nasal cavity by removing the mucosa and bone layers between them
- There are two main approaches: External and Endoscopic
  - The external approach requires a skin incision
  - The endoscopic approach creates the ostium from within the nose without the need for a skin incision
  - Both have similar success rates, with their own advantages and disadvantages

Congenital Nasolacrimal Duct Obstruction

Congenital nasolacrimal duct obstruction (NLDO) is a common condition that may affect up to 50% of newborns. It is caused by a membranous blockage of the valve of Hasner at the nasal end of the nasolacrimal duct. Most of these obstructions resolve within the first 4 to 6 weeks of life. By the first year of life, approximately 90% of these will resolve.

Clinical Features

- Tearing in an infant
- Matting of the eyelashes
- Usually no conjunctival injection
- A dacryocystocoele may be present (a soft cystic lump located at the lower medial part of the eyelid), which is a non-infective collection of mucus in the lacrimal sac

Management

- Most cases are treated conservatively with Crigler's massage (downward pressure movements over the external skin region over the lacrimal sac). This is typically performed 10 times per day.
- If a dacryocystocoele is present, topical antibiotics can be used, along with Crigler's massage, or probing
- When the NLDO fails to resolve with conservative measures, surgical intervention may be required
- Probing of the nasolacrimal duct to perforate the membrane of the Valve of Hasner, re-establishing the flow of tears. It is usually not done until the age of 6–12 months because spontaneous canalisation may occur.
- Less commonly, other surgical procedures are required for persistent NLDO after probing. The probing can be repeated and also combined with other procedures, such as infracture of the nasal turbinates, intubation of the nasolacrimal duct, balloon dacryoplasty and even dacryocystorhinostomy for refractory cases of tearing due to NLDO.

Take Home Messages

- Acquired NLDO is surgically treated by endoscopic or external DCR.
- Congenital NLDO is a common condition that often spontaneously resolves with time.
- Conservative treatments, such as massage and topical therapy, are the mainstay of treatment.
- Surgical treatment is only indicated in a minority of cases, for refractory disease.

7.4 Facial Nerve Palsy

Patients with facial nerve palsy commonly require review by ophthalmologists. This is because a significant part of their acquired deficit is the inability to blink or close their eye well, which may lead to visual complications that can be severe.

In this chapter, we will go through the anatomy of the facial nerve, talk about the different aetiologies that can result in a facial nerve palsy, and touch on the examination and management of such patients.

Revisit of Facial Nerve Anatomy

(Refer to Chapter 1: Basic Anatomy of the Eye, Adnexa and Visual Pathways)

The anatomy of the facial nerve is complex, owing to the many branches it has, which, in turn, transmit a combination of sensory, motor and parasympathetic fibres. Anatomically, the course of the facial nerve can be divided into 2 parts — an intracranial portion, as well as extracranial.

Within the skull, the facial nerve nucleus arises from the pons, ventrolateral to the CN VI nucleus and medial to the spinal nucleus of CN V. It starts its course as 2 main roots — a large motor root and a smaller sensory root. Both roots run through the internal acoustic meatus (IAM), which is an opening within the petrous part of the temporal bone. The roots then leave the IAM and traverse the facial canal to finally exit the cranium via the stylomastoid foramen. Within the facial canal, the 2 roots fuse and then give rise to different facial nerve branches, including the greater petrosal nerve (containing parasympathetic fibres to the lacrimal gland), the nerve to the stapedius, and the chorda tympani.

After exiting the cranium, the posterior auricular nerve branches off from the facial nerve, becoming the first extracranial branch of CN VII. The facial nerve then continues anteriorly and inferiorly into the parotid gland, and splits into 5 terminal branches, which provide motor innervation for the various facial muscles. They are:

- Temporal branch
- Zygomatic branch
- Buccal branch
- Marginal mandibular branch
- Cervical branch

Function

Branches of the facial nerve serve 2 main functions:

- Motor innervation: muscles of facial expression, the superficial platysma muscles and the stapedius ear muscles
- Secretory and sensory innervation: greater superficial petrosal nerve innervates the lacrimal gland to mediate tearing; chorda tympani innervates the tongue to mediate taste

Causes of Facial Nerve Palsy

There are various aetiologies for facial nerve palsy, but they can be best remembered by dividing the causes into supranuclear, nuclear and infranuclear causes. Another way of classifying the different causes would be to group them accordingly via the various aetiologies, as illustrated in Table 7.2.

Supranuclear causes — These refer to lesions before the facial nuclei in the pons, and will result in contralateral paralysis of voluntary facial movement, with the facial muscles of the lower face affected while the function of the upper face remains preserved.

Nuclear causes — these are lesions at the brainstem where the facial nerve nucleus arises from. This will result in an ipsilateral facial weakness involving both the upper and lower face. Evidence of other neurological signs should also be assessed; for example, a concomitant CN VI palsy may point towards a pontine lesion.

Infranuclear causes — this also results in ipsilateral facial weakness involving both The upper and lower face. If other cranial nerve palsies are present, for example, CN V or VIII palsy, it may indicate a lesion at the cerebellopontine angle.

Table 7.2. Classification of Causes of Facial Nerve Palsy by Location

Location	Example
Supranuclear	Cerebral Palsy
Nuclear	Brainstem/pontine infarct Moebius syndrome
Infranuclear	Cerebellopontine angle tumour (e.g. vestibular schwannoma) Skull-base tumours (e.g. nasopharyngeal carcinoma) Temporal bone fractures Parotid tumours Bell's palsy

Remember that in **upper motor neuron lesions** (supranuclear), the upper facial muscles still function normally (i.e. the patient is able to raise both eyebrows) due to the bilateral innervation of the upper facial muscles, while the **contralateral** lower facial muscles will be affected. In **lower motor neuron lesions** (nuclear and infranuclear), both upper and lower facial muscles on the **ipsilateral** side will be affected.

Table 7.3. Classification of Causes of Facial Nerve Palsy by Aetiology

Aetiology	Example
Idiopathic	Bell's palsy
Congenital	Moebius syndrome
Neoplasm	Pontine glioma Cerebellopontine angle tumour Parotid gland tumour
Infection	*Herpes zoster* (Ramsay-Hunt) Otitis media Lyme disease
Demyelination	Multiple sclerosis (affecting pons)
Vascular causes	Pontine infarct or haemorrhage
Trauma	Base of skull/Temporal bone fracture

Bell's palsy

- 70% of patients have complete recovery within 6 weeks, while 85% will fully recover eventually
- Poor prognostic signs include complete facial paralysis at presentation and advanced age
- Aberrant regeneration is more common in cases of incomplete recovery

Clinical Examination

Look for the following when examining a patient with facial nerve palsy:

- Lagophthalmos (incomplete closure of the eyelids) (Fig. 7.22)
- Paralytic ectropion (outward turning of the eyelid margin)
- Corneal surface abnormalities

- Other cranial nerve abnormalities, including CN V (corneal sensation), CN VI (abduction deficit), and CN VIII (hearing)
- Signs and symptoms of aberrant regeneration, e.g. reverse jaw-winking (blinking leading to mouth twitching) and gustatory epiphora (tearing during mealtimes)

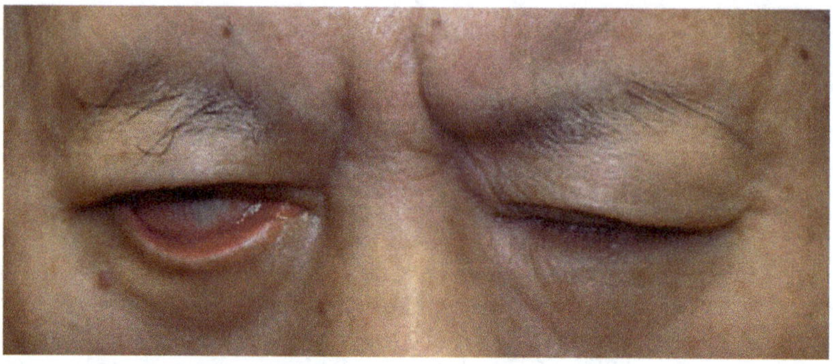

Fig. 7.22. A patient with right facial nerve palsy with significant lagophthalmos on forced eye closure and weakness of the orbicularis, resulting in a paralytic ectropion of the right lower eyelid.

Grading

Grading systems have been developed to allow clinicians to objectively grade the severity of the patient's signs and symptoms, allow proper communication between reviewing physicians, and monitor patients for improvement or deterioration. The grading system familiar to most is the House-Brackmann scale. However, a more practical grading system for the ophthalmologist is the CADS grading scale, which is ophthalmic specific. It encompasses both objective and subjective measures for grading and is based on these 4 areas of examination in the periorbital region:

- Corneal involvement
- Resting or static asymmetry
- Dynamic function
- Synkinesis

Table 7.4. House-Brackmann Scale

Grade	Characteristics
1 – normal	Normal facial function
2 – mild dysfunction	Normal symmetry and tone at rest Slight weakness noticeable on close inspection
3 – moderate dysfunction	Obvious weakness and asymmetry, but not disfiguring Complete eye closure with effort
4 – moderately severe dysfunction	Disfiguring asymmetry Incomplete eye closure
5 – severe dysfunction	Barely perceptible motion Asymmetry at rest
6 – complete paralysis	No movement seen

Table 7.5. CADS Grading Scale

<table>
<tr><th colspan="2">Cornea</th><th colspan="2">Static asymmetry</th><th colspan="2">Dynamic Function</th><th colspan="2">Synkinesis</th></tr>
<tr><td>No staining</td><td>0</td><td>▸ No brow ptosis
▸ No ectropion
▸ No upper or lower eyelid retraction</td><td>0</td><td>▸ No blink lagophthalmos</td><td>0</td><td>Absent</td><td>0</td></tr>
<tr><td>PEE <5</td><td>1</td><td>▸ Mild brow ptosis
▸ Medial ectropion
▸ Upper eyelid at limbus
▸ Mild lower eyelid retraction ≤2 mm inferior scleral show
▸ LMBD >5 mm shorter than contralateral slde</td><td>1</td><td>▸ Lagophthalmos on blink <5 mm
▸ Brow elevation reduced but present</td><td>1</td><td>▸ Mild eye closure when smiling/ speaking/ eating
▸ Gustatory epiphora: not bothersome</td><td>1</td></tr>
<tr><td>PEE ≤½ cornea</td><td>2</td><td rowspan="3">▸ Severe brow ptosis
▸ Significant ectropion
▸ Superior scleral show
▸ >2 mm inferior scleral show</td><td rowspan="3">2</td><td>▸ Lagophthalmos on blink ≥5 mm
▸ Lagophthalmos on gentle closure ≤5 mm
▸ Brow elevation: none or twitch</td><td>2</td><td rowspan="3">2 ▸ Significant eye closure when smiling/ speaking/ eating
▸ Gustatory epiphora: bothersome</td><td rowspan="3">2</td></tr>
<tr><td>PEE >½ cornea or epithelial defect</td><td>3</td><td rowspan="2">▸ Lagophthalmos on gentle closure >5 mm
▸ Lagophthalmos on forced closure >2 mm</td><td rowspan="2">3</td></tr>
<tr><td>▸ Absent corneal sensation
▸ Absent/ reduced Bell's phenomenon
▸ Schirmer's ≤5 mm*
▸ Affected eye is the only eye</td><td>3a</td></tr>
</table>

**Schirmer's test with anaesthetic, and if the lower eyelid is apposed to the globe. LMBD, lid margin-to-brow distance; PEE, punctate epithelial erosion.*

Management

Management of a patient with facial nerve palsy depends on the severity of the symptoms and prognosis for recovery. The treatments are aimed at protecting the cornea and aiding with eyelid closure. They can be divided into conservative as well as surgical options.

Conservative

- Lubricants: intensive preservative-free eyedrops in the day and eye ointment at night

- Eyelid-taping at night
- Temporary lid weights
- Botox to induce an upper eyelid ptosis
- Oral prednisolone for cases of Bell's palsy presenting acutely

Surgical

- Tarsorrhaphy, either temporary or permanent, to reduce palpebral aperture and obviate the risk of exposure keratopathy
- Implanted gold weight to the upper eyelid
- Ectropion correction surgery (if paralytic ectropion does not improve)
- Brow lift or mid-face lift

Newer surgical approaches to facial nerve palsies that have poor recovery include neurotisation procedures (nerve-transfers and cross-facial nerve grafts) and muscle transpositions. More emphasis is now also placed on rehabilitation and neuromuscular retraining, as increasing evidence shows that it can help in the recovery of patients with facial nerve palsy.

References

1. Bergin DJ. (1992) Lumps and bumps of the eyelids and their management. *J Dermatol Surg Oncol* **18(12)**:1042–1048.
2. Ellis E 3rd. (2012) Orbital trauma. *Oral Maxillofac Surg Clin North Am* **24(4)**: 629–648.
3. Lim NC, Sundar G, Amrith S, *et al.* (2015) Thyroid eye disease: a Southeast Asian experience. *Br J Ophthalmol* **99(4)**:512–518.
4. Sliverman N and Shinder R. (2017) What's new in eyelid tumors. *Asia-Pac J Ophthalmol* **6**:123–152.
5. Tailor TD, Gupta D, Dally RW, *et al.* (2013) Orbital neoplasms in adults: Clinical, radiologic and pathologic review. *Radiographics* **33(6)**:1739–1758.

Chapter 8

PAEDIATRIC OPHTHALMOLOGY AND STRABISMUS

Janice Lam Sing Harn, Cheryl Ngo Shufen

8.1 Assessment of Vision in Children

Learning Objectives

- Understand visual milestones — from infancy to childhood.
- How to assess vision in an infant or child.
- How to recognise signs that may be a cause for concern.

Normal Visual Development in Children

Changes in Visual Acuity with Age

Born with an immature visual system, visual development begins within the first few weeks of life and continues to develop till the age of 8. Myelination of the optic nerves and maturation of the visual cortex occurs over the first 2 years of life. The fovea, the most visually sensitive part of the retina, reaches maturity at approximately 4 years of age.

Birth to 4 Months of Age

A *normal newborn* is usually born with poor vision due to immature visual centres in the brain and gradually develops the ability to focus on an object in front of him/her in the first few weeks of life. Development of good vision is dependent on well-focused images on the retina.

- At 1 month of age, a baby should be able to focus briefly on objects up to 1 metre away
- By 2 months of age, infants should be able to track and follow moving objects, as their visual coordination and depth perception improves. However, it is not uncommon to notice a child's eyes deviating inwards or outwards up to 8 weeks of life, as their movements are still not well coordinated.
- By 3–4 months of age, distance vision continues to develop, and an infant should be able to reach for objects around them and smile when they recognise a familiar face, e.g. a parent across the room

Colour vision usually starts developing at birth, and at one month of age, an infant can recognise intense colours and contrasting patterns (Fig. 8.1). By 4 months of age, they can differentiate and respond to the full range of shades and colours.

Fig. 8.1. Teller acuity cards — a type of forced preferential looking test for visual acuity.

5–12 Months of Age

- During these months, the control of ocular movements and eye-body coordination skills continues to improve
- Beyond 9 months of age, infants can start to judge distances fairly well and throw objects with precision

1–2 Years of Age

During this period, a child's hand-eye coordination and depth perception should be well developed.

The visual system in children continues to be flexible throughout the first 8 years of life, thus treatment of amblyopia is best attempted before the age of 8. Any obstruction to focusing a clear image on the retina may lead to decreased vision and the development of amblyopia.

How to Assess Visual Acuity in a Young Infant

Children have low attention spans, hence it is important to use objects that are attractive, high contrast, or colourful to get their attention.

It is difficult to assess vision in an infant, but an estimation of gross visual function can be made. This is achieved by assessing an infant's ability to:

- **Fixate** on a visual object, **follow** it and maintain **steady** fixation. We usually record this as normal if an infant's gaze is **central, steady** and **maintained**.
- Blink/shy away from ***bright light***
- By 3–4 months, look for an infant's ability to **fixate on familiar faces**
- The presence of ***nystagmus*** during this time usually indicates poorer vision
- If there is objection to occlusion in either eye, it can be inferred that vision is fairly equal in both eyes (Fig. 8.2). However, if the baby objects only when one eye is covered, a difference in vision between both eyes — with the better vision in the eye that objects to occlusion — must be suspected.
- A drum that induces physiological optokinetic response (***OKN drum***, Fig. 8.3) can be used to assess normal vision. A horizontal OKN response is present by 3 months of age and a vertical OKN response should be expected by approximately 6 months of age.

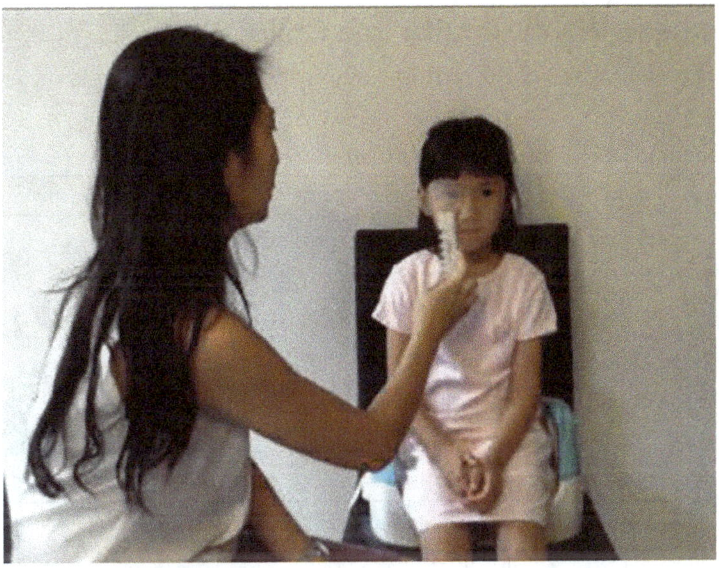

Fig. 8.2. Using an occluder to assess monocular vision in either eye.

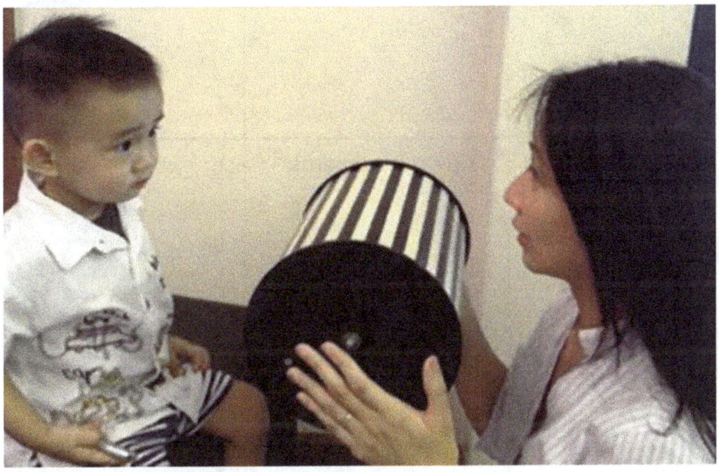

Fig. 8.3. Vertical optokinetic nystagmus testing using an OKN drum. If a vertical nystagmus can be elicited, vision is 6/120 or better.

Table 8.1. Normal Visual Development in Children

Normal Visual Development in Children — Expected Range of Visual Acuities According to Age	Causes for Concern, if Present
• Birth → 6/300 • 1 month → 6/200–6/90 • 3 months 6/90–6/60 • 6 months → FPL 6/60–6/36 • 9 months → FPL 6/36–6/24 • 1 year → FPL 6/12 • 2 years → FPL 6/12–6/9 • 3 years → FPL 6/9–6/6 • 4 years → FPL 6/6	• Wandering eyes/roving gaze • Presence of nystagmus • Lack of response to familiar faces, e.g. parents • Staring straight at bright lights • Oculodigital reflex

How to Assess Visual Acuity in a Child

Assessment of vision in a child requires age-appropriate methods of testing.

Table 8.2. Methods of Vision Testing for Children of Different Ages

Type of Test	Age Tested	Name of Test	Example
Forced preferential looking (FPL) **Not suitable for children under the age of 6 months, uncooperative, has motor abnormalities, e.g. nystagmus*	3 to 9 months	• Teller cards (grating) ▪ Increasing	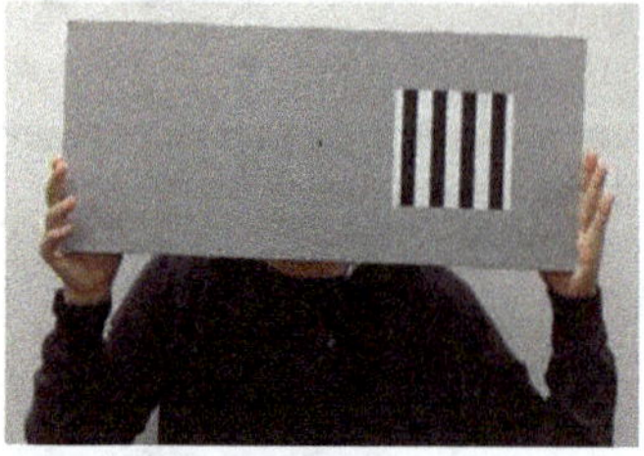 **Fig. 8.4**
	9 months to 2 years	• Cardiff cards (picture)	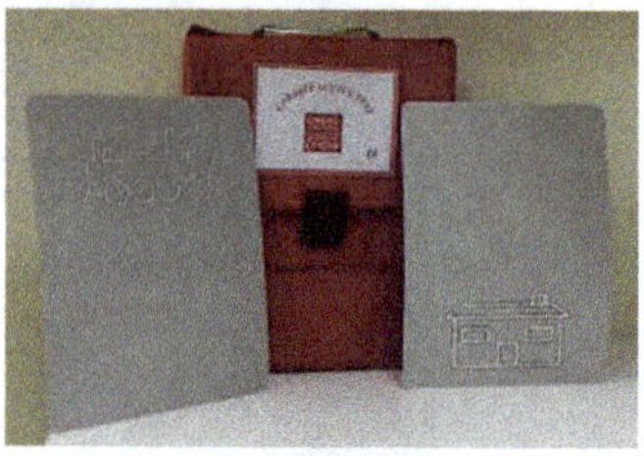 **Fig. 8.5**
Matching tests	2 to 4 years	• Kay picture cards	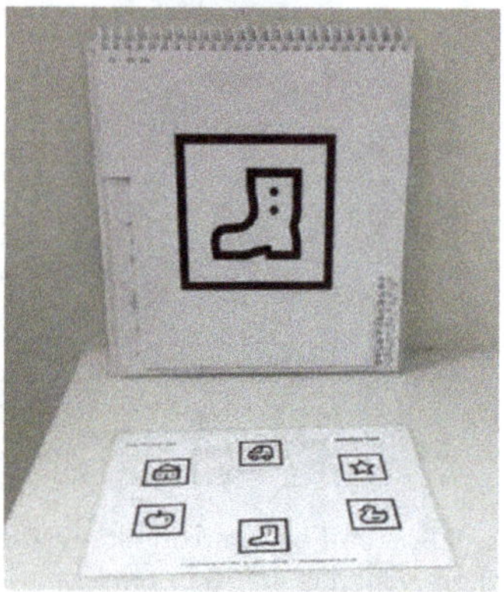 **Fig. 8.6**
	3 to 4 years	• Sheridan Gardiner (tests letters HOTUVXA)	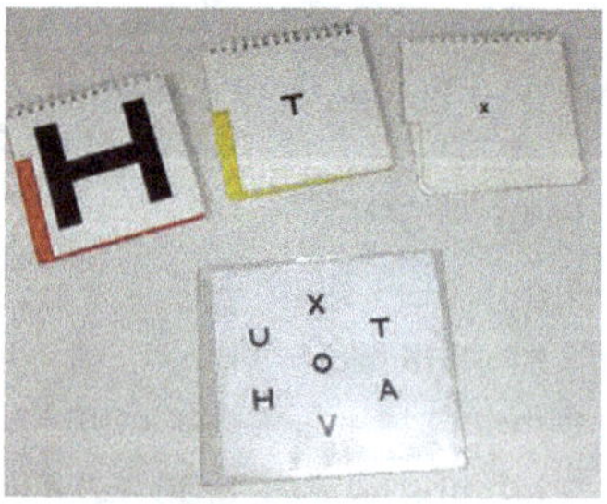 **Fig. 8.7**

Type of Test	Age Tested	Name of Test	Example
Resolving ability of the eye	When a child is able to recognise letters/ numbers	• Snellen chart ▪ Using letters, numbers or tumbling E	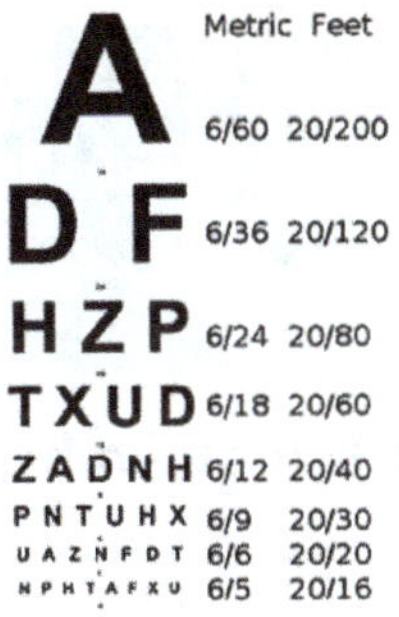 **Fig. 8.8**
		• Bailey Lovie (ETDRS, LogMAR)	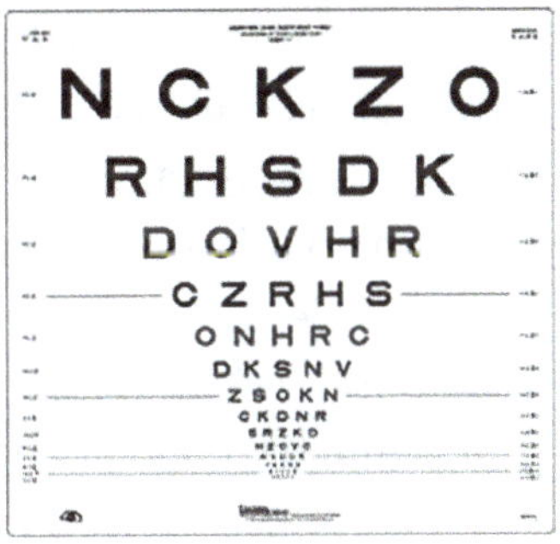 **Fig. 8.9**

Take Home Messages

- Normal newborns have poor vision and visual development occurs in the first few weeks of life.
- Assessment of vision in INFANTS
  - Fix + Follow, Gaze central, steady, maintained.
  - Light → should blink/shy away from bright light.
  - Faces → fixates on faces.
  - Objection to Occlusion.
  - Older infant → forced preferential looking.
- Assessment of vision in CHILDREN
  - Forced Preferential Looking.
  - Matching tests.
  - Resolving ability of the eye → Snellen's chart, Bailey-Lovie chart.

8.2 Amblyopia

Learning Objectives
- Understand what amblyopia is.
- Note the causes of amblyopia.
- Understand the management of amblyopia.

Definition of Amblyopia "Lazy Eye"

- Decreased vision in one or both eyes due to abnormal development of vision in infancy or childhood
- Visual acuity in either eye worse than 6/12 or if there is more than 2-line difference in visual acuity between the 2 eyes
- There may not be an obvious problem of the eye
- Vision loss occurs because nerve pathways between the brain and the eye are not properly stimulated
- The brain "learns" to see only blurry images with the amblyopic eye even when glasses are used
- As a result, the brain favours one eye more, usually due to poorer vision in the other eye

Causes of Amblyopia

- Strabismus or squint
- Vision deprivation, e.g.
  - Ptosis obscuring the visual axis
    i. Congenital ptosis
    ii. Capillary haemangioma
  - Congenital cataract
- Refractive error
  - Large refractive error or unequal amount of refractive error between two eyes
    i. Large refractive error in both eyes → isoametropic amblyopia
    ii. Unequal amount of refractive error between two eyes → anisometropic amblyopia
    iii. High astigmatism causing amblyopia → meridional amblyopia

The end result of all forms of amblyopia is reduced vision in the affected eye(s)

Congenital Ptosis

- A drooping eyelid that is present at birth (Fig. 8.10)

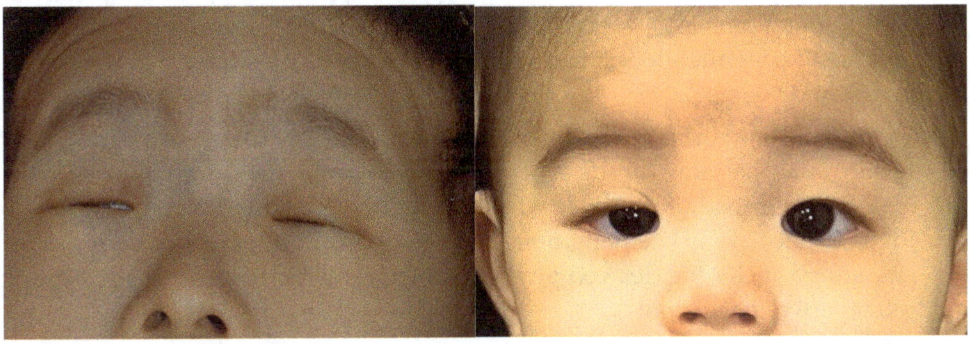

Fig. 8.10. Congenital ptosis. **Left**: Child with bilateral ptosis and chin up head position. **Right**: Child with right-sided partial ptosis that is not obscuring the visual axis. There is loss of the right upper eyelid crease with overaction of the frontalis muscle, as shown by the more pronounced forehead creases on the right.

- The drooping eyelid can cover part or all of the pupil and interfere with vision, resulting in amblyopia
- Ptosis may also cause astigmatism, resulting in amblyopia as well
- Partial ptosis may be left alone; however, if ptosis causes astigmatism and occlusional/deprivation amblyopia, spectacle correction is necessary as well as treatment of congenital ptosis, either with taping up of the eyelid or surgery to relieve the ptosis
- Types of ptosis repair surgeries:
  - Levator muscle resection
    i. Shortening of the levator-aponeurosis complex through a lid-crease incision in those with moderate levator function
  - Frontalis suspension procedure
    i. Augment the patient's lid elevation through brow elevation, using tissue from other parts of the body (autologous graft, e.g. fascia lata) or artificial materials. The procedure is indicated when the levator function is poor.
  - Frontalis flap procedure
    i. A minimally invasive surgery using a single incision in the crease of the eyelid and requires no grafting of the patient's tissue or external materials, with minimal scarring. This procedure is indicated when the levator function is poor.

Capillary/strawberry Haemangioma

- Benign tumour consisting of an abnormal overgrowth of tiny blood vessels
- May not be present at birth, but appears within the first 6 months of life
- Usually begins to decrease in size between 12 and 15 months of age. Most regress nearly completely by 5 or 6 years of age.
- Eyelid haemangiomas may result in amblyopia by causing ptosis that obscures the visual axis or astigmatism in the affected eye, leading to meridional amblyopia
- Orbital haemangiomas can compress the globe, eye muscles or optic nerve

- Treatment
  - No treatment may be necessary if there are no associated complications
  - Propranolol is taken orally, but in some patients, it can be applied topically if the haemangioma is very small and thin. Propranolol can affect the heart rate and blood pressure, hence, careful monitoring at the beginning of treatment is required.
  - Steroids can stop the progression of haemangiomas by causing the blood vessels to shrink. Depending on the size and location of the haemangioma, steroids may be prescribed orally, injected directly into the haemangioma, or applied to the surface of the haemangioma. Steroid medications can have undesirable side effects, including delayed physical growth, cataract, glaucoma and central retinal artery occlusion.
  - Laser treatments can sometimes be used on superficial haemangiomas to prevent growth, diminish their size, or lighten their colour
  - Traditional surgery to remove haemangiomas around the eye is generally reserved for small, well-defined haemangiomas that are located under the skin surface

Assessment of Amblyopia

- Assessment of best corrected vision in a child requires age-appropriate methods of testing, as outlined in Section 8.1
- Any refractive error should be tested using cycloplegic retinoscopy, corrected for and vision-tested
- Ocular alignment should be assessed
- Full ophthalmologic assessment, including dilated fundus examination, should be carried out to rule out ocular pathologies that may contribute to decreased vision

Management of Amblyopia

- Early treatment is always best, before the age of 7– 8
- If necessary, children with refractive errors (nearsightedness, farsightedness or astigmatism) can wear glasses
- Children with cataracts, squints or other "amblyogenic" conditions are usually treated promptly
- SOME improvement in vision may be attained with amblyopia therapy initiated in younger teenagers (through age 14 years)
- Patching of the better-seeing eye to allow the weak eye to get stronger
- "Penalise" or blur the stronger (good) eye with atropine eye drops temporarily

Take Home Messages

- Amblyopia is decreased vision in one or both eyes due to abnormal development of vision.
- Causes include strabismus, vision deprivation or refractive errors.
- Management
  - Patching of the better-seeing eye to allow the weak eye to get stronger.
  - "Penalise" or blur the stronger (good) eye with atropine eye drops.

8.3 Strabismus

Learning Objectives

- How to assess strabismus.
- Causes and management of eso- and exo-deviations.
- Principles of strabismus management.

Assessment of Strabismus

Strabismus

- Misalignment of the eyes, which may be
  - Horizontal
  - Vertical
  - Torsional
- Nomenclature (Fig. 8.11)
  - Orthophoria (straight)
  - Esotropia (manifest convergent strabismus; seen on cover test)
  - Esophoria (latent convergent strabismus; seen only on alternate cover test)
  - Exotropia (manifest divergent strabismus; seen on cover test)
  - Exophoria (latent divergent strabismus; seen only on alternate cover test)
  - Intermittent exotropia (manifest divergent strabismus, which occurs at times; seen on cover test)
  - Right hypertropia (named after the higher eye; seen on the cover test)

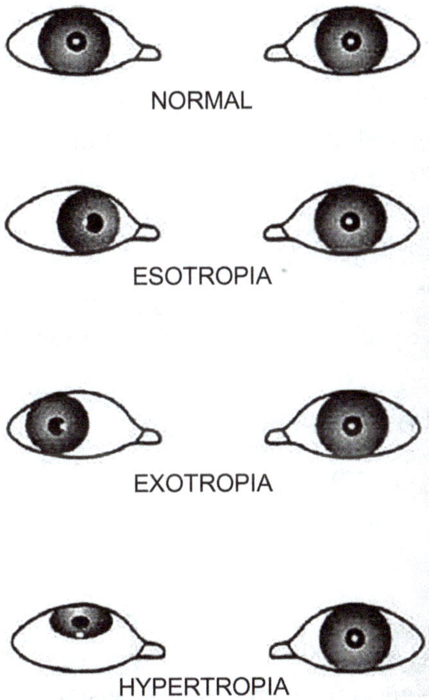

Fig. 8.11. Hirschberg test using a bright co-axial light source.

- Clinical presentation
  - Abnormal head posture
  - Head tilt
  - Face turn
  - Facial asymmetry
- Binocular red reflex (Bruckner)
  - A bright coaxial light source, such as a direct ophthalmoscope, is used. Both eyes of the patient are simultaneously illuminated from approximately one metre in distance. When strabismus is present, the deviated eye may appear to have a brighter red reflex.
- Hirschberg test (corneal light reflex)
  - A bright coaxial light source, such as a direct ophthalmoscope, is used. The position of the corneal light reflex is evaluated (Fig. 8.11 and Fig. 8.12).
  - Normal: slight symmetrical nasal displacement of 5 degrees

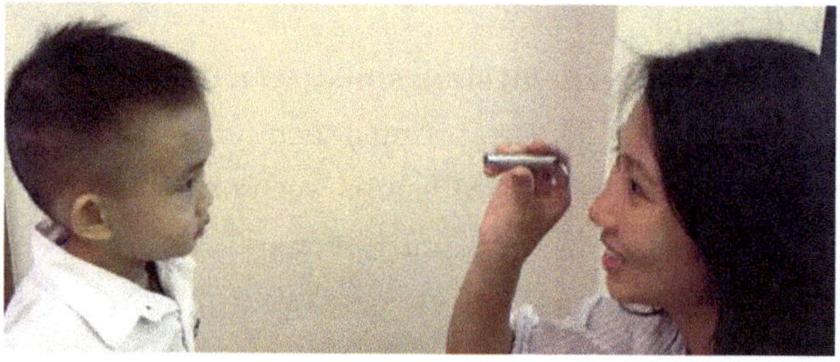

Fig. 8.12. Hirschberg test — checking for the corneal light reflex using a bright pentorch.

- Cover test/Uncover test
  - Used to detect tropias/manifest squints
  - Patient needs to be able to fixate on an object
  - Cover the normal eye (1–2 sec) and observe if the deviating eye shifts towards the midline
- Alternate cover test
  - Dissociates binocular fusion to determine full deviation (detects both tropias and phorias (latent squints))
  - Alternately occlude each eye, observe for refixation shift of the uncovered eye towards the midline

Esodeviation (Inward Deviation of the Eye)

Infantile Esotropia (Fig. 8.13)

- Onset first 6 months of age
- Large angle
- Amblyopia in 50%
- Early surgery usually required
- Poor prognosis for high-grade stereopsis/3D vision
- Usually requires a second surgery for other associated motor anomalies

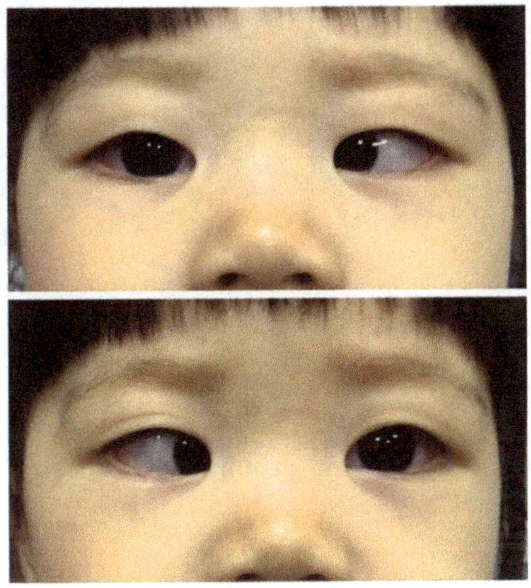

Fig. 8.13A. Alternating infantile esotropia, before surgery.

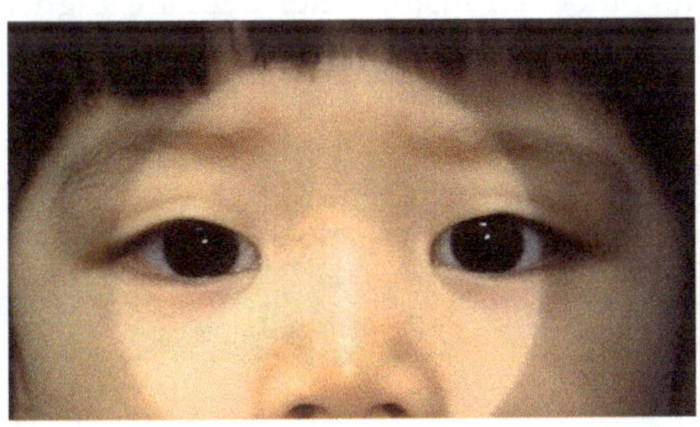

Fig. 8.13B. The same child after strabismus surgery. The eyes appear straight now, with the Hirschberg corneal light reflex well-centred in each eye.

Accommodative Esotropia

- Far-sighted (Fig. 8.14A)
- Increase focusing effort to see clearly
- Acquired between 6 months and 5 years of age
- Hypermetropic glasses
  - Straight after hypermetropic glasses (fully accommodative esotropia, Fig. 8.14B)
    i. Good prognosis for stereoacuity and binocular fusion
  - Residual ET after full hypermetropic glasses (partially accommodative esotropia, Fig. 8.14C) — surgery needed

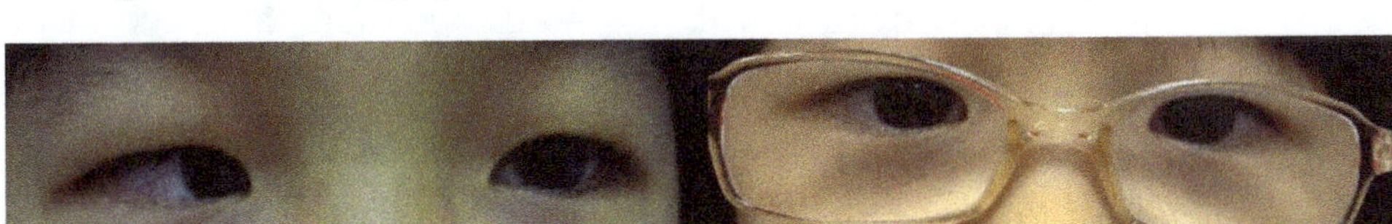

(A) (B)

Fig. 8.14A & B. In this child with accommodative right esotropia, the right esotropia resolves with fitting the child with a pair of hyperopic glasses to relax the accommodation.

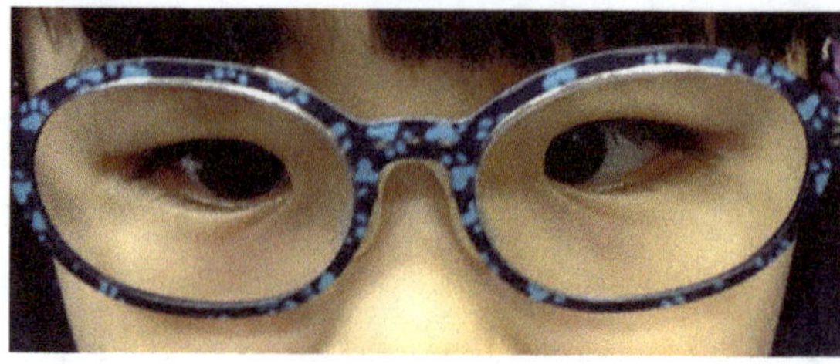

(C)

Fig. 8.14C. Residual left esotropia is seen in the child with partially accommodative esotropia.

Exodeviation

- Intermittent exodeviation is the most common form of strabismus (Fig. 8.14E)
- Between ages 2 and 8
- Occurs when the child is tired/day dreaming
- Vague eye discomfort, photophobia, squinting
- Good stereopsis and binocular fusion when eyes are aligned (Fig. 8.14D)
- Requires surgery if poorly controlled

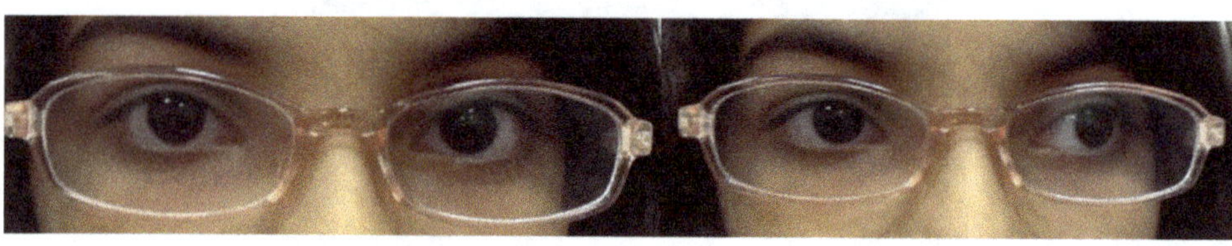

(D) (E)

Fig. 8.14D and E. Intermittent exotropia.

Sensory Deviation

- Loss of vision causes an eye to drift
- Visual loss <2 years of age usually leads to esotropia (Fig. 8.14F)
- Visual loss >2 years of age usually leads to exotropia (Fig. 8.14G)

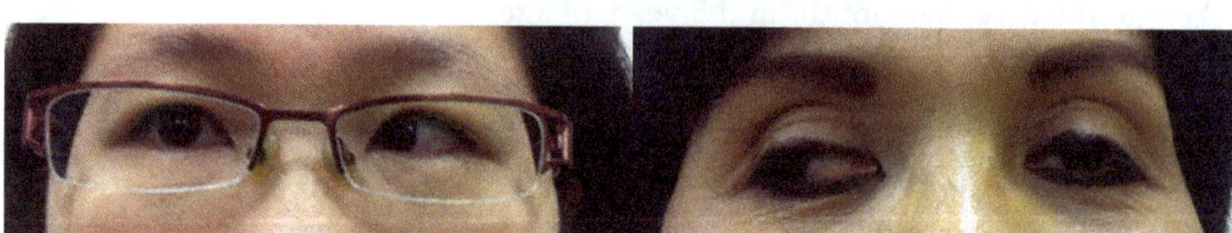

(F) (G)

Fig. 8.14F and G. Esodeviations and exodeviations may result from poor vision in the deviating eye.

Complications of Strabismus

- Acquired: diplopia/double vision
- Before age 6: cortical suppression of image from the deviated eye
  - Strabismic amblyopia
  - Loss of binocular fusion and stereopsis

- Dangerous strabismus
    - Acquired strabismus
    - Associated with diplopia
    - Limited eye movements
    - Ptosis or other neurological signs
    - Poor vision
    - Abnormal red reflex

Principles of Strabismus Management

- Prescribe glasses if necessary
- Manage any strabismic amblyopia "lazy eye" as appropriate:
    - patching of the better-seeing eye
    - atropine penalisation of the better-seeing eye (in children who are non-compliant to patching)
- Orthoptic exercises
- Prisms to relieve diplopia
- Strabismus surgery
    - Aims:
        i. Achieve binocular single vision
        ii. Eliminate head posture
        iii. Cosmesis
    - Types of surgery
        i. Slacken/weaken the muscle (e.g. recession)
        ii. Tighten/strengthen the muscle (e.g. resection, plication)
        iii. Reduce the length of the moment arm (Faden)
        iv. Change the vector of muscle force by moving the muscle's insertion site (transposition)

Take Home Messages

- Strabismus can be detected using the Hirschberg test (corneal light reflection test) as well as cover tests.
- Acquired strabismus or those associated with neurological signs and poor vision must be investigated urgently.
- Management of strabismus should start with conservative/non-surgical options first, such as optimising their vision with glasses and patching, if necessary. Orthoptic exercises may be implemented for the management of intermittent exotropia and prisms may be used to relieve diplopia.
- Surgery for strabismus can be considered for diplopia, abnormal head posture, worsening angles of deviation of strabismus or decreasing stereopsis, or cosmetically unacceptable strabismus.

8.4 Leukocoria

Learning Objectives

- Understand important causes of leukocoria.
- Understand the presentation and assessment of retinoblastoma.
- Understand the presentation and assessment of congenital cataracts.

Approach to Leukocoria

Presence of a "white pupil", the name given to the clinical finding of a white pupillary reflex (Fig. 8.15), when the path of light is obstructed in the eye.

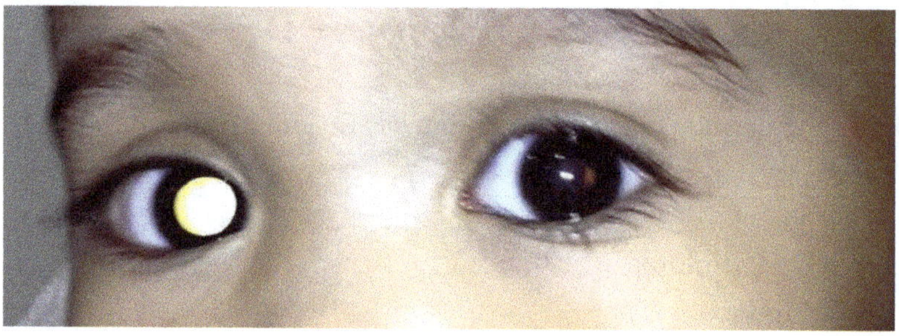

Fig. 8.15. Right eye leukocoria.

Causes of Leukocoria

- Lens
  - Cataract
- Vitreous
  - Persistent foetal vasculature
- Retina
  - Retinoblastoma
  - Non accidental injury
  - Coats' disease
  - Retinopathy of prematurity
  - Optic disc abnormalities
  - Congenital infections (toxoplasmosis, toxocara)

Assessment of Leukocoria

- **All children with newly discovered leukocoria should be urgently referred to an ophthalmologist**
- History
  - Prenatal exposures (toxins, infection, medications) and complications
  - Birth history
  - Postnatal course (infection, oxygen exposure, medications)
  - Medical history, growth pattern, development, and review of systems

   - Recent exposures to possible infective sources (puppies, kittens, medications)
   - Family history (particularly for retinoblastoma or other eye diseases, eye loss, osteogenic sarcoma, and foetal loss or miscarriage)
- Physical examination, including dysmorphic features, growth parameters, signs of coagulopathy, trauma or neurocutaneous disorders, and organomegaly
   - Age-appropriate vision assessment and external examination (See Section 8.1)
   - Anterior segment and dilated fundoscopic examination
- Radiologic investigation
   - Ophthalmic ultrasonography is routinely used to determine the presence or absence of an intraocular mass with associated intralesional calcium, which is indicative of retinoblastoma

Retinoblastoma

Epidemiology

- Most common intraocular malignancy (Fig. 8.16) in children
- Incidence of one in 15–20,000 live births
- Average age of presentation — 18 months
   - Bilateral — 13 months
   - Unilateral — 24 months
   - Family history — 11 months

Genetics

- 40% hereditary
- Autosomal dominant germline mutation of RB1 gene (tumour suppressor gene) on 13q14
- Two active copies of the retinoblastoma gene are normally carried in human cells. Both copies must be mutated to lead to the development of retinoblastoma.

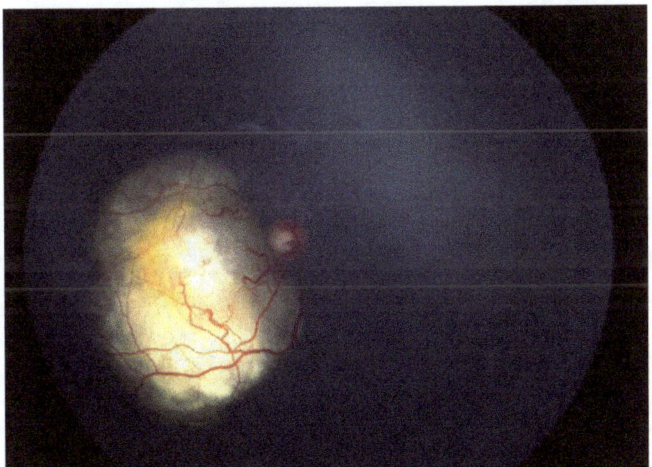

Fig. 8.16. Retinoblastoma of the right eye involving the macula.

- The initial mutation inactivates one copy of the gene. This mutation may occur in somatic or germline cells. The second mutation occurs in somatic cells.

Presentation

- Leukocoria in 50% — most common presentation
- Strabismus
- Change in eye appearance (heterochromia or red, painful or watery eyes)
- Reduced visual acuity

Assessment

- MRI (Fig. 8.17) to look for:
  - Involvement of optic nerve
  - Pineal gland (PNET) involvement
  - Other eye involvement
- Evaluate cerebrospinal fluid (CSF) and bone marrow when the child is at risk for metastatic disease
- Examination under anaesthesia (EUA) — staging
  - Retcam
  - Ophthalmic ultrasonography (B scan; Fig. 8.18)
  - Fundus fluorescein angiogram
- Genetic testing/counselling

Management

- Aims of management are to:
  - Preserve life
  - Save globe
  - Save vision
  - Managing any complications arising from treatment

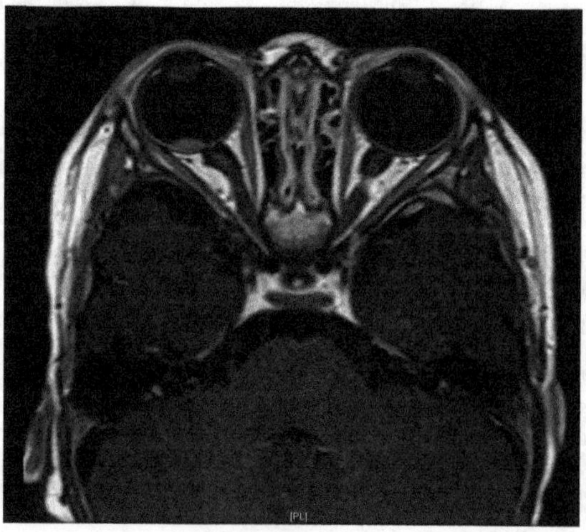

Fig. 8.17. MRI showing retinoblastoma of the right eye not involving the optic nerve.

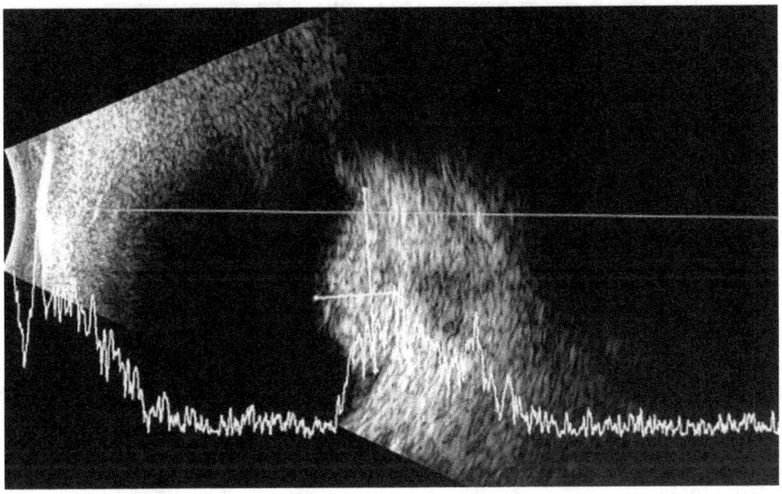

Fig. 8.18. B scan of eye showing an intraocular mass.

- Multimodal multidisciplinary management
  - Enucleation
  - Chemo reduction (systemic, local, intra-arterial, intravitreal)
  - Local (laser photocoagulation, cryotherapy)
  - Genetic testing

Congenital Cataracts (Fig. 8.19)

Aetiology

1. Primary — idiopathic or hereditary
2. Secondary

- Systemic
  - Genetic (Down syndrome, trisomy 13/15)
  - Metabolic (Lowe syndrome, galactosaemia)
  - Infections (Rubella, CMV, HSV, Toxoplasmosis)
- Ocular
  - developmental (anterior segment dysgenesis, aniridia, nanophthalmos, persistent fetal vasculature)
  - diseases (ocular trauma, uveitis, retinoblastoma)
- Toxic
  - Steroids
  - Radiation

Assessment

- VA — Does the child fixate on light? Any objection to occlusion?
- Red reflex
- Ophthalmoscopy through an undilated pupil
  - Central opacity or surrounding cortical distortion >3 mm is visually significant

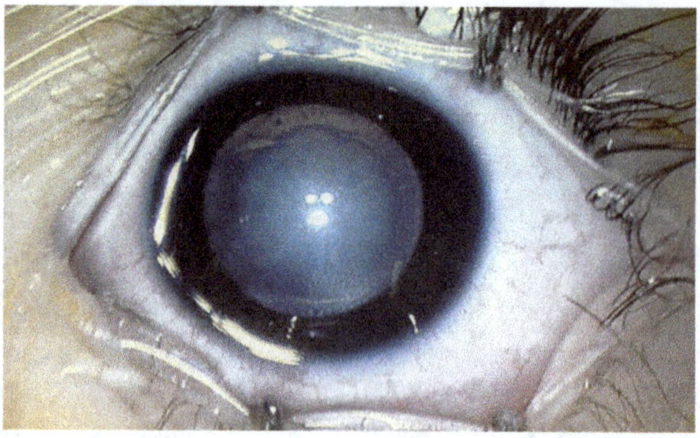

Fig. 8.19. Intraoperative photograph showing the presence of a lamellar cataract in a young infant.

- Laboratory tests
  - TORCH (toxoplasma, rubella, CMV, herpes) and varicella titres
  - VDRL (for syphilis)
  - Serum calcium, phosphorus, glucose and ferritin
  - Urine for reducing substance, galactose 1-phosphate uridyltransferase, galactokinase, amino acids

Management

- Surgery
  - Visually significant cataract
  - Between 4 and 6 weeks of age
  - If bilateral, second eye surgery 1 week after the first, or can be done on the same day under general anaesthesia
- Post-op
  - Refractive correction
    - i. Glasses (bilateral)
    - ii. Contact lens
  - Aggressive amblyopia treatment if unilateral

Non-Accidental Injury/Shaken Baby Syndrome

- Suspect when
  - Injury is unexplained
  - Severity of the injury is incompatible with history
  - History keeps changing
  - Injury is inconsistent with the developmental age
  - Delay in seeking medical care following an injury
  - Suspected abuse needs to be thoroughly investigated with the assistance of child protection services

Associated Features

- Bruising
- Burns
- Fractures
- Abusive head trauma
  - Intracranial haemorrhage
  - Diffuse retinal haemorrhage (Fig. 8.20)
    i. Often multilayered
    ii. Occur in 60–85% of non-accidental head injuries
    iii. Uncommon in accidental head trauma
  - Diffuse brain injury
    i. Signs and symptoms may be non-specific, such as vomiting, poor feeding, irritability or lethargy
  - May have no external signs of injury

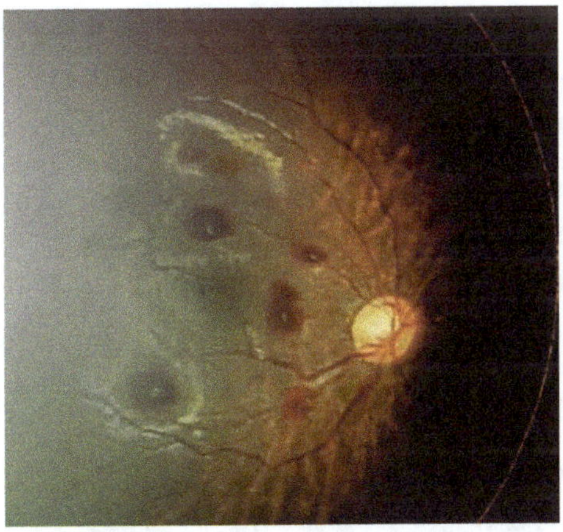

Fig. 8.20. Fundus photograph of the right eye in a child who sustained multiple retinal haemorrhages after a non-accidental injury.

Retinopathy of Prematurity (ROP)

- Retinal vascularisation on the internal retinal surface begins at the optic nerve at 16 weeks gestation and proceeds anteriorly towards the ora serrata
  - Reaches the nasal ora serrata by 36 weeks
  - Reaches the temporal ora serrata by 40 weeks
- Screening
  - All premature babies <1500 g, <32 weeks gestation age
  - 1st check 4–6 weeks after birth, or at 31 weeks gestational age, whichever is later
- Risk Factors
  - Small for gestational age
  - Low birth weight

- Longer duration of artificial ventilation
- Multiple births
- Respiratory distress
- Congenital heart disease
- Post-natal anaemia
- Intracranial haemorrhage
- Apnoea of prematurity
- Exchange transfusion
- Perinatal hypoxia
- Sepsis
- Intrauterine growth retardation

- Zones and extent (Fig. 8.21)
  - Zone I is a circle, the radius of which extends from the centre of the optic disc to twice the distance from the centre of the optic disc to the centre of the macula
  - Zone II extends centrifugally from the edge of zone I to the nasal ora serrata
  - Zone III is the residual temporal crescent of the retina anterior to zone II
  - Stage 1: Demarcation Line
    i. Line that separates the avascular retina anteriorly from the vascularised retina posteriorly

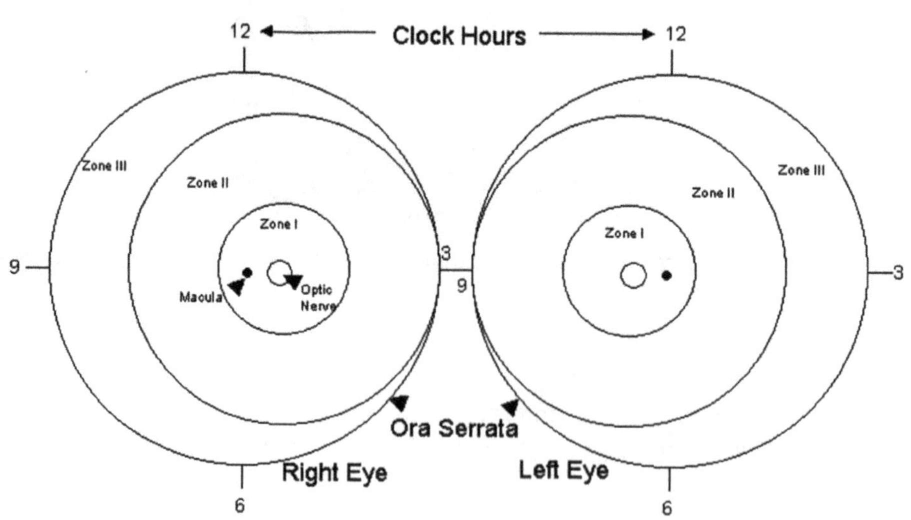

Fig. 8.21. Diagram detailing the zones and extent of retinopathy of prematurity.

- Stage 2: Ridge
  i. The ridge arises from the demarcation line and has height and width
- Stage 3: Extraretinal fibrovascular proliferation
  i. Neovascularisation extends from the ridge into the vitreous.
- Stage 4: Partial retinal detachment (Fig. 8.22)
- Stage 5: Total retinal detachment

Fig. 8.22. Left eye of the infant showing stage 4 retinopathy of prematurity with a partial retinal detachment.

- Treatment
  - Laser therapy
  - Intravitreal anti-VEGF (vascular endothelial growth factor)

Take Home Messages

- Prompt diagnosis and treatment are important in leukocoria.
- All children with newly discovered leukocoria should urgently be referred to an ophthalmologist.
- The most important cause of leukocoria is retinoblastoma, as it can be life-threatening.

8.5 Tearing and Discharge in an Infant/Young Child

Learning Objectives

- Understand the common and sight-threatening causes of tearing in an infant or young child.
- How to assess tearing in an infant or young child.

Approach to Tearing in an Infant/Young Child

Nasolacrimal duct obstruction (NLDO) is the most common cause of persistent tearing in an infant/young child and can lead to infection and ocular discharge. Other causes range from mild, self-limiting conditions (e.g. allergic conjunctivitis) to severe sight-threatening ocular emergencies (e.g. ophthalmia neonatorum).

Causes of Tearing in an Infant/Young Child

Aetiology of tearing in a child can be congenital or acquired and occur secondary to either ***hypersecretion*** of the tear glands or ***obstruction*** of the tear drainage system (Fig. 8.23).

The causes of tearing can also be classified as follows:

Table 8.3. Classification of the Causes of Tearing

Sight-threatening causes	Congenital glaucoma Ophthalmia neonatorum
Common causes	NLDO Conjunctivitis, frequently allergic
Others	Corneal or conjunctival foreign body/abrasion Eyelid abnormalities Epiblepharon causing lash-corneal touch Trichiasis/distichiasis Entropion Blepharitis

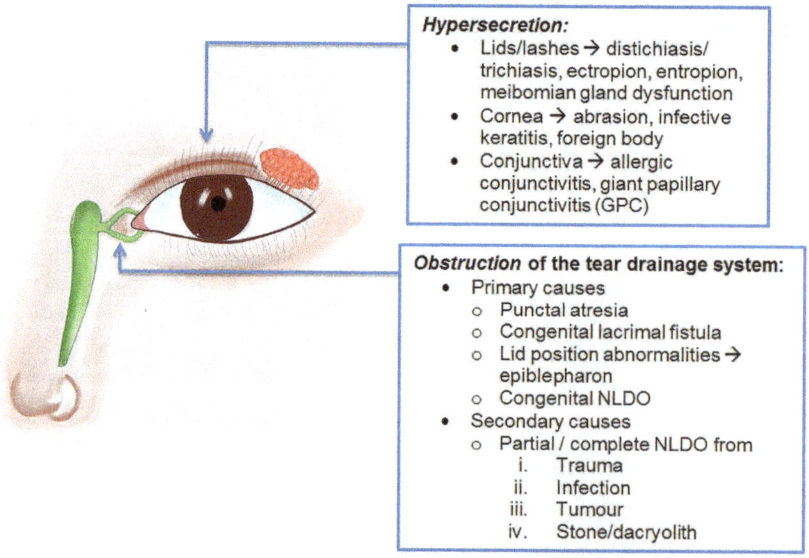

Fig. 8.23. Causes of tearing in an infant or young child.

Assessment of Tearing in an Infant/Young Child

History

- Onset (acute/gradual), progression
- Type of discharge: watery, purulent
- Past medical history: previous sinus surgery/disease, trauma, dacryocystitis
- Previous surgery/radiation

Examination

Examine the patient under the slit lamp, looking for:

- Eyelids: entropion, ectropion, distichiasis, trichiasis, lid laxity
- Punctum: well-apposed to tear lake/globe, atresia
- Tear film — oily, high or low
- Cornea/Conjunctiva — ulcers, infiltrates, punctate epithelial erosions, abrasions, giant papillary conjunctivitis
- Intraocular pressure (IOP) — suggestive of glaucoma

Fluorescein Tests

- Level of tear film
- Fluorescein dye disappearance test (FDDT)
  - Instil 2% fluorescein eyedrop
  - After 5 minutes, check for dye to disappear
  - Delay in disappearance → problem lies in the tear drainage system
- Jones I test
  - Check for fluorescein in the nose with a cotton swabstick
  - Lack of fluorescein in the nose would suggest a partial/complete NLDO

Other Investigations

- Nasal endoscopy → look for dye under inferior turbinate within the inferior meatus (may be difficult in young children)
- Syringing and probing
  - Done under general anaesthesia in young children
  - Check for the presence of punctal atresia/stenosis
  - Soft/hard stop
    - i. Soft stop → suggestive of proximal NLDO
    - ii. Hard stop → suggestive of distal NLDO
  - Presence of reflux

Congenital Nasolacrimal Duct Obstruction

Please refer to Section 7.3 in Chapter 7: Oculoplastics.

Congenital Glaucoma

Please refer to Section 4.2 in Chapter 4: Glaucoma.

Ophthalmia Neonatorum

Causes

- Infections:
  - Bacterial
    - i. Most common: *Neisseria gonorrhoea, Chlamydia trachomatis*
    - ii. Others: *Staphylococcus aureus, Streptococcus pneumoniae, Streptococcus viridans, Staphylococcus epidermidis, Haemophilus influenzae, Enterococcus, Escherichia coli, Klebsiella, Serratia, Pseudomonas aeruginosa*
  - Viral:
    - i. Herpes simplex virus (1–2 weeks after birth: vesicles on the face, herpetic dendritic keratitis)
- Chemical:
  - Usually presents within the first 24 hours
  - Types:
    - i. Silver nitrate
    - ii. Erythromycin, tetracycline
  - Self-limiting, resolves within 1–2 days
- Trauma

Time frame of signs/symptoms following the birth of a child can play an important role in determining the most likely aetiology in ophthalmia neonatorum.			
Chemical conjunctivitis	*Neisseria gonorrhoea*	*Chlamydia trachomatis*	Herpes simplex virus (HSV)
Within 24 hours after birth	3–5 days after birth	5–14 days after birth	1–2 weeks after birth

Assessment

- Things to ask for in history
  - Symptoms/signs, e.g. eye redness, discharge
  - Duration, laterality, progression
  - Visual behaviour — normal or abnormal?
  - Maternal infections, e.g. vaginal discharge
  - Mode of delivery — ophthalmia neonatorum commonly acquired through passage of the baby through the birth canal
  - Any birth complications

- Things to look out for in an examination
  - Take conjunctival scrapings before performing eye lavage
  - Examine the eye for
    - Conjunctival redness, chemosis
    - Corneal epithelial defect, infiltrate, perforation
    - Purulent discharge
    - Anterior segment for hypopyon
    - Dilated fundal examination
  - Check the child systemically
    - Signs of meningitis — fever/sepsis/neck stiffness
- Investigate for the cause
  - Send the conjunctival scrapings for microbiological diagnosis
    - Gram stain
    - Cultures and sensitivities
    - *Chlamydia* immunofluorescence/polymerase chain reaction (PCR)
    - *Neisseria gonorrhoea* PCR
  - Blood cultures if the child is septic
  - Conjunctival scrapings for mother if she has symptoms suggestive of pelvic inflammatory disease

Management

- Co-manage this patient with a paediatrician to rule out systemic involvement → refer to Paediatrics Infectious Disease
- Counsel the mother about the need to start topical broad-spectrum antibiotics, e.g. Tobramycin eyedrops
- Teach the mother to perform eye toileting hourly with saline lavage to reduce bacterial/viral load
- Close follow-up → review the child daily until cultures are available
  - Tailor treatment according to culture results/sensitivity
- Treat the child and parents
  - Child
    1. Chlamydia: Oral erythromycin 50 mg/kg/day in divided doses Q6H x 2 weeks
    2. Gonorrhoea: IV/IM ceftriaxone 50 mg/kg/day in divided or single dose x 7 days
    3. Herpetic: Oral acyclovir 30 mg/kg/day in 3 divided doses x 2 weeks
       - Admit
       - Topical acyclovir as well

- Adult
  - i. Chlamydia
    - Oral azithromycin 1 g x (1 dose) or
    - Oral doxycycline 100 mg BD x (7 days)
  - ii. Gonococcal
    - IM ceftriaxone 250 mg x (1 dose) + oral azithromycin 1 g (1 dose) or
    - Oral doxycycline 100 mg BD x (7 days)

Systemic Manifestations

Ophthalmia neonatorum may be associated with systemic manifestations if due to a bacterial cause.

- Gonorrhoea
  - Meningitis
  - Arthritis
  - Septicaemia
  - Stomatitis, rhinitis
- Chlamydia
  - Pneumonitis
  - Otitis media
  - Pharyngeal
  - Rectal colonisation

Orbital Cellulitis in Children

Please refer to Section 7.2 in Chapter 7: Oculoplastics.

Take Home Messages

- Glaucoma in an infant/young child can present with tearing and can lead to blindness if left untreated.
- The *most common cause* of excessive tearing in an infant is nasolacrimal duct obstruction.
- *Important sight-threatening causes* of tearing in a young child/infant are congenital glaucoma, orbital cellulitis and ophthalmia neonatorum.

8.6 Refractive Error

Learning Objectives

- Understand how to prescribe refractive correction for children.
- Know the definitions of emmetropia, ametropia, hyperopia, myopia and astigmatism.
- Know how to read a refraction prescription.

Prescribing for Children

- In adults, the correction of refractive errors has 1 measurable endpoint: the best corrected visual acuity
- In children, however, the correction of refractive errors has 2 goals:
  - Provide a focused image on the retina
  - Achieve optimal balance between accommodation and convergence
- Techniques of refraction in children:
  - Subjective refraction
    i. Can be performed in older children
    ii. Difficult in infants and young children due to their inability to cooperate with subjective refraction techniques
  - Objective refraction
    i. Optimal technique of refraction in infants and small children
    ii. Requires paralysis of accommodation with complete cycloplegia, also known as cycloplegic refraction

Definition of Emmetropia, Ametropia, Hyperopia, Myopia and Astigmatism

Emmetropia (Fig. 8.24)

- Refractive state in which parallel rays of light from a distant object are brought to focus on the retina in the non-accommodating eye

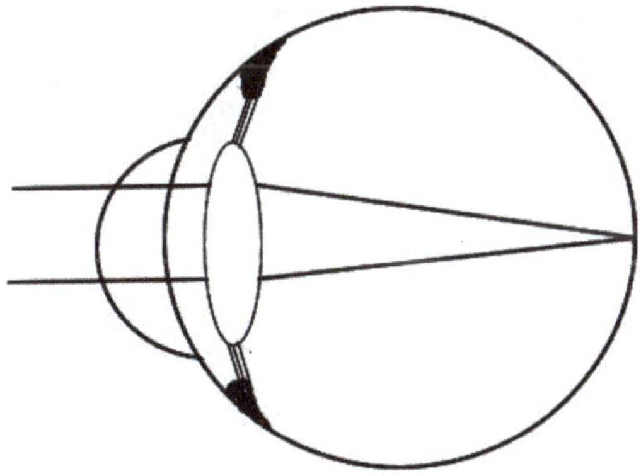

Fig. 8.24. Emmetropia with accommodation relaxed.

Ametropia

- Absence of emmetropia
- Can be classified as axial or refractive
  - i. Axial ametropia — the eyeball is either unusually long (axial myopia) or short (axial hyperopia)
  - ii. Refractive ametropia — the eyeball is statistically normal, but the refractive power of the eye (cornea and/or lens) is abnormal, being either excessive (refractive myopia) or deficient (refractive hyperopia)

Hyperopia (Fig. 8.25)

- Can be axial or refractive

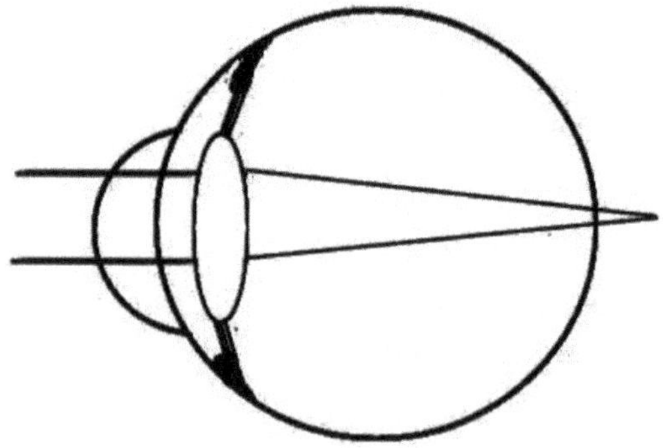

Fig. 8.25. Hyperopia with accommodation relaxed.

- Eye possesses insufficient optical power for its axial length, hence in the non-accommodating eye, the light rays from an object at infinity attempts to focus light ***behind*** the retina
- Usually expressed with a "plus" sign in dioptres (D)

Myopia (Fig. 8.26)

- Can be axial or refractive
- Eye possesses too much optical power for its axial length, hence in the non-accommodating eye, the light rays from an object at infinity converge and focus ***in front*** of the retina
- Usually expressed with a "minus" sign in dioptres (D)

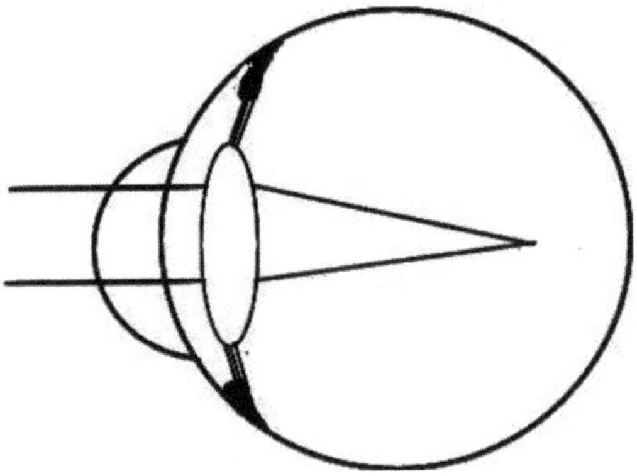

Fig. 8.26. Myopia with accommodation relaxed.

Astigmatism

- Optical condition of the eye in which light rays from an object do not focus to a single point because of variations in the curvature of the cornea or lens at different meridians, resulting in a set of 2 focal lines
- Usually expressed with a "minus" sign in dioptres (D), with an axis ranging from 0 to 180 degrees (orientation of meridian of greatest curvature)

How to Read a Refraction Prescription

- Looking at a prescription for refraction, numbers are listed under the headings of **Right or Left eye, or OD and OS** (Latin abbreviations)
  - OD — oculus dextrus — means right eye
  - OS — oculus sinister — means left eye
  - Occasionally, a notation for OU may be seen, which means involving both eyes
- **Spherical (SPH) Component**
  - Plus sign — signifies hyperopia
  - Minus sign — signifies myopia
  - Numbers represent dioptres, the unit used to measure the refractive correction or focusing power that the eye requires
    i. Dioptre: often abbreviated as "D"
- **Cylinder (CYL) Component**
  - A measure of the amount of astigmatism one has
  - Axis: ranges from 0 to 180 degrees
    i. Reveals the orientation of the astigmatism to the meridian of the greatest curvature (usually referring to the cornea)
- **Near Add Component**
  - Needed when the accommodative amplitude is insufficient for the patient to read or carry out near-vision tasks, usually in adults who have developed presbyopia
  - Can also be given to children who have a high accommodative convergence to accommodation ratio (AC:A ratio)
  - Usually expressed with a "plus" sign as convex lenses are needed for correction

Example of a refraction prescription:

Cylinder: Presence of 1 dioptre of cylinder with axis of greatest curvature at 180 degrees

Near Add: This patient requires 2.50 dioptres of convex lenses to achieve a near vision of N5

Right Eye (OD)					
Sph (D)	Cyl (D)	Axis (degrees)	VA (visual acuity)	Near Add (D)	VA (visual acuity)
+3.00	–1.00	180	6/6	+2.50	N5

Sphere: Signifies this patient requires 3 dioptres to correct the hyperopia

Best corrected visual acuity that patient can see with this refractive correction

Take Home Messages

- Refraction in children may be achieved by either subjective or objective refraction techniques.
- Reading a refraction prescription:
  - Has both Spherical and Cylindrical components.
  - Plus (+) sign — signifies hyperopia.
  - Minus (–) sign — signifies myopia.
  - Numbers represent dioptres, the unit used to measure the refractive correction or focusing power that the eye requires.
    i. Dioptre — often abbreviated as "D".

References

1. American Academy of Ophthalmology (AAO). 2016–2017 Edition. Paediatric Ophthalmology and Strabismus, and Orbit, Eyelids and Lacrimal system chapters.
2. American Academy of Ophthalmology (AAO). 2016–2017 Edition. Clinical Optics & Paediatric Ophthalmology and Strabismus chapters.
3. American Optometric Association. www.aoa.org.
4. Approach to the child with persistent tearing. www.uptodate.com.
5. Normal Vision Development in Babies and Children. www.aao.org.
6. Wilson FM. *Practical Ophthalmology — A manual for Beginning Residents* (AAO), 4th edn.
7. Wong TY. *The Ophthalmology Examinations Review*, 2nd edition.

Chapter 9

NEURO-OPHTHALMOLOGY

Lin Hui'en Hazel Anne, Clement Tan Woon Teck

Neuro-ophthalmology is a challenging and fascinating branch of ophthalmology as the clinical cases are diverse in presentation. Good knowledge of neuro-anatomy (Chapter 1), ophthalmology, neurology, neurosurgery, general medicine and radiology are required to determine the site and elucidate the cause of the disease.

This chapter aims to provide an overview of and approach to the important neuro-ophthalmic conditions that non-ophthalmologists may encounter.

9.1 Optic Neuropathy

Learning Objectives

- To be able to recognise optic neuropathy as a possible cause of visual loss.
- To be able to clinically determine normal, swollen and pale optic discs(s), and to list differentials for each.

Evaluation of a Patient with Suspected Optic Neuropathy

The term "optic neuropathy" refers to dysfunction of the optic nerve(s), without specifically describing the cause (or aetiology). Many conditions can cause optic neuropathy, and these can present in a variety of ways. Patients may report loss of vision, darkening of vision, change in colour saturation or something that "does not feel right". Patients with optic neuropathies are typically found to have a loss of visual acuity, visual field defects, dyschromatopsia and a relative afferent pupillary defect in varying combinations. When evaluating patients with possible optic neuropathy, it is crucial to take a thorough history and perform a complete ophthalmic and neurological examination. In addition, investigations are usually needed to aid the clinician with diagnosis and subsequent follow-up.

History

- Visual loss — onset, progression, severity
- Pain — headache, presence of pain on eye movement
- History of trauma
- Past medical history — vascular risk factors, malignancy, family history
- Dietary and medication history, including supplements and traditional medicines
- Social history — smoking, alcohol consumption, illicit drugs

Examination

- Vital signs of optic nerve function:
  - Visual acuity
  - Pupillary function (Is there a *RAPD?)
  - Colour vision
  - Visual fields

*Note that a RAPD is practically always present when there is a unilateral optic neuropathy unless there is equally severe loss of vision from the retina or macular disease in the fellow eye.

- Anterior and posterior segment examination: particularly of the optic disc
- Intraocular pressure
- Neurological examination (particularly the cranial nerves): Is this an isolated optic neuropathy or are other parts of the nervous system involved?

Investigations

- Perimetry — Humphrey visual fields (static perimetry) or Goldmann visual fields (kinetic perimetry)
- Optical coherence tomography (OCT) of the disc and macula
- Ganglion cell analysis
- Neuroimaging — magnetic resonance imaging (MRI) with contrast and fat suppression/computed tomography (CT), with or without accompanying vascular studies
- Imaging of the fundus/optic disc is useful for documentation and follow-up

The appearance of the optic disc, though important, does not usually give a direct indication of the underlying pathology. Optic neuropathies can present with a normal-looking disc (Fig. 9.1), a swollen disc, a pale disc, or a cupped disc (Fig. 9.2). Disc swelling may indicate inflammation, ischaemia or raised intracranial pressure. A pale disc simply indicates a past or chronic, ongoing insult to the optic nerve. Optic disc cupping is typically seen in glaucoma but may also be the result of other diseases. An outline of the causes of the swollen or pale disc is given in Table 9.1.

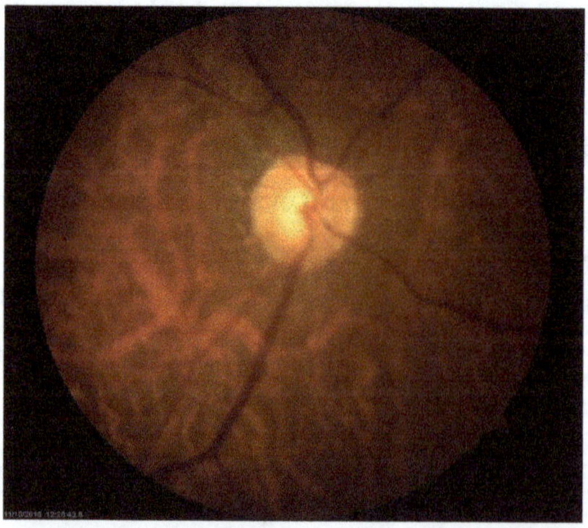

Fig. 9.1. A normal optic disc. The disc is pink, with clear margins, and a cup:disc ratio of approximately 0.4.

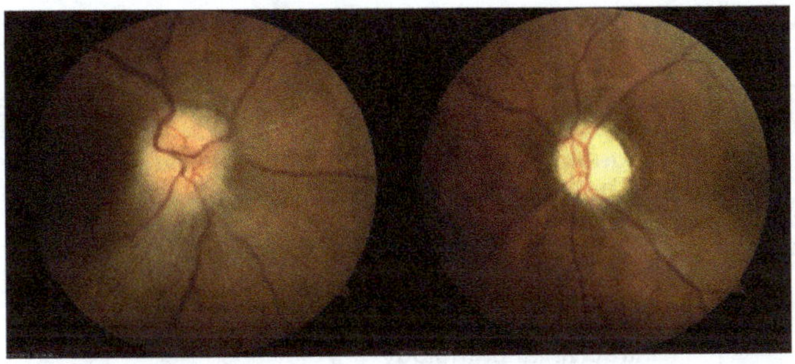

Patient 1 – right swollen disc and left pale disc from sequential ischaemic optic neuropathies.

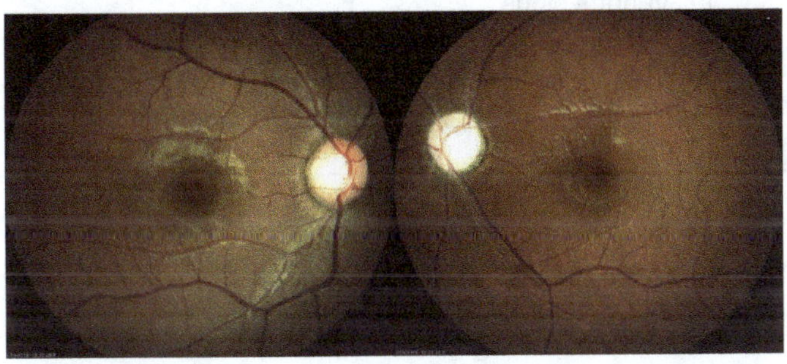

Patient 2 – bilateral slightly cupped discs and left pale disc from an optic disc glioma

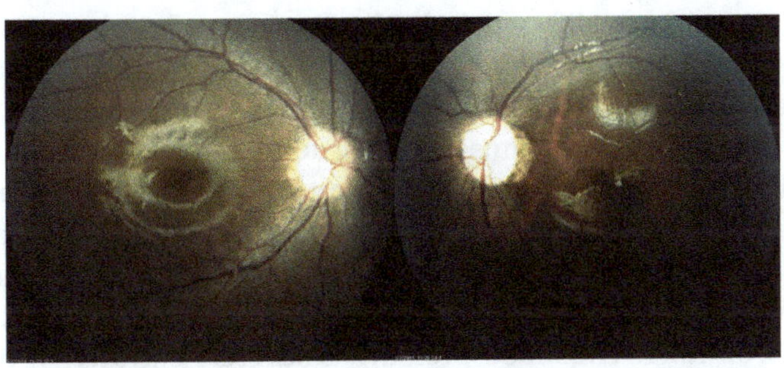

Patient 3 – bilateral pale discs from inflammatory optic neuropathy.

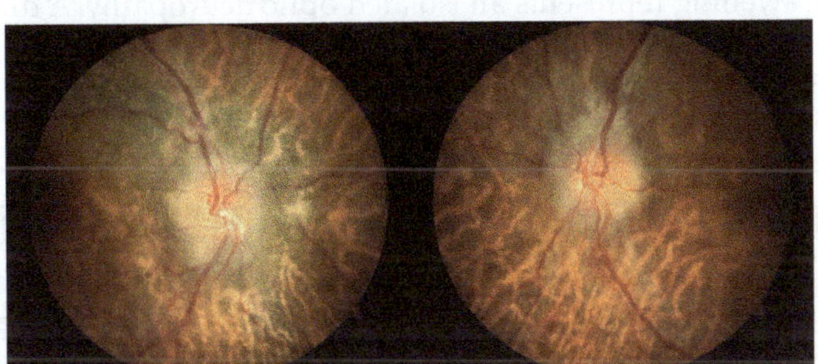

Patient 4 – bilateral swollen discs from raised intracranial pressure.

Fig. 9.2. Various presentations of optic neuropathies.

Table 9.1. Causes of Swollen and Pale Optic Discs

Swollen Disc(s)		Pale Disc(s)	
Unilateral	**Bilateral**	**Unilateral**	**Bilateral**

• Ischaemic
• Inflammatory*
• Compressive*
• Infiltrative*
• Radiation*
• Others: CRVO
	• Malignant hypertension#
	• Raised intracranial pressure (ICP)#
	  ▪ Identifiable intracranial pathology
	  ▪ Idiopathic
	• Venous sinus thrombosis#
		• Compressive
		• Traumatic
		• Ischaemic∞
		• Inflammatory∞
		• Infiltrative∞
		• Radiation
			• Hereditary
			• Toxic/nutritional
			• Compressive
			• Radiation

*May occasionally be bilateral	#May also cause unilateral disc swelling	∞Sequential past insult may result in bilateral pale discs	

Clinical Presentation of Optic Neuropathies

Optic Disc Swelling

A swollen disc is due to nerve oedema from the obstruction of axoplasmic flow, which may result from ischaemia, inflammation, compression, metabolic, or toxic disorders. Signs of disc swelling include obscuration of vessels crossing the optic disc, blurring of disc margins, hyperaemia, haemorrhages and exudates.

Patient presentation is dependent on the cause of optic disc swelling. Disc swelling from ischaemic or inflammatory optic neuropathies (optic neuritis) usually presents with acute visual loss. Disc swelling from compressive or infiltrative optic neuropathies may present with painless, progressive visual loss. Patients with papilloedema (disc swelling caused by raised intracranial pressure (ICP)) often present with transient visual obscuration, or symptoms of raised ICP such as headache and vomiting. The blood pressure is severely elevated in patients with malignant hypertension.

Not all disc swelling represents an isolated optic neuropathy. A dilated fundus examination is necessary in all patients to determine if there is other intraocular pathology. Figure 9.3 illustrates three patients who had optic disc swelling secondary

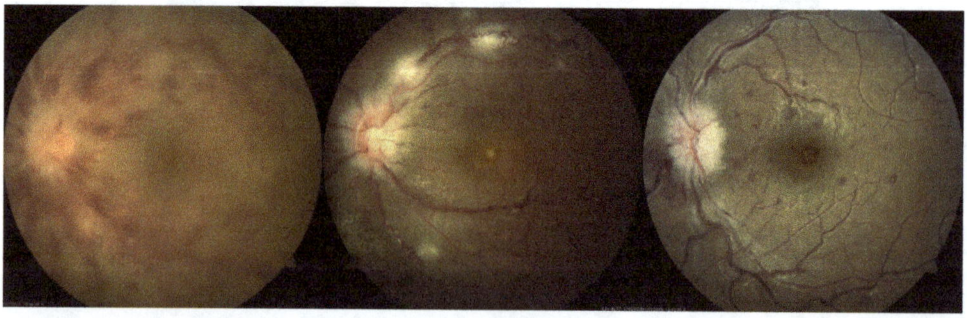

Fig. 9.3. From left to right: central retinal vein occlusion, retinal vasculitis and lymphoproliferative disorder.

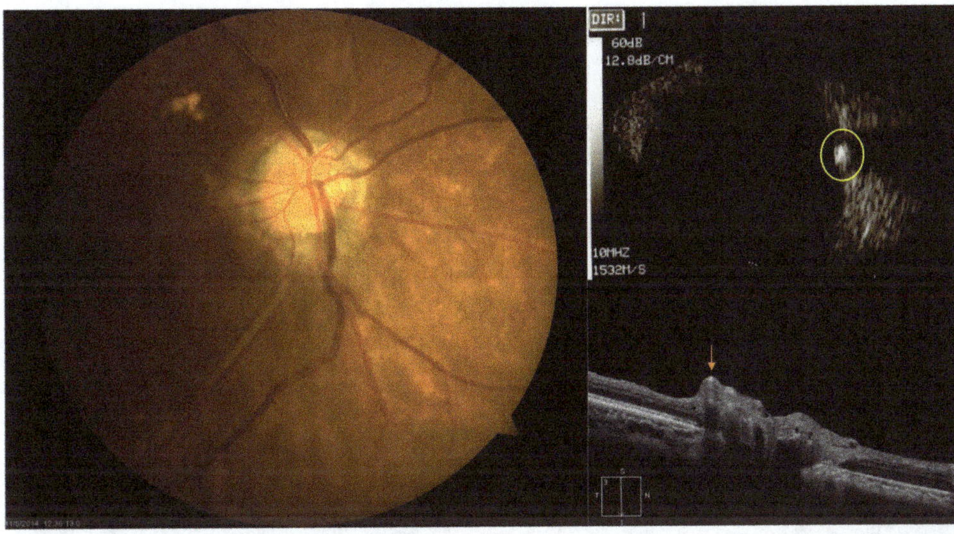

Fig. 9.4. Lumpy appearance of an optic nerve head secondary to disc drusen, which can give the impression of a swollen disc. On B scan imaging, a hyper-reflective spot is seen (yellow circle). This high signal is obtained with a reduction in the gain setting. Drusen can also be seen (orange arrow) on the OCT.

to other intraocular diseases. The optic disc may sometimes appear on fundoscopic examination to be swollen, even though there is no actual thickening of the retinal nerve fibre layer. Such pseudo disc swelling may be the result of a congenitally small, crowded disc or optic disc drusen. Figure 9.4 illustrates a patient who has optic nerve head drusen.

Before attributing the appearance of a swollen optic disc to pseudo-swelling, it is necessary to ensure that there are no signs and symptoms of visual loss or raised intracranial pressure and preferably obtain imaging of the retinal nerve fibre layer to monitor for progression.

Optic Disc Pallor

A pale disc represents a previous optic nerve injury. It is generally held that disc pallor sets in 6 weeks or more after insult to the optic nerve.

The management of patients with optic disc pallor is, in the first instance directed at determining the cause of the pallor and begins with a thorough history and physical examination elucidating the onset and tempo of progression of visual loss and the presence of other neurological or systemic symptoms and signs.

Some of the causes of such optic neuropathy also cause significant morbidity or mortality. Examples of these are intracranial tumours, infections and inflammations. It is essential to sufficiently investigate optic disc pallor to exclude these.

Optic Disc Cupping

When faced with a cupped disc, it is essential to exclude glaucoma as a cause (see Chapter 4: Glaucoma). Other optic neuropathies may uncommonly cause disc cupping, and should be considered as part of the differentials. In addition, if the patient has normal optic nerve function, which remains static over time, with no change in the optic disc appearance, this may represent physiological cupping.

Clinical Case Examples of Optic Neuropathies

Optic Neuritis

A 28-year-old woman presents with right eye blurring of vision for 2–3 days. This is associated with a mild ache on eye movements, and she reports that the apple she was eating did not appear as red when seen with the right eye compared with her left eye. Her visual acuity is 6/24 on the right and 6/6 on the left. There is a right RAPD and she can only read 3 of 15 plates on the Ishihara charts. Confrontation visual fields reveal a central visual field defect. Figure 9.5 shows the optic nerve appearance and corresponding MRI scans of the orbits. The left eye is normal on examination.

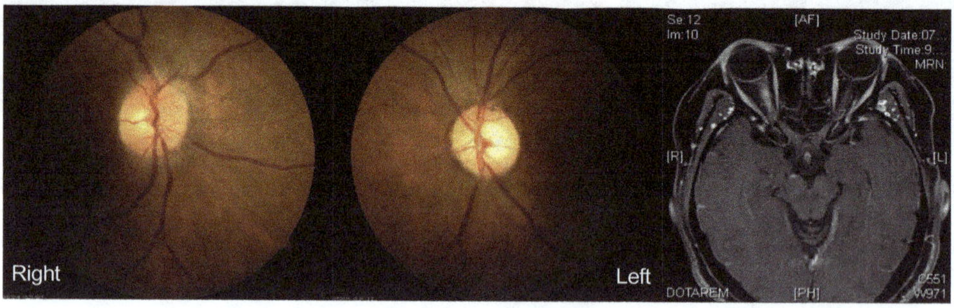

Fig. 9.5. The left eye is normal, and the right optic disc is swollen. Thickening and enhancement of the right optic nerve on T1 with contrast, axial cut of her MRI orbits and anterior visual pathway.

How Else May Optic Neuritis Present?

1. Optic neuritis may be subclinical and present later as a pale disc (Fig. 9.6(a))
2. Retrobulbar involvement, with the absence of optic disc swelling
3. Bilateral optic nerve involvement, with or without disc swelling (Fig. 9.6(b))

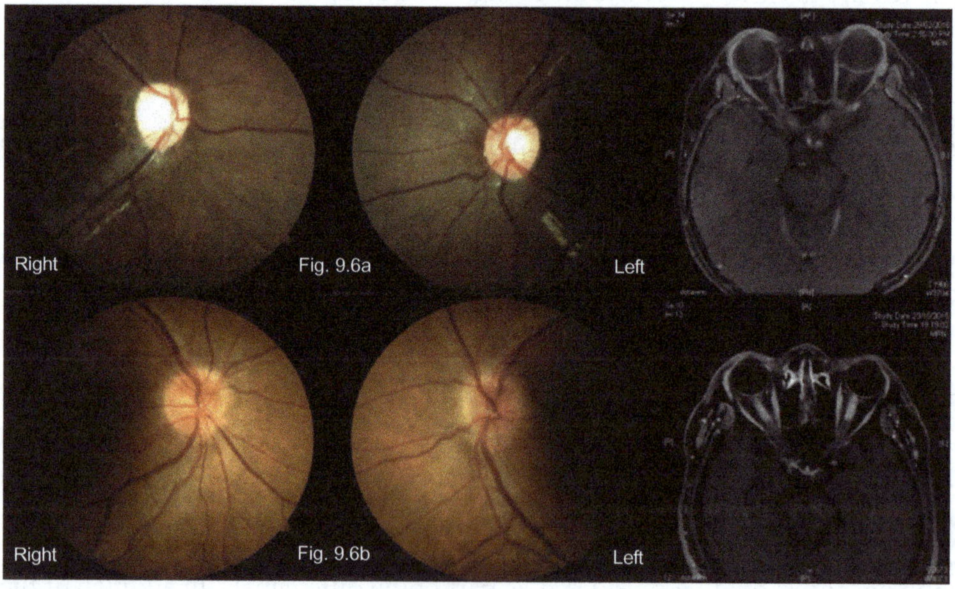

Fig. 9.6. (a) Right pale disc from previous optic neuritis, with corresponding atrophy on imaging; (b) bilateral swollen discs, which are thickened, and enhanced with contrast on imaging, implying active inflammation of both optic nerves.

What are the Possible Causes of Optic Neuritis?

Neuromyelitis Optica (NMO) or NMO Spectrum Disorder (NMOSD), Myelin Oligodendrocyte Glycoprotein antibody-associated disease (MOGAD) and Multiple Sclerosis (MS). Other autoimmune diseases, such as sarcoidosis and systemic lupus erythematosus, can also cause an optic neuritis.

How Should We Manage this Patient?

This patient should have the following investigations:

a) Lumbar puncture to exclude infections and abnormal cells such as malignant cells. Oligoclonal bands (paired with serum study) should be tested as well.
b) Serology to test for aquaporin 4 antibodies (AQP4), myelin oligodendrocyte glycoprotein antibody (anti-MOG) and other diseases such as systemic lupus erythematosus and sarcoidosis
c) Pre-steroid work-up
d) Consider MRI spine after discussion with Neurologist

Subsequently, if there are no contraindications to systemic steroids, the patient should be offered intravenous corticosteroids (methylprednisolone) for 3–5 days. During this time, regular visual function assessment should be performed to determine the response to steroids. For severe diseases and poor responders, plasma exchange should be considered, particularly for NMOSD.

Patients with NMOSD are also considered for long-term immunosuppression/ immunomodulation[7], and those with MOGAD may also be following a recurrence. If a patient has MS, long-term treatment will include other disease-modifying drugs.

What is the Risk of Developing Multiple Sclerosis in a Patient Who Presents for the First Time with Optic Neuritis?

The risk of MS depends on the presence of brain lesions in demyelinating optic neuritis. The presence of any brain lesion suggests the patient has a 72% risk of MS over 15 years compared to 15% if there are no brain lesions.

Ischaemic Optic Neuropathy

A 65-year-old man presents with a sudden onset of blurring of vision of the right eye, which he noticed when he woke up in the morning. He has a past medical history of ischaemic heart disease, diabetes mellitus, hypertension, and smokes 1 packet of cigarettes a day. On examination, visual acuity is 6/12 on the right and 6/9 on the left. There is a right RAPD, and inferior altitudinal defect on confrontational visual field testing of the right eye. His right optic disc is swollen, as seen in Fig. 9.7.

What is the Diagnosis, and What Forms of this Condition are there? How do You Tell Them Apart?

This patient has an ischaemic optic neuropathy (ION). This can affect the anterior portion of the optic disc, characterised by disc swelling, or the posterior portion, where the disc looks normal.

Ischaemic optic neuropathy can be arteritic or non-arteritic (NA), and can affect the anterior of posterior portion of the nerve.

Ophthalmologists use the term NAAION for non-arteritic anterior ischaemic optic neuropathy.

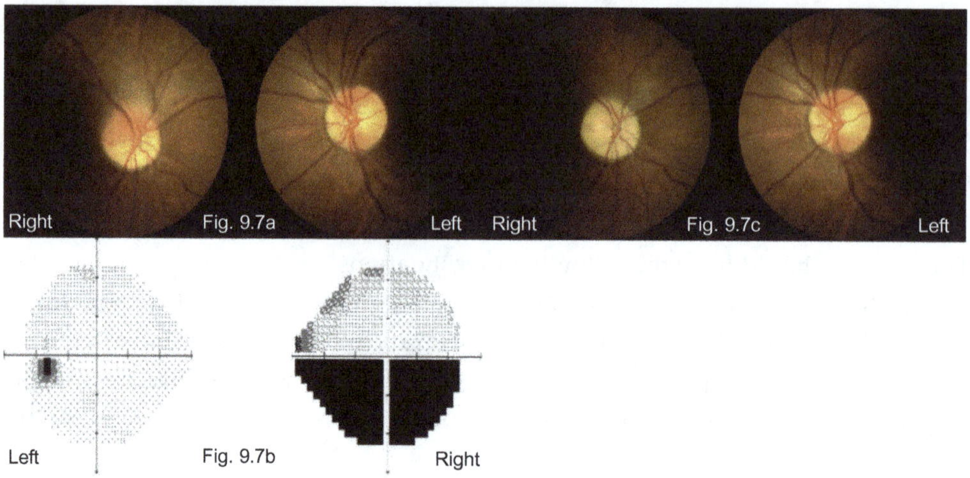

Fig. 9.7. (a) Right optic disc swelling secondary to NAAION; (b) corresponding visual fields showing an inferior altitudinal defect; (c) 3 months later, a right optic disc pallor is seen.

What are the Risk Factors for NAAION?

- Ocular — small, crowded disc
- Systemic — hypertension, diabetes mellitus, hyperlipidaemia, ischaemic heart disease, carotid artery disease, sleep apnoea and smoking

How Should this Patient be Managed?

- Exclude arteritic AION
  - Take a good history for the symptoms described in Table 9.2
  - Test ESR, CRP, platelets (one or more of these three, particularly the ESR, is typically elevated)

Table 9.2. Features of AAION and NAAION

	Arteritic Ischaemic Optic Neuropathy	Non-arteritic Ischaemic Optic Neuropathy
Patient	Typically >70 years old	Typically >50 years old
Onset	Acute	Acute
History	May have the features of giant cell arteritis — headaches, jaw claudication, scalp tenderness, hip and shoulder pain, and fever	Risk factors as described above No specific systemic symptoms
Examination	Severe drop in visual acuity RAPD Any visual field defect Typically, pallid swelling of optic disc	Normal VA to HM RAPD Typically, altitudinal field defect Swelling of the optic disc
Investigations	Urgent ESR, CRP, FBC Temporal artery biopsy Coronary studies Pre-steroid work up Ultrasound of temporal and axillary arteries	Blood pressure Fasting glucose, HbA1C Fasting lipids Sleep apnoea studies
Treatment	Co-management with Rheumatologist and urgent steroids	Treatment of vascular risk factors

- Modification of lifestyle — smoking, diet
- Investigate for risk factors — fasting glucose and lipids, blood pressure, studies for sleep apnoea

Raised Intracranial Pressure (ICP)

A 35-year-old woman presents with headaches for 2 months, associated with blurring of vision on waking. She has a background history of a brainstem tumour, which was treated with radiotherapy. Her visual acuity is 6/6 in both eyes, and there is no RAPD. Colour vision is normal. Optic discs, OCT of the disc and visual fields are shown in Fig. 9.8.

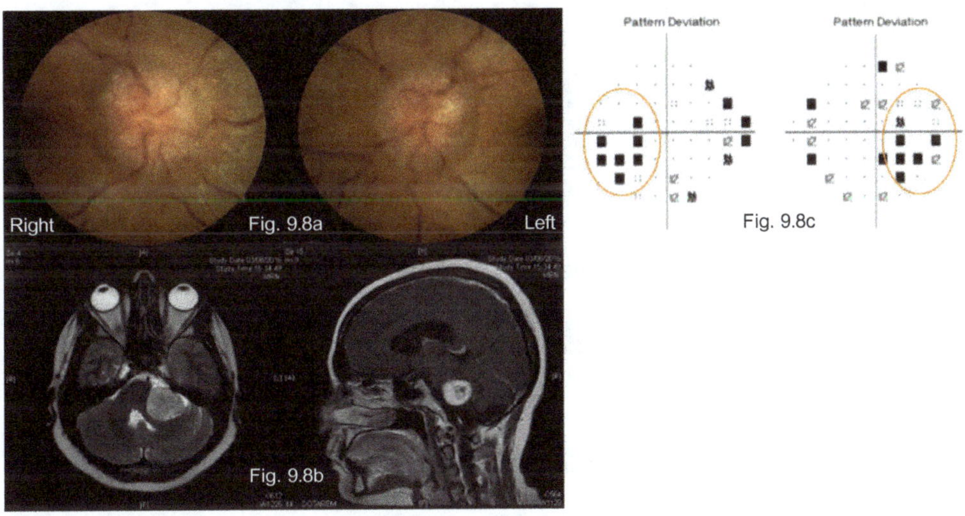

Fig. 9.8. (a) Bilateral severely swollen discs; (b) neuroimaging showing a space-occupying lesion compressing the fourth ventricle; (c) perimetry demonstrating enlarged blind spots (orange circles).

What are the Life-threatening Considerations in a Patient with Bilateral Swollen Discs?

- Malignant hypertension
- Raised intracranial pressure, e.g. masses, meningitis, intracranial haemorrhage
- Cerebral venous thrombosis

What Investigations Should You Order?

- Urgent blood pressure check
- Urgent neuroimaging: MRI brain with contrast and Magnetic Resonance Venogram (MRV)
- If above are normal, a lumbar puncture (LP) for opening pressure and CSF studies is indicated

What are the Causes of Raised Intracranial Pressure?

- Space-occupying lesions
- Infections/inflammations, e.g. meningitis
- Haemorrhage — spontaneous bleed or secondary to trauma
- Idiopathic

What is Idiopathic Intracranial Hypertension (IIH)/Pseudotumour Cerebri (PTC)?

IIH/PTC is a spectrum of disorders, with several associations (see below), which results in raised ICP, with no intracranial pathology found. These patients may present with headaches, transient visual obscurations, and/or disc swelling, with a corresponding decrease in optic nerve function.

What are the Risk Factors/Associations for IIH/PTC?

- Obesity
- Hormones — hormonal imbalance from gynaecologic disease, medications (e.g. oral contraceptives)
- Medications — steroids (use or withdrawal), vitamin A, tetracycline

What are the Diagnostic Criteria for IIH/PTC (Modified Dandy Criteria)?

- Awake and alert patient
- Symptoms of raised ICP — headaches, blurring of vision
- Normal MRI
- Normal neurological examination except for Abducens Nerve (CN6 palsy) and/or optic disc swelling
- Raised opening pressures of >25 mm H_2O found on LP performed in the lateral decubitus position
- Normal CSF composition
- No other explanation for the raised ICP

How are Patients with IIH/PTC Managed?

- Treat/remove any associations
- Lifestyle modifications — weight loss and management of other metabolic diseases
- Pain relief — analgesia for headaches
- Reduce ICP — acetazolamide, topiramate, surgical interventions (CSF stents or shunts), and optic nerve sheath fenestration

Take Home Message

Optic neuropathies can present as pale or swollen discs and could be classified as unilateral or bilateral.

9.2 Visual Field Defects

Learning Objectives

- To detect visual field defects on confrontational visual field.
- To recognise patterns of monocular and binocular visual field defects and the site of the lesions causing these defects.

Detection of Visual Field (VF) Defects

Visual field examination should be performed for ALL patients who have visual complaints. Visual field defects may be monocular or binocular. While the cause of the visual field defect is not always apparent on ocular or neurologic examination, the pattern of the visual field defect is often suggestive of the site of insult to the visual pathway.

Figure 9.9. illustrates the common visual field defects that one may encounter with lesions along the visual pathway. Table 9.3 summarises the common VF defects that we encounter in our practice and a guide to further investigations that we perform.

Patients with visual field defects may have normal central visual acuity, and have non-specific complaints of general blurring, darkening of vision, presenting with unexplained falls or bumping into objects. Some others may be completely asymptomatic and found to have visual field defects when being screened for other conditions.

In general, monocular field defects tend to suggest lesions in one eye or optic nerve, while certain patterns of binocular defects suggest lesions of the visual pathway beyond the optic nerves.

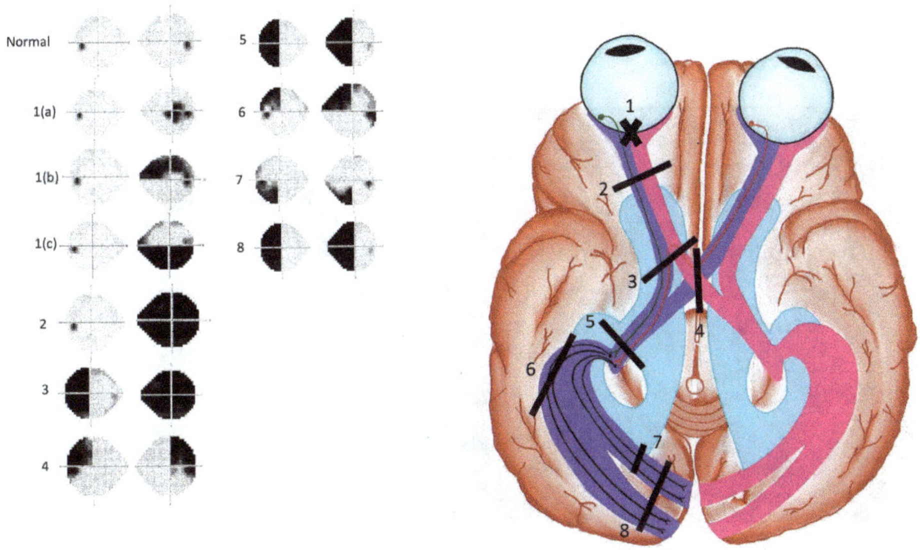

Fig. 9.9. Lesions of the visual pathway at various levels and their corresponding field defects.

Table 9.3. Examples of Commonly Encountered Visual Field Defects

Monocular visual field defects	Cause/site of lesion	Further investigations (guide)
1. Central scotoma 2. Inferior altitudinal defect 3. Arcuate defect arising from blind spot	1. Macula, optic nerve (e.g. optic neuritis) 2. Optic nerve (ischaemic optic neuropathy) 3. Optic nerve (glaucoma)	• Macula OCT • Fluorescein angiogram • OCT RNFL • MRI of the orbits and anterior visual pathway ± brain

Binocular visual field defects		
1. Pattern of monocular visual loss, which presents bilaterally 2. Bitemporal hemianopia 3. Homonymous hemianopia 4. Homonymous superior quadrantanopia 5. Homonymous superior quadrantanopia	1. Bilateral optic neuropathies or retinopathies 2. Optic chiasm 3. Contralateral retrochiasmal visual pathway 4. Contralateral temporal lobe* 5. Contralateral parietal lobe* *Suggestive but not exclusive	MRI of the orbits and anterior visual pathway ± brain Lumbar puncture if indicated

Monocular Visual Field Defects

Monocular visual field defects are usually ocular in origin. However, at times, visual pathway disorders can present as monocular visual field defects, either because they are asymmetrical or because only the central visual fields were examined.

When dealing with a monocular visual field defect, it is important to consider both optic neuropathies, as well as retinopathies (which include maculopathies) as differential diagnoses. Retinal causes of visual loss will be discussed in Chapter 6.

Figure 9.10 shows a superior arcuate defect secondary to glaucomatous damage to the optic nerve.

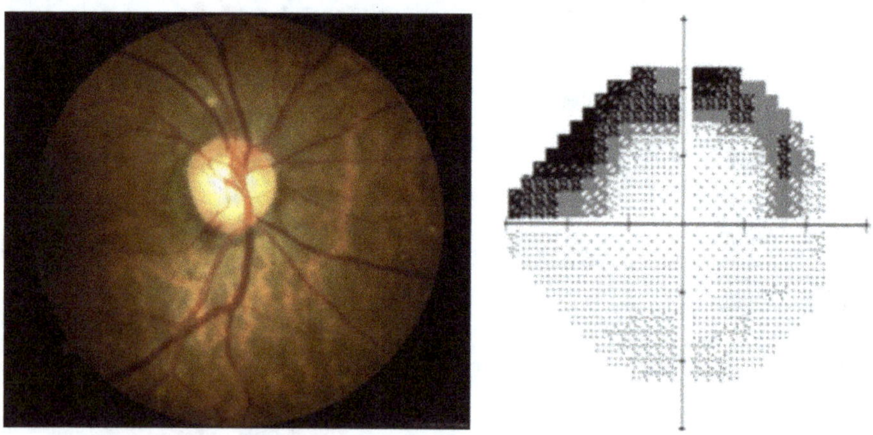

Fig. 9.10. Thinning of the optic nerve rim inferiorly with associated drance haemorrhage secondary to glaucoma.

Binocular Visual Field Defects

Binocular visual field defects can occur because of bilateral optic neuropathies or retinopathies (Fig. 9.11) or from a lesion anywhere along the visual pathway from the optic chiasm to the occipital lobe. Because of the way the fibres of the visual pathway are arranged, visual field defects tend to be more congruous if the lesion is more posterior. For example, an occipital lobe lesion (Fig. 9.12) will give rise to a visual field defect that is more congruous than that of a pre-geniculate optic tract lesion.

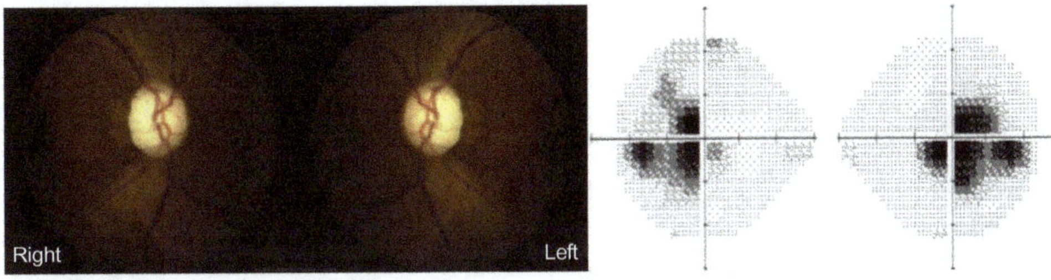

Fig. 9.11. Bilateral optic disc cupping and temporal pallor, with corresponding cecocentral visual field defects, likely secondary to hereditary optic neuropathy.

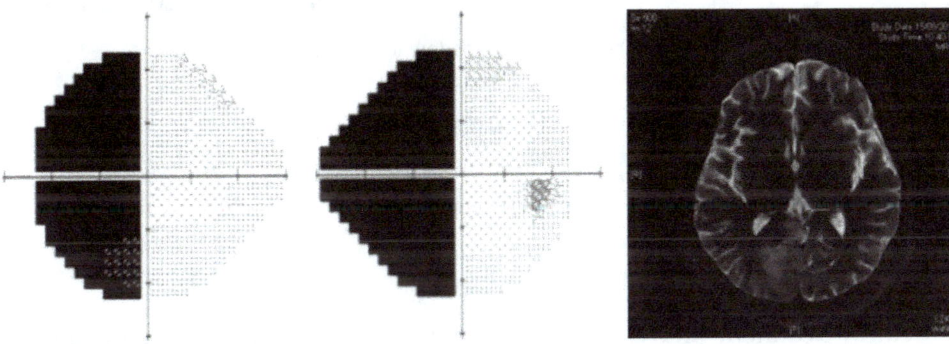

Fig. 9.12. Congruous homonymous hemianopia secondary to occipital lobe infarction.

As patients may report blurring of vision as their chief complaint, it is crucial to enquire if they occluded one eye to determine the side of blurring. Often, hemianopias or quadrantanopias may be thought to be blurring of vision of the side of the visual field defect.

Clinical Case Examples of Visual Field Defects

Bitemporal Hemianopia

A 28-year-old man was referred after an optometrist noticed disc pallor during screening. He was otherwise asymptomatic, but on further questioning revealed that he had breast enlargement. His visual acuity was 6/6 bilaterally and he had normal colour vision. There was no RAPD. On clinical examination, he was found to have bow tie pallor of his optic discs (Fig. 9.13) and a bitemporal hemianopia. MRI scan showed a pituitary macroadenoma, compressing on the optic chiasm (Fig. 9.14).

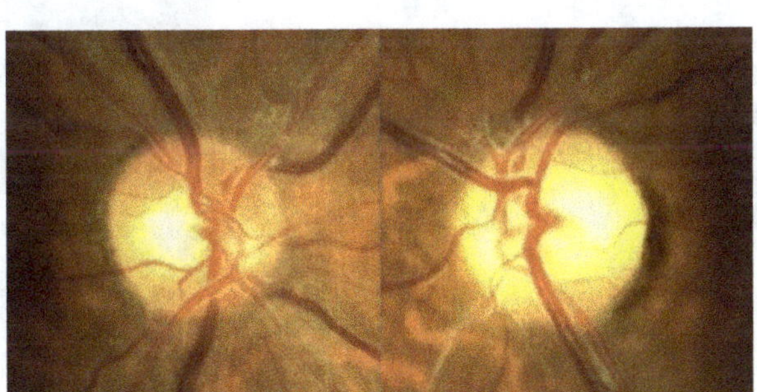

Fig. 9.13. Bow-tie optic disc pallor, which is more evident on the left.

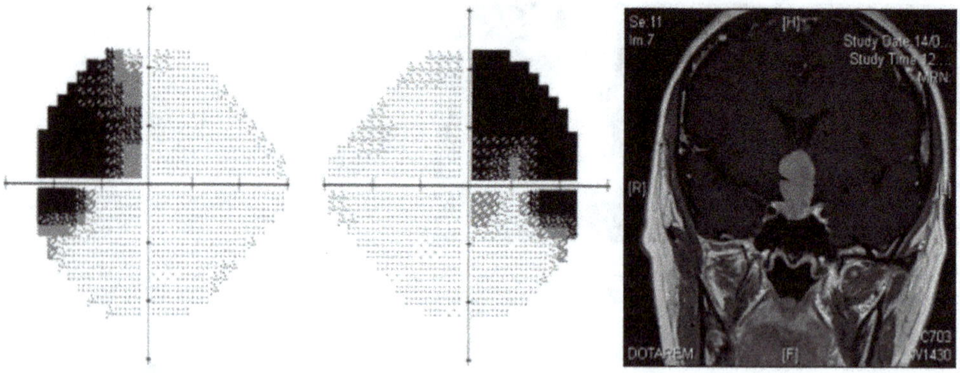

Fig. 9.14. Bitemporal hemianopia secondary to a pituitary macroadenoma.

What Other Investigations Should be Performed?

In addition to neuroimaging, investigation of the pituitary hormones should be performed.

How Should You Manage Patients with Pituitary Adenomas?

- Co-manage with endocrinologist and neurosurgeon
- Medical treatment (individualised) — hormone supplements, cabergoline or bromocriptine (for prolactinoma)
- Surgical intervention is indicated if there is evidence of compressive optic neuropathy, progressive enlargement of tumour and/or invasion of the cavernous sinus

Homonymous Hemianopia

A 70-year-old Chinese man with a background of diabetes mellitus and hypertension presented with right-sided blurring of vision for 2 days. He was still able to drive and read the newspapers. Visual acuities were 6/6 in either eye, and ocular examination was unremarkable apart from age-related cataracts. His colour vision and pupil examination were normal, and he was found to have right homonymous hemianopia on visual field testing. Urgent neuroimaging confirmed the presence of a stroke of the left occipital lobe (Fig. 9.15).

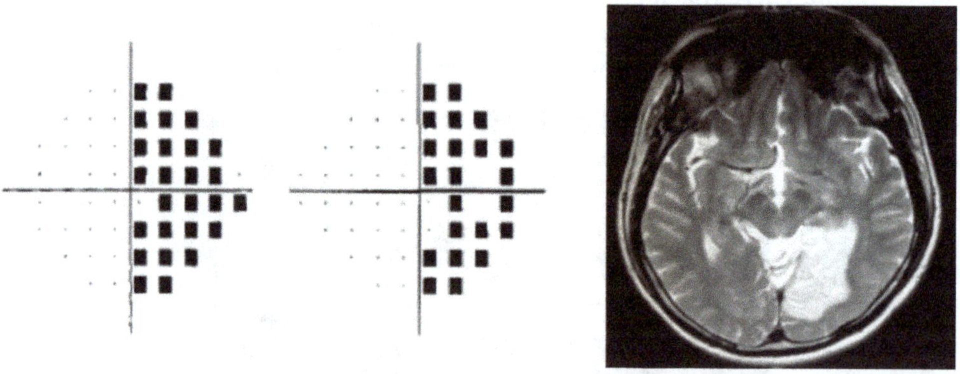

Fig. 9.15. Macular sparing right homonymous hemianopia secondary to a left occipital infarct.

How Will You Manage this Patient?

- Determine risk factors for stroke — investigate for hypertension, diabetes mellitus, hyperlipidaemia and sources of emboli
- Co-manage with neurologist
- Treat underlying risk factors

Take Home Message
The pattern of visual field defect can help to localise the lesion.

9.3 Ocular Motility Disorders

Learning Objectives

- Understand the innervation of the extraocular muscles and identify motility disorders (limitations).
- Understand the use of a cover test in the context of strabismus resulting from neuro-ophthalmic disease.
- Recognise common patterns of ocular motility abnormalities.

History

Ocular motility disorders frequently present with diplopia. However, some patients may not complain of any visual symptoms, and some may report slight blurring of vision rather than double vision. When faced with a patient who has diplopia, it is important to determine the following:

The important details to determine in the evaluation of a patient with diplopia are:

- Is the diplopia monocular or binocular? (Table 9.4)
- Is the diplopia vertical, horizontal or oblique (torsional)? This refers to the location and orientation of the second image.
- Is the diplopia the same in all directions of gaze? This refers to the separation and orientation of the images.
- Is the diplopia constant or intermittent?
- Has the diplopia been static since onset or progressive?

Table 9.4. Causes of Diplopia

Monocular	Binocular		
Tends to be ocular in nature	Paretic		Restrictive
	Supranuclear	Nuclear/Infranuclear/ NMJ/Muscle	
1. Cornea* 2. Lens* 3. Macula 4. Cerebral polyopia (rare)		1. Cranial nerve palsies (single/multiple) 2. Myasthenia gravis 3. Myopathies	1. Thyroid eye disease 2. Orbital inflammatory disease 3. Orbital wall fractures

*Monocular diplopia from disturbances in the optical media typically resolves when looking through a pinhole.

Ocular Motility Examination

The ocular motility examination is directed at elucidating the site and cause of the ocular motility defect. It begins with determining if there is any limitation in ocular motility, whether it is restrictive or paretic, and the nerve(s) and/or muscle(s) involved. The innervation of the extraocular muscles is shown in Table 9.5.

The basic eye movement examination consists of examining pursuit (slow) movements to determine the range (extent) of eye movements into the different positions of gaze. The eyes are first observed in the primary position (looking straight ahead) using the corneal light reflex (Hirschberg test) to determine the relative position of the eyes. The patient is then asked to track a target into the nine cardinal positions of gaze (including primary position) to determine how far the eyes move into each of those positions. Figure 9.16 shows a normal ocular motility examination.

Table 9.5. Innervation of and Movements Produced by the Extraocular Muscles

	Primary Action	Secondary Action	Tertiary Action	Innervation
Medial rectus	Adduction	—	—	3rd (oculomotor) cranial nerve
Lateral rectus	Abduction	—	—	6th (abducens) cranial nerve
Superior rectus	Elevation	Intorsion	Adduction	3rd (oculomotor) cranial nerve
Inferior rectus	Depression	Extorsion	Adduction	3rd (oculomotor) cranial nerve
Superior oblique	Intorsion	Depression	Abduction	4th (trochlear) cranial nerve
Inferior oblique	Extorsion	Elevation	Abduction	3rd (oculomotor) cranial nerve

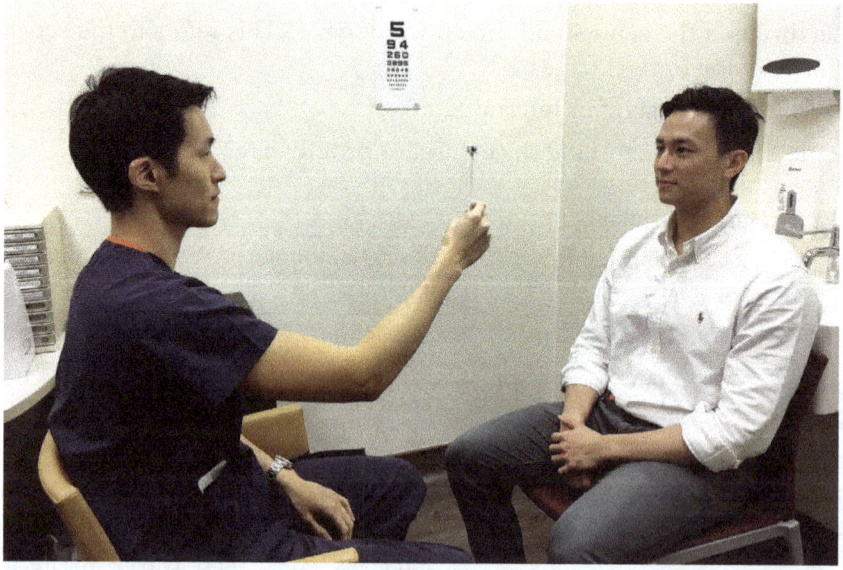

Fig. 9.16. (a) Performing the ocular motility examination with an accommodative target.

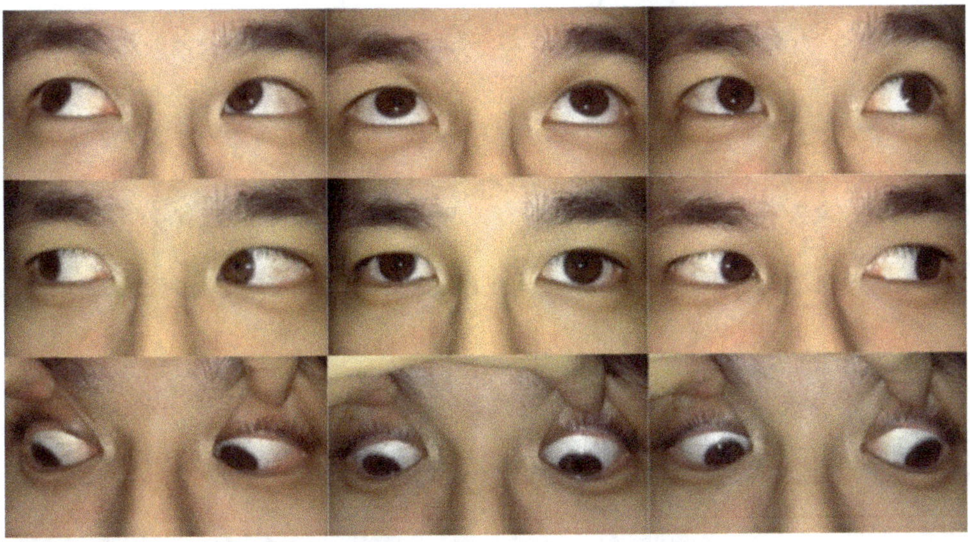

Fig. 9.16. (b) Shows the normal range of ocular motility.

Further Eye Movement Testing Includes:

- Saccadic (fast) eye movements
- Cover test in the different gaze positions (primary position, right, left, up and down-gaze as well as right and left head tilts). The alternate cover test dissociates the eyes and allows for small angles of deviation to be detected by the examiner. This allows subtle ocular motility defects to be elucidated. The angle of deviation can also be measured using prisms, and this is important for diagnosis and follow up. (See Chapter 8: Paediatric Ophthalmology.)

Clinical Case Examples of Ocular Motility Disorders

Oculomotor Nerve Palsy

A 59-year-old man with a past medical history of diabetes mellitus, hypertension and ischaemic heart disease presented acutely with dizziness and difficulty opening his eyes. His eye movements in 9 positions of gaze (Fig. 9.17) are shown below. There was no anisocoria, and the remainder of the ocular examination, including optic nerve function, was otherwise normal.

What is the Diagnosis?

Nuclear oculomotor nerve palsy (CN3 Palsy). The presence of bilateral ptosis can be explained by the innervation of a central subnucleus (in the midbrain) (Fig. 9.18) supplying the bilateral levator palpebrae superioris, and the contralateral elevation deficit is due to contralateral innervation of the superior recti muscle.

Should this Patient have Neuroimaging?

Yes. Urgent neuroimaging in the form of MRI brain with contrast and MR angiogram should be performed.

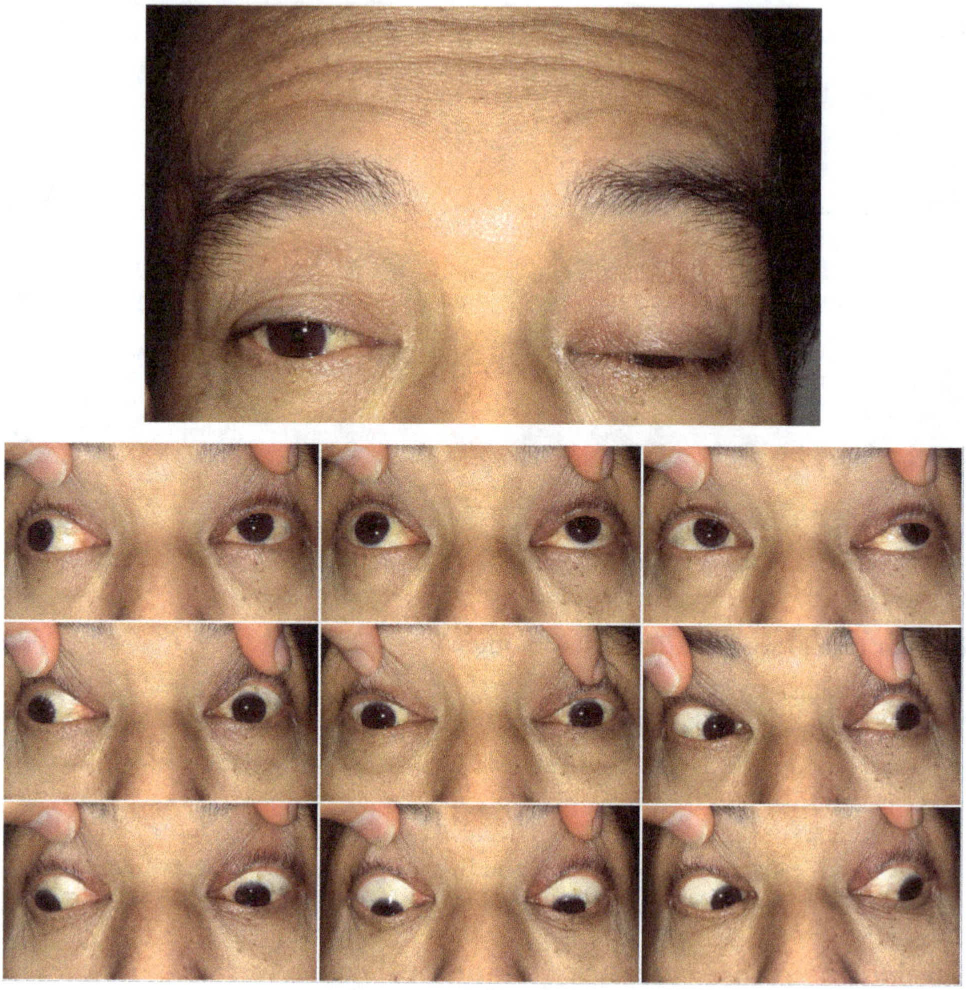

Fig. 9.17. Ocular motility.

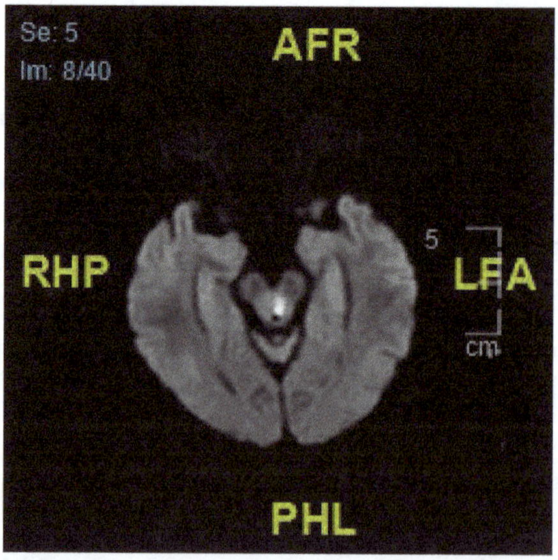

Fig. 9.18. MRI brain shows an infarct in the midbrain, affecting the oculomotor nucleus.

How Should this Patient be Managed?

Co-management with a physician and neurologist is critical for the control of risk factors. Additional investigations include an ultrasound of the carotid and vertebral arteries and a 2D echocardiogram of the heart.

Abducens Nerve Palsy

A 63-year-old man with a background history of diabetes mellitus and hypertension presents with a 2-day history of acute, binocular, horizontal diplopia. His visual acuity is 6/6 bilaterally and the pupillary examination is unremarkable. His range of eye movements is shown in Fig. 9.19.

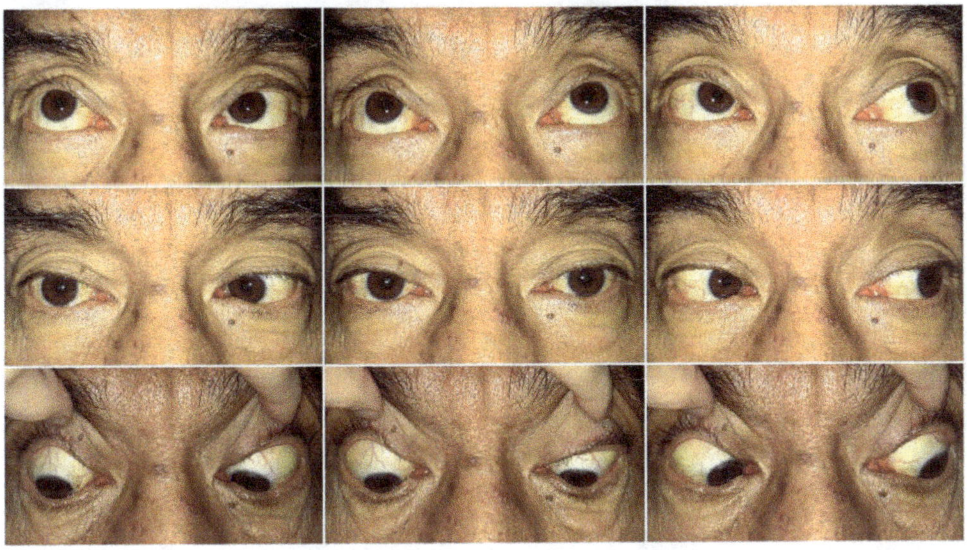

Fig. 9.19. Ocular motility.

What are the Possible Causes of an Abduction Deficit?

Paretic	Restrictive
Abducens nerve palsy Myasthenia gravis Miller Fisher syndrome	Medial wall fractures Thyroid eye disease Muscle fibrosis from longstanding palsy

What Does this Patient Have? What Else is Important in His Examination?

- Right abduction deficit, possibly due to an abducens nerve palsy (CN6 palsy)
- CN6 palsy may be a false localising sign in raised intracranial pressure. All patients with a CN6 palsy should have a dilated fundus examination to exclude optic disc(s) swelling secondary to raised ICP.

How Should He Be Managed?

- Co-manage ischaemic risk factors with the internist
- ENT review to exclude nasal pathology such as nasopharyngeal carcinoma
- Conservative management with monocular occlusion or prisms. If the cause is ischaemic, there is a chance of spontaneous recovery over weeks to months.

- Surgery should only be considered after AT LEAST 6 months of observation, with stable prism cover test measurements

Myasthenia Gravis

A 60-year-old man presents with 2 weeks' history of worsening diplopia throughout the day. Ocular examination reveals cataract and limitation of eye movements in multiple directions of gaze (Fig. 9.20). In addition, there is an improvement of his ocular motility following a neostigmine test (Fig. 9.21).

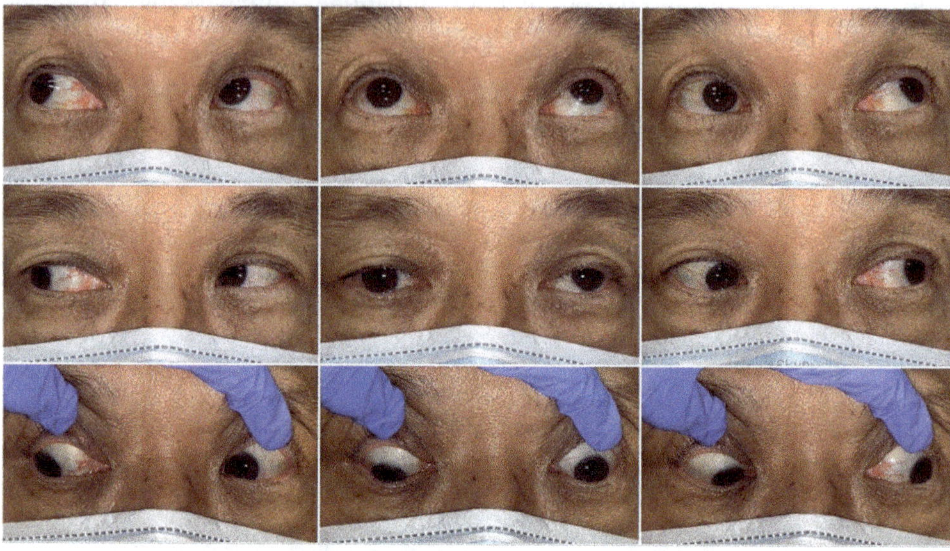

Fig. 9.20. Ocular motility of a patient with myasthenia gravis.

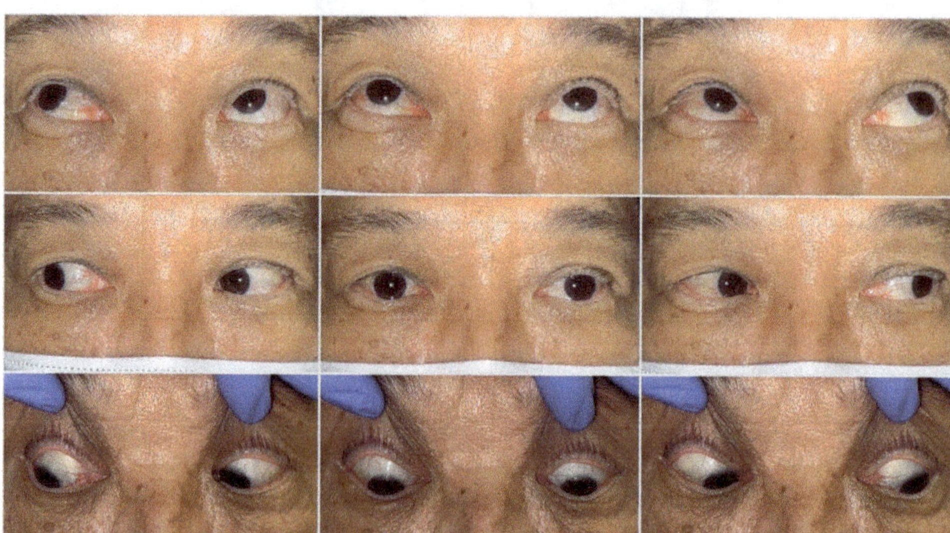

Fig. 9.21. Improvement in ocular motility following a neostigmine test.

What are the Differential Diagnoses?

- Myasthenia gravis
- Cranial nerve palsy
- Myopathies, e.g. myotonic dystrophy, chronic progressive external ophthalmoplegia

What is the Pathology in Myasthenia Gravis (MG)?

The muscle weakness that occurs in MG is secondary to antibodies at the neuromuscular junction (NMJ), which interfere with normal interaction between acetylcholine and its receptors (Fig. 9.22).

How is the Diagnosis of Myasthenia Gravis Made?

- Clinical — ice pack test, neostigmine test, edrophonium test
- Biochemical — anti-acetylcholine receptor antibody, anti-muscle specific kinase antibody

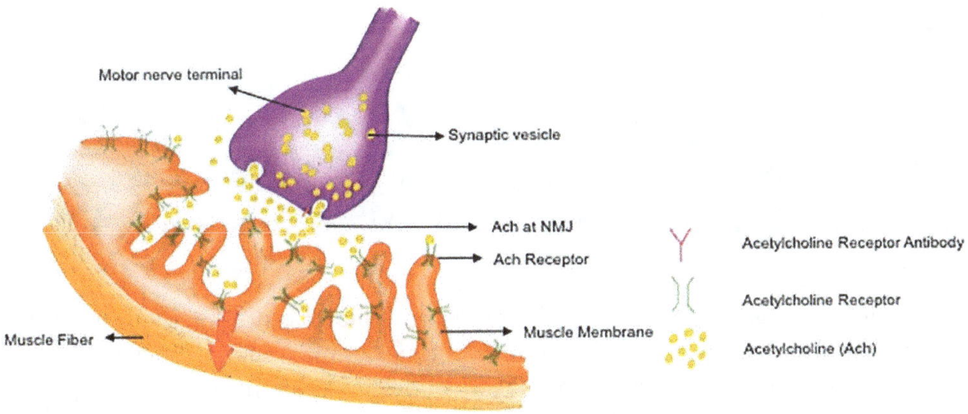

Fig. 9.22. (a) Normal neuromuscular junction (NMJ). Ach release and its interaction with nicotinic receptors on the muscle membrane.

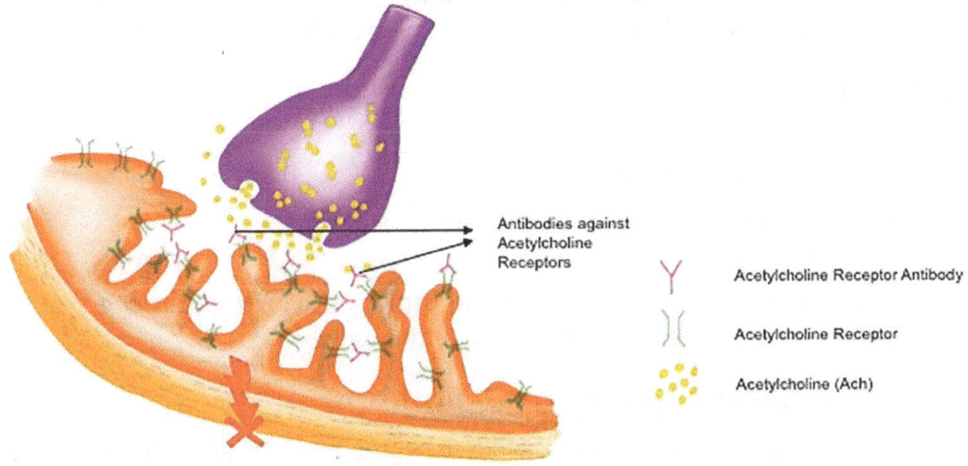

Fig. 9.22. (b) NMJ in myasthenia gravis. In myasthenia gravis, the normal interaction between the Ach and its receptors is affected by the presence of antibodies, which compete with Ach to bind with the receptors, causing weakness of muscle contraction.

- Electrophysiology — single-fibre electromyogram and repetitive nerve stimulation
- Imaging (supporting test) — in patients with myasthenia, a CT thorax should be performed to exclude a thymoma

How is Myasthenia Gravis Treated?

- Anti-cholinesterase, e.g. pyridostigmine
- Corticosteroids and/or steroid-sparing agents
- Thymectomy (if there is a thymoma)
- Plasmapheresis and intravenous immunoglobulin (typically for generalised myasthenia or myasthenic crisis)

Take Home Message

Consider myasthenia gravis in all ocular motility deficits.

9.4 Pupillary Abnormalities

Learning Objectives

- To be able to perform a complete an examination of the pupils.
- To appreciate the various abnormalities in relation to afferent and efferent pathway disorders.

History

Pupillary abnormalities may be discovered incidentally by the patient or family member or during an ocular examination. At times, pupil abnormalities present as part of another ophthalmic problem that was brought to attention; for example, in the case of a pupil involving CN3 palsy.

Important questions to ask in the history depend on the type of pupillary abnormality found. In addition, questions pertaining to general health, existing comorbidities, medication (topical and systemic) as well as a history of trauma are important in all patients. More specific questions are listed below.

Anisocoria

- How was it noticed?
- Any pain — including headache, neck pain
- History of trauma?
- Use of medications
- Presence of other symptoms, including diplopia (which might suggest an oculomotor nerve palsy), limb weakness or numbness

Relative Afferent Pupillary Defect (RAPD)

- Any preceding visual loss? (Important to examine the optic nerve function)
- Neurological deficits

Light-near Dissociation

- History of diabetes mellitus
- Sexual history/known history of syphilis or herpetic infection
- Others: alcohol consumption, recent illness

Case Example of Pupillary Abnormality

Horner's Syndrome

A 68-year-old Chinese man complains of right-sided mild ptosis. He also has a background history of weight loss and epistaxis. He had no prior history of eyelid trauma, cataract surgery or contact lens use and he denied the use of any topical medications. Visual acuity was 6/9 bilaterally, and apart from nuclear sclerotic cataracts, examination of the anterior and posterior segments was unremarkable. He was noted to have anisocoria, which was worse in the dark. Apraclonidine eye drops reversed the anisocoria (Fig. 9.23).

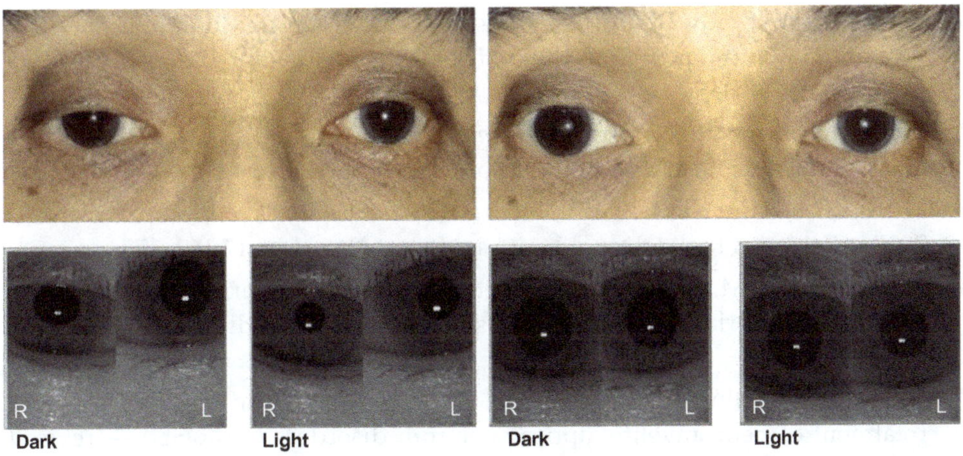

Fig. 9.23. Pre- and post-apraclonidine test, demonstrating right eyelid elevation and reversal of anisocoria.

What is Horner's Syndrome?

Horner's syndrome refers to the constellation of findings (partial ptosis, miosis and/or anhidrosis) resulting from a lesion affecting any part of the sympathetic pathway.

In this patient, it was secondary to the nasopharyngeal carcinoma, which invaded the cavernous sinus.

What are the Potential Life-threatening Causes of Horner's Syndrome?

- Intracranial pathology — strokes, compressive lesions
- Neck pathology — pancoast tumour, enlarged thyroid, lymphadenopathy, trauma

- Vascular — carotid artery dissection, cavernous sinus infiltration

How Do You Diagnose Horner's Syndrome?

- Confirmatory tests — cocaine test, apraclonidine test
- Localisation tests — hydroxyamphetamine test, phenylephrine test
- Appropriate imaging

Take Home Message

Horner's syndrome comprises a triad of partial ptosis, miosis and anhidrosis.

References

1. American Academy of Ophthalmology, *Neuro-ophthalmology* **87**:2014–2015.
2. Digre KB and Corbett JJ. (2001) Idiopathic intracranial hypertension (pseudotumor cerebri): A reappraisal. *Neurologist* **7**:2–67.
3. Optic Neuritis Study Group. (2008) Visual function 15 years after optic neuritis: A final follow-up report from the optic neuritis treatment trial. *Ophthalmology* **115(6)**:1079–1082 e5.
4. *Walsh and Hoyt's Clinical Neuro-ophthalmology: The Essentials*, 2nd ed. Nuclear and Infranuclear Ocular Motility Disorders, Chapter 18, p. 391.
5. Thomson A, Banwell BL, Barkhof F, *et al.* (2018) Diagnosis of multiple sclerosis: 2017 revisions of the McDonald criteria. *Lancet Neurology* **17**:162–173.
6. Wingerchuck DM, Banwell BL, Bennett JL, *et al.* (2015) International consensus diagnostic criteria for neuromyelitis optica spectrum disorders *Neurology* **85**:177–189.
7. Kümpfel T, Giglhuber K, Aktas O, *et al.* (2024) Update on the diagnosis and treatment of neuromyelitis optica spectrum disorders (NMOSD) — revised recommendations of the Neuromyelitis Optica Study Group (NEMOS). Part II: Attack therapy and long-term management. *Journal of Neurology* **271**:141–176.
8. Banwell BL, Bennett JL, Marignier R, *et al.* (2023) Diagnosis of myelin oligodendrocyte glycoprotein antibody-associated disease: International MOGAD Panel proposed criteria. *Lancet Neurology* **22**:268–282.

Chapter 10

PRINCIPLES AND PRACTICE OF LOW VISION REHABILITATION

Danial Bohan

Learning Objectives

- Understand the role of low vision care in ophthalmology.
- Identify patients with low vision.
- Understand the functional impact of low vision.
- Understand low vision evaluation and management.
- Refer the patient for low vision rehabilitation services.

The number of elderly living with vision loss will increase over the decades, with the ageing population and increasing longevity in Singapore and globally. Therefore, understanding the principles of low vision care and practice is critical and relevant.

10.1 What is Low Vision?

Low vision is vision impairment that is not corrected by standard eyeglasses or by medical or surgical treatment. It may result from many different ocular and neurological disorders.

A person with low vision is one who has:

- An impairment of visual functioning even after treatment and/or standard refraction correction
- A visual acuity of less than 6/18 to light perception
- A visual field of less than 10° from the point of fixation, but who
- Uses, or is potentially able to use, vision for the planning and/or execution of a task

Lighthouse International revised this definition of visual impairment to include aspects of functioning:

Functional visual impairment is a significant limitation of visual capability resulting from disease, trauma or congenital condition, which cannot be fully ameliorated by standard refractive correction, medication or surgery, and is manifested by one of the following:

- Insufficient visual resolution (worse than 6/12 in the better eye with the best correction of ametropia)
- Inadequate field of vision (20° or worse along the widest meridian in the eye with the more intact central field; homonymous hemianopia)

- Reduced peak contrast sensitivity (<1.7 log CS binocularly)
- Insufficient visual resolution or peak contrast sensitivity at high or low luminances within the range typically encountered in everyday life

This expanded definition takes a functional perspective and compels us to consider any patient who has difficulty performing a visual task as potentially in need of low vision care and rehabilitation.

The American Academy of Ophthalmology's Smartsight Model of Vision Rehabilitation similarly adopts this functional definition of low vision and calls for ophthalmologists to refer patients with low vision for rehabilitation at two levels:

- Level 1 asks all ophthalmologists who see patients with less than 6/12 visual acuity in the better eye, contrast sensitivity loss, scotoma or field loss to "recognise" and "respond" by assuring patients that much can be offered with rehabilitation
- Level 2 incorporates comprehensive multidisciplinary vision rehabilitation care processes as part of the continuum of ophthalmic care

10.2 Functional Impact of Low Vision

In low vision care, it is crucial to understand pathology from a functional perspective and explains visual deficits and complaints. The pathological process correlates with the patient's functional status. It also influences management decisions, the types of optical aids and vision rehabilitation services needed, and the patient's ability to respond to those interventions.

Faye *et al.* classified three types of visual deficits based on the effects of functional vision, which is paramount when approaching the patient with low vision — cloudy media (Fig. 10.1), central field deficit (Fig. 10.2) and peripheral field deficit (Fig. 10.3).

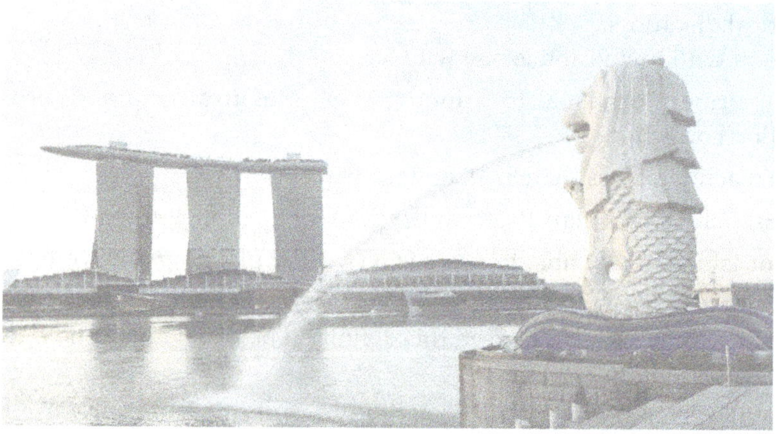

Fig. 10.1. Cloudy media.

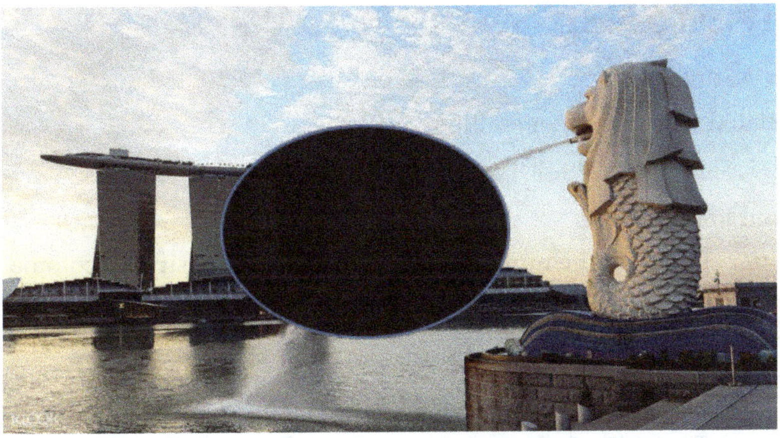

Fig. 10.2. Central field deficit.

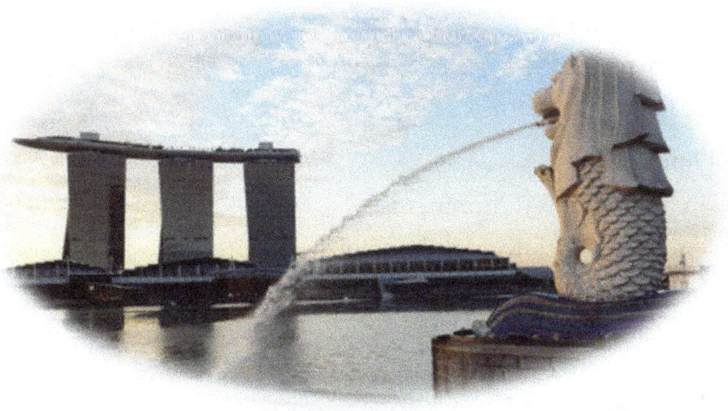

Fig. 10.3. Peripheral field deficit.

Cloudy Media

Common Aetiology

- Corneal scars, dystrophy and oedema
- Pupil/iris atrophy, polycoria and iridectomy
- Inoperable cataract
- Vitreous inflammation and haemorrhage

Functional Implications

- Blurred vision for distance and near tasks
- Faded colours
- Glare disability
- Reduced contrast sensitivity

Central Field Deficit

Common Aetiology

- Age-related macular degeneration
- Macular scar and ischaemia

Functional Implications

- Varies depending on the number, size, location and density of scotoma
- Reduced central vision for distance, intermediate and near tasks; reading and facial recognition
- Reduced retinal illuminance

Peripheral Field Deficit

Common Aetiology

- Advanced glaucoma
- Retinitis pigmentosa
- Neurologic (stroke, tumours)

Functional Implications

- Mobility in unfamiliar environments
- Anxiety and bumping into peripheral objects
- Mobility at night and under poor illumination
- Locating objects

Low Vision Evaluation

The low vision evaluation takes a functional and clinical approach to optimise patient performance in daily living tasks and include the following components:

- History
- Visual acuity and refraction
- Visual field testing
- Contrast sensitivity function
- Magnification evaluation

History

The history aims to uncover the patient's chief complaint and functional loss. Therefore, it is important to think not just in terms of anatomical lesions but also in terms of the patient's loss of ability to perform daily living tasks. The history covers the following aspects:

- Chief complaint
- Visual/ocular history
- General health review
- Activities of daily living
- Lifestyle, education and career history

- Social history and support systems
- Psycho-social issues, adjustment and coping
- Functional and task-related history
- Priorities and goals of rehabilitation

Visual Acuity and Refraction

Visual acuity and refraction are performed to establish the patient's residual vision and to determine visual disability. Assessing visual acuity and refraction is critical to:

- Monitor the effect, progression and treatment of eye diseases
- Determine the magnification of optical low vision aids for reading
- Verify a patient's visual fitness to drive
- Classify patients as "legally blind" for assistance schemes, support services, benefits and exemptions

The Early Treatment Diabetic Retinopathy Study (ETDRS) chart is widely used in low vision assessment as it incorporates accepted principles of chart design (Fig. 10.4).

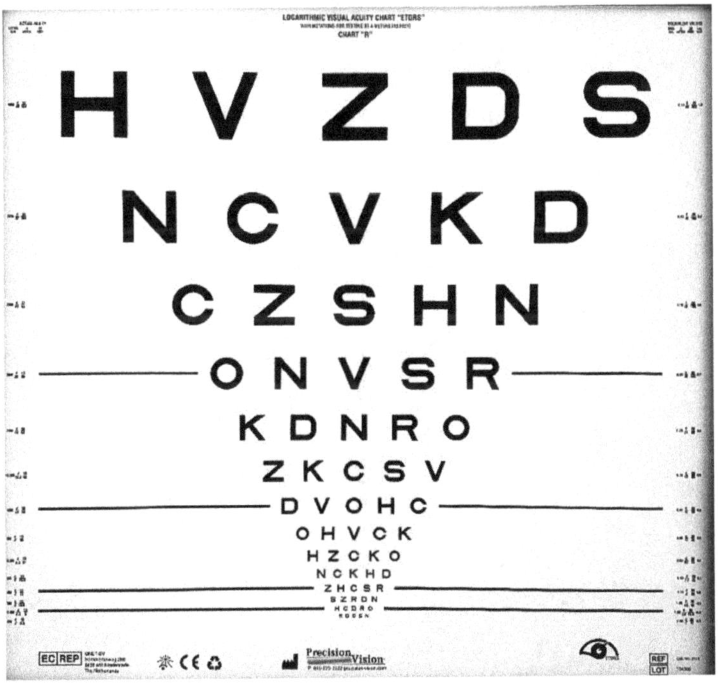

Fig. 10.4. ETDRS chart.

Visual Field Testing

Perimetry, or visual field testing, aims to evaluate the depth and breadth of a patient's field of view. For absolute peripheral field defect, dynamic visual field testing such as a Tangent screen or Goldmann perimetry is useful (Fig. 10.5). For central field defect, threshold testing such as the Humphrey visual field analyser or California Central Field Test is more appropriate (Fig. 10.6). The purpose of undertaking visual field testing in low vision is to explain the nature of disability described or noted by the patient.

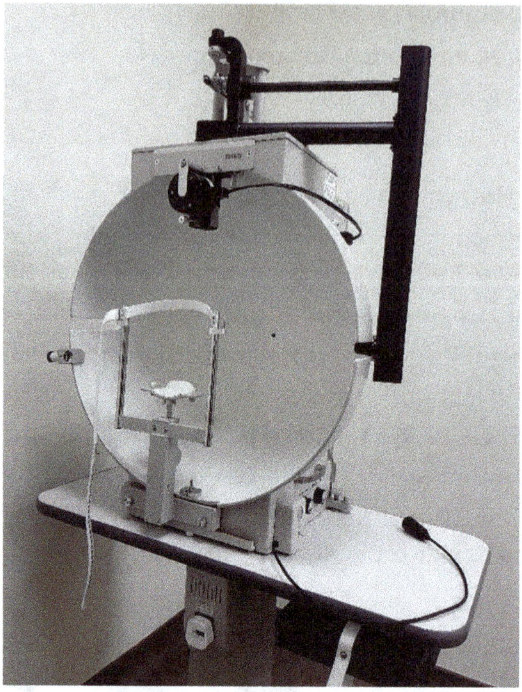

Fig. 10.5. Goldmann perimeter.

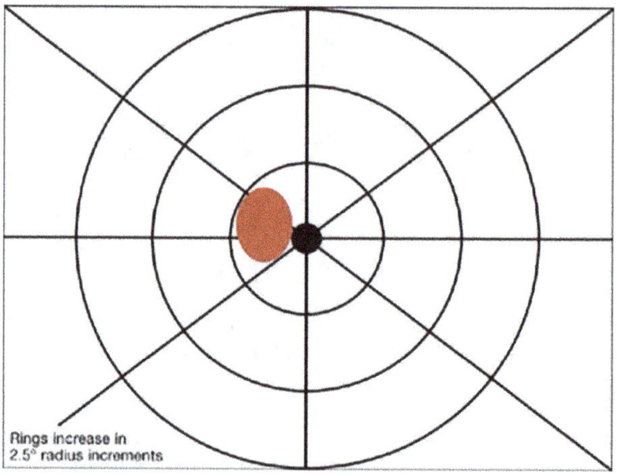

Fig. 10.6. California Central Field Test.

A recent development in low vision evaluation is an assessment of scotomas (blind spots within the visual field) and training patients to use healthy retinal areas to optimise viewing.

Visual field testing is important for the following reasons:

- Provide objective information about scotomas and correlate with poor task performance
- Show patterns of peripheral field loss for the indication of orientation and mobility training and rehabilitation planning

- Follow disease progression and explain functional visual change that does not correlate with acuity or contrast test

Contrast Sensitivity Function

Contrast sensitivity function is critical in activities such as face recognition and navigating steps. The Pelli-Robson Chart (Fig. 10.7) is commonly used to assess contrast sensitivity. This test is valuable to help the patient gain a greater understanding of the nature of their visual impairment and why certain adaptive strategies can be adopted to optimise vision.

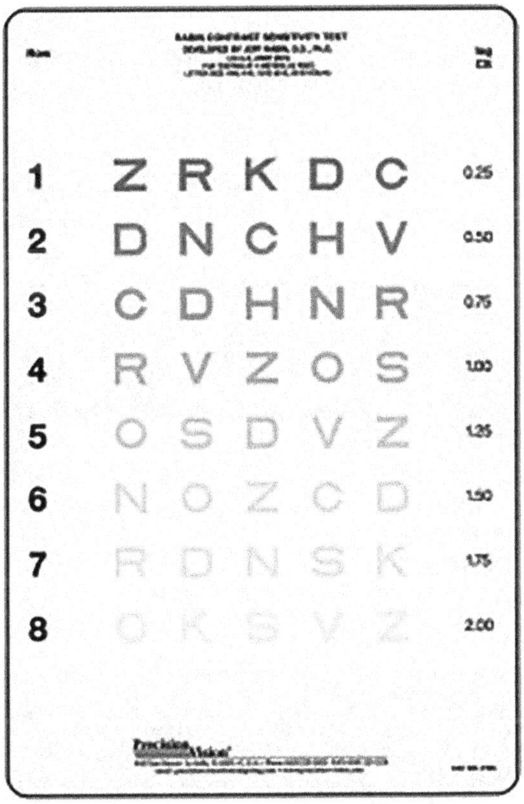

Fig. 10.7. Pelli-Robson chart.

Contrast sensitivity is useful for:

- Determining magnification need
- Assessing the ability to use optical low vision aids
- Determining the optimal illumination level to maximise vision
- Monitoring disease progression
- Understanding the overall functioning of the patient and plan rehabilitative strategies

Magnification Evaluation

The primary management for low vision is to optimise residual vision through magnification — the process of optically enlarging the retinal image with an optical device. After a low vision evaluation and complete assessment of the patient's needs and visual abilities, an optical device is prescribed to enhance function and critical tasks in everyday life, education and work. Magnification can be achieved using four different methods:

- Relative size magnification
- Relative distance (approach) magnification
- Angular magnification
- Electronic magnification

Relative size magnification involves physically enlarging texts or using large print devices (Fig. 10.8).

Relative distance magnification is achieved by bringing objects closer (approaching) to the eyes and focussing the image with a magnifier (Fig. 10.9).

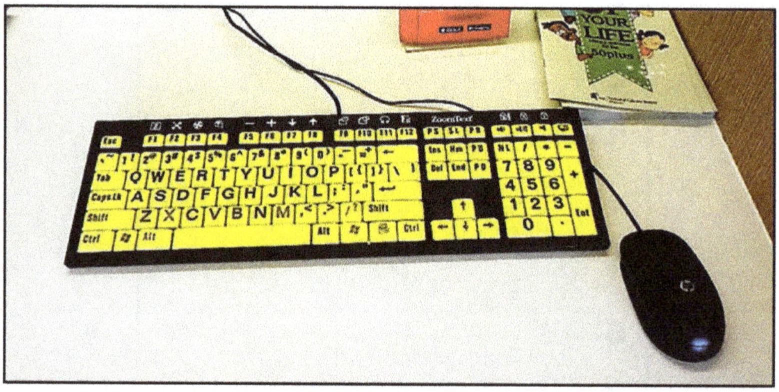

Fig. 10.8. Large keyboard.

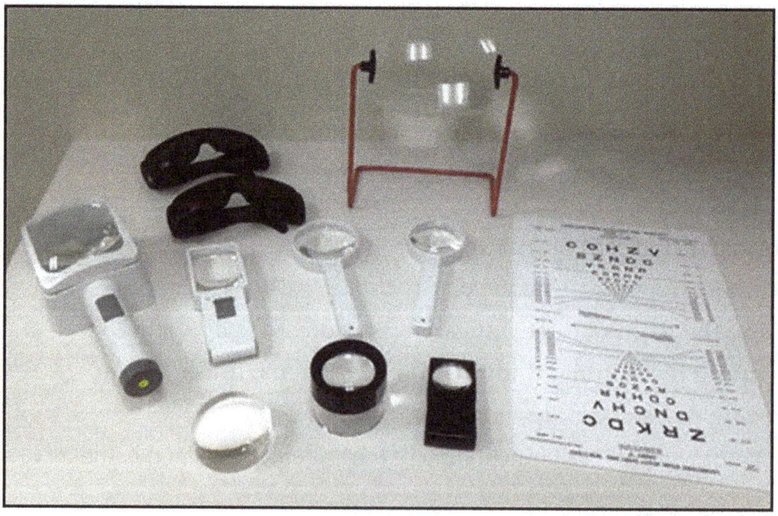

Fig. 10.9. Optical devices.

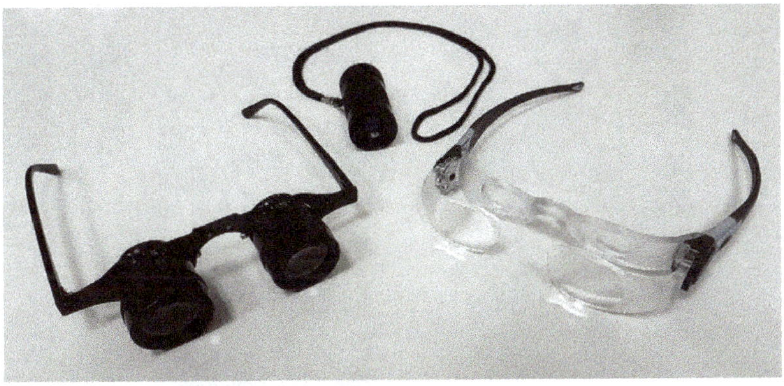

Fig. 10.10. Binocular spectacles and telescope.

Angular magnification is enlargement when the patient looks through a telescopic device (Fig. 10.10).

Electronic magnification combines relative size and relative distance magnification, with the use of electronic magnification devices (Fig. 10.11).

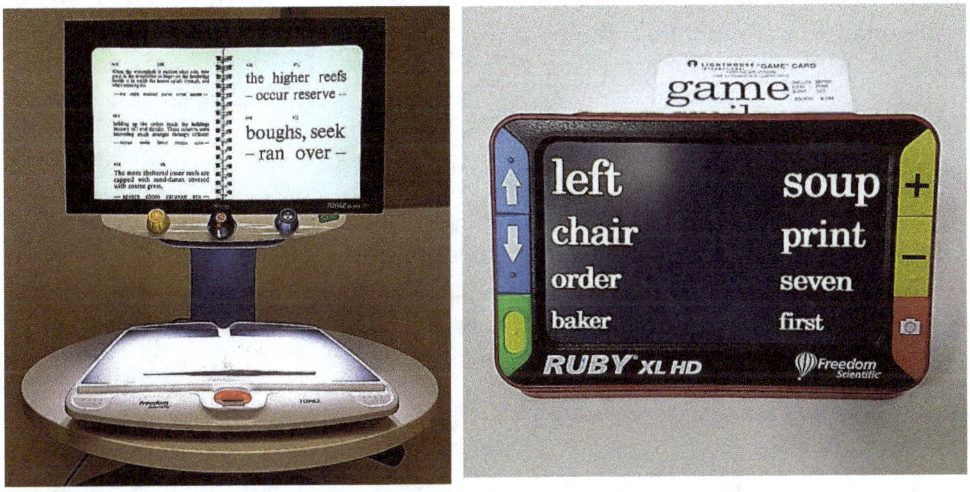

Fig. 10.11. Desktop and portable electronic magnifier.

Visual Substitution

When visual impairment progresses to a severe stage, optical devices may be inappropriate or impractical. At this stage, patients are taught to compensate with their other senses, such as touch, hearing, taste and smell, and by using sensorial devices such as Braille, tactile watches, talking clocks, liquid level indicators and audiobooks (Fig. 10.12).

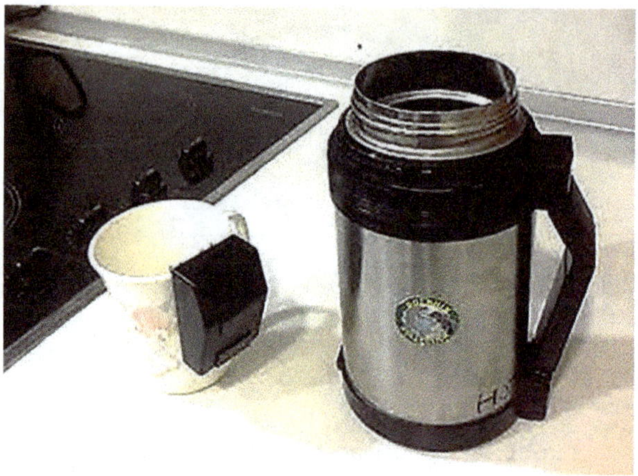

Fig. 10.12. Liquid level indicator.

Comprehensive Low Vision Rehabilitation

Comprehensive low vision care and rehabilitation involves a team-based, multidisciplinary and integrated approach, and includes:

- Occupational therapy — training the patient to perform activities of daily living
- Orientation and mobility training — teaching navigation skills
- Counselling and mental health services
- Career and assistive technology services

Take Home Messages

- Low vision rehabilitation plays a significant role in minimising disability and improving quality of life for patients with low vision.
- All ophthalmic professionals involved in clinical practice have a responsibility to be informed about it and to refer patients appropriately and seamlessly.

References

1. American Academy of Ophthalmology. Vision Rehabilitation Committee. (2013) *Preferred Practice Pattern® Guidelines. Vision Rehabilitation for Adults.* San Francisco, CA: American Academy of Ophthalmology.
2. Arditi A, Rosenthal B. (1996) *Developing an Objective Definition of Visual Impairment.* New York: Arlene R. Gordon Research Institute, The Lighthouse Inc.
3. Colenbrander A. (2010) Assessment of functional vision and its rehabilitation. *Acta Ophthalmol* **88**:163–173.
4. Colenbrander A, Goodwin L, Fletcher DC. (2007) Vision rehabilitation and AMD. *Int Ophthalmol Clin* **47**:139–148.
5. Dickinson C. (1998) *Low Vision: Principles and Practice.* Oxford: Butterworth-Heinemann.
6. Faye EE. (1976) *Clinical Low Vision,* 1st ed. New York: Little Brown and Company.

7. Fletcher DC, Schuchard RA. (1997) Preferred retinal loci relationship to macular scotomas in a low vision population. *Ophthalmology* **104**:632–638.
8. Jackson AJ, Wolffsohn JS. (2007) *Low Vision Manual*. Philadelphia, USA: Butterworth-Heinemann.
9. Markowitz S. (2006) Principles of modern low vision rehabilitation. *Can J Ophthalmol* **41**:289–312.
10. National Research Council, National Academy of Sciences. (1980) Recommended standard procedures for the clinical measurement and specification of visual acuity. *Adv Ophthalmol* **41**:103–148.
11. Pelli DG, Robson JG, Wilkins AJ. (1988) The design of a new letter chart for measuring contrast sensitivity. *Clin Vis Sci* **2**:187–199.
12. Whittaker SG, Scheiman M, Sokol-McKay DA. (2016) *Low Vision Rehabilitation. A Guide for Occupational Therapists*, 2nd ed. New Jersey, USA: Slack Incorporated.
13. World Health Organization. (1993) *Management of Low Vision in Children*. Geneva, Switzerland: World Health Organization.

Chapter 11

ELECTROPHYSIOLOGICAL TESTING

Graham E Holder

Learning Objectives

To understand the role of electrophysiological testing in ophthalmology

Gain an understanding of how electrophysiological tests, such as electroretinography (ERG) and visual evoked potentials (VEP), are used to assess the function of the visual pathways objectively, facilitating the diagnosis and management of retinal and optic nerve disorders.

To appreciate how the different tests enable the assessment of different parts of the visual system

Learn about the various types of ERG tests (Full-Field ERG, Pattern ERG, Multifocal ERG) and their specific uses in evaluating retinal and macular function, as well as how VEPs can help diagnose intracranial visual pathway dysfunctions.

To gain a basic comprehension of result interpretation

Understand how the results of electrophysiological tests are placed in clinical context to facilitate accurate diagnosis, how different waveforms have different pathophysiological significance, and how these findings guide clinical decision-making and patient management.

Electrophysiology involves objective recording of the function of the visual pathways and can have a significant impact on diagnosis and patient management. But when and why to order? The presentation may suggest the possible site of dysfunction, such as night blindness in retinal rod system abnormality, or photophobia in generalised retinal cone system dysfunction, but symptoms such as reduced visual acuity may have multiple possible causes, including optic nerve disease; an abnormal fundus appearance may or may not explain the nature and/or severity of the symptoms; a child with nystagmus may or may not have a progressive blinding disorder; the efficacy of treatment in inflammatory disease of the retina may be unclear. These are some of the issues that can be addressed by electrophysiology.

The process involves presenting controlled stimuli to the patient and measuring the electrical responses generated at a retinal or cortical level. The retina is highly complex, with multiple layers and cell types (see chapter 1), and "translates" images of the outside world into electrical signals that are transmitted to the brain for the process of "seeing". Both retinal and cortical responses can be measured. They have known characteristics in normal individuals in terms of size, timing and shape, which may be altered in a predictable way in disease. Interpretation usually involves placing the data in clinical context as electrophysiological data are rarely in themselves diagnostic.

When a flash of light strikes the retina a very complex set of biochemical reactions occurs consequent upon photoisomerisation of the photopigment, rhodopsin. This is known as the phototransduction cascade and results in hyperpolarisation of the photoreceptors. The signals are then transmitted to the bipolar cells. Rods and short wavelength cones have On-bipolar cells (depolarising), whereas long and medium wavelength cones also have Off-bipolar cells (hyperpolarising). Transmission then occurs to the retinal ganglion cells, whose axons form the optic nerves, which convey the signal, now in digital form (spikes) from the retina to the brain, where vision occurs.

11.1 Retinal Function Testing

The main test of retinal function is electroretinography. The (full-field) electroretinogram (ERG) is a massed retinal response to a luminance (flash) stimulus and reflects the transmission of signals from the photoreceptors to the bipolar cells. It is usually recorded using electrodes in contact with the bulbar conjunctiva, to stimuli delivered by a Ganzfeld bowl, an integrating sphere enabling uniform whole field illumination; the Ganzfeld can also provide a diffuse background for photopic adaptation. The separation of the function of different cell types and layers within the retina is achieved by modification of the adaptive state of the eye (dark adapted or scotopic; light adapted or photopic) and the nature of the stimulus. As the recordings are influenced by many factors, standardisation of procedures and techniques is mandatory for meaningful scientific and clinical communication between laboratories. This standardisation is enabled by the International Society for Clinical Electrophysiology of Vision (ISCEV), which regularly publishes and revises minimum standards for the performing of all the main electrophysiological tests.

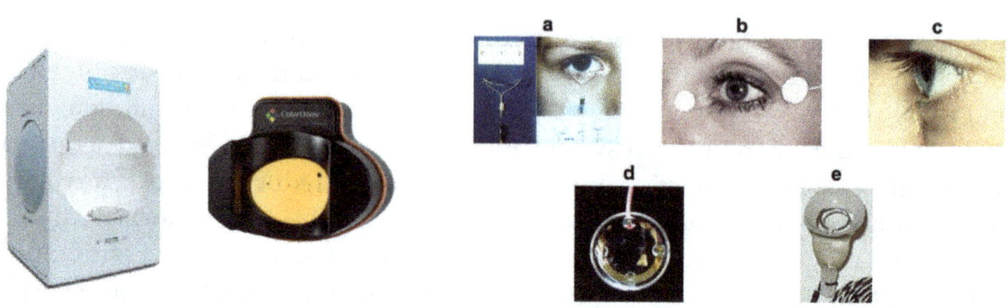

Fig. 11.1. Two commercially available Ganzfeld stimulators are shown on the left, with different ERG electrodes on the right. The H-K loop (a), the DTL (b) and the gold foil (c) electrodes preserve the optics of the eye and can be used for all types of ERG. The Jet or Burian-Allen contact lens electrodes (d, e) are unsuitable for pattern ERG recording.

11.2 Clinical ERG

The patient is maximally dilated and is dark-adapted for 20 minutes. Stimulation commences with dim flashes, followed by brighter flashes. Background illumination in the Ganzfeld bowl then restores photopic adaptation (10 minutes) and a 30 Hz flicker ERG and single flash photopic ERG are recorded. Many laboratories perform a scotopic intensity series and a scotopic red flash ERG as routine, but although often important to diagnosis, they are not part of the minimum standard. There is both inter-individual variability and a dependence upon stimulus and recording techniques, and it is therefore necessary for each laboratory to establish their own normative references series. Age, pupil size, electrode type and refractive error will all influence the data obtained. Note that each ERG type is replicated; with good techniques ERGs are highly reproducible.

The nomenclature of the waveforms in Fig. 11.2 refers to the adaptive state of the retina (dark-adapted; light-adapted), and stimulus strength in cd.s/m^2. The DA 0.01 stimulus, a dim flash, is below the cone threshold and the response arises in the rod On-bipolar cells. The DA 0.01 response is a measure of sensitivity within the rod system. Specificity is provided by the bright flash dark-adapted response (DA 10), as most of the a-wave in a normal subject arises in the rod photoreceptors, with responses from the cones not being visible (there are perhaps 120 million rods but only 6–7 million cones). Visualisation of dark-adapted cone function is enabled by the DA 0.3 red flash; there is an early cone response (c) followed by a later rod system response (r). Photopic adaptation is then restored by the background light within the Ganzfeld (a standardised background strength for a standardised time) and stimuli are presented upon that background. In addition to the presence of the rod-suppressing background, the rod system has poor temporal resolution and cannot follow a 30 Hz flicker, and the 30 Hz response is a pure cone system response. However, it has inner retinal origins and gives a measure of cone system sensitivity; specificity is enabled by the LA 3.0 response in which the a-wave arises in the cone photoreceptors modified by Off-bipolar cells, and the b-wave is a synchronised response from On- and Off- bipolar cells.

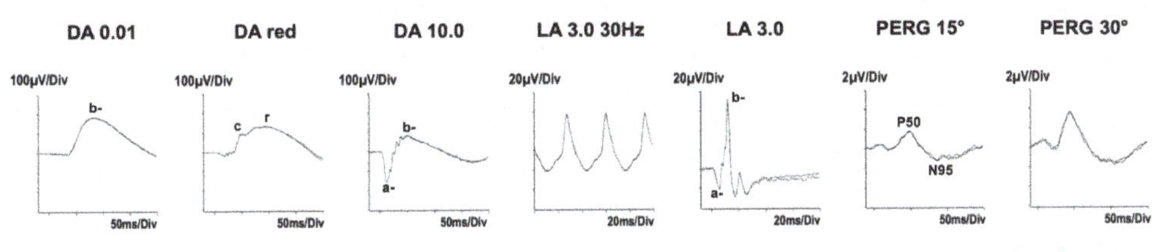

Fig. 11.2. Example ERGs and pattern ERGs (PERG) recorded in a normal subject.

Table 11.1. The Main ERG Responses and their Clinical Value

Dark Adapted (Scotopic) Stimuli	Clinical Utility
DA 0.01	Signal arises from inner retinal rod system. Cones do not usually contribute to the response.
DA 0.3 red flash	Early component from dark-adapted cones, later component from rods
DA 10.0	Clearly defined a-wave facilitates assessment of photoreceptor function.

Light Adapted (Photopic) Stimuli	Clinical Utility
30 Hz flicker	Inner retina derived pure cone system response
LA 3.0	a-wave: cone photoreceptors and off-bipolar cells b-wave: On- and Off- cone bipolar cells

As the (full-field) ERG is a massed retinal response, no abnormality is present when dysfunction is confined to small retinal areas, and that is also true if dysfunction is confined to the macula (although the macula is cone-dense the majority of retinal cones lie outside the vascular arcades). The macula is fundamental to high level visual functions such as colour vision and visual acuity, and techniques for testing macular function are needed. This is performed with either a pattern ERG (PERG) or a multifocal ERG (mfERG). The PERG is a contrast response generated by isoluminant reversal of a black and white checkerboard. PERGs are small signals and computerised signal averaging is used in conjunction with many stimulus reversals to record the PERG. Using a standard rate of ~4 reversals/second, the PERG has two main components; a prominent positive component, P50, at approx. 50 ms, followed by a larger negative component, N95, at approx. 95 ms. The N95 component has origins in the central retinal ganglion cells (RGCs); P50 is approximately 70% from RGCs, but is consequent upon activation of the macular photoreceptors and acts objectively as a measure of macular function.

The mfERG stimulus consists of multiple hexagons (see Figure 3), often 61 in number, that flash on/off in a pseudo random binary sequence. Complex mathematics derives the responses relating to each individual hexagon and generates multiple cone system waveforms despite using only a single recording electrode. The patient needs to be able to maintain accurate fixation for mfERG data to be meaningful. The mfERG is a luminance response and, as such, gives data that are complimentary to the contrast related PERG.

Table 11.2. The Main Test Modalities and their Clinical Use

Protocol	Functional Assessment
Full Field ERG (FFERG)	General retinal assessment
Pattern ERG (PERG)	Macula (central vision) and central retinal ganglion cell assessment
Multifocal ERG (mfERG)	Spatial distribution of central retinal function

11.3 Clinical Interpretation

ERGs in a variety of inherited disorders are shown below. There are many proteins involved in the process of phototransduction and subsequent intraretinal signalling, and genetically determined retinal disease, with altered protein structure and function, is not uncommon. The underlying pathophysiology in the disorders shown below is known and enables the ERG signals to be appropriately related to their cellular origins.

The upper 3 disorders affect the photoreceptors. The patient with rod-cone dystrophy (retinitis pigmentosa, RP) shows a subnormal DA 0.01 response, indicative of rod system sensitivity, but the markedly subnormal photoreceptor-derived DA 10 a-wave localises the dysfunction to the photoreceptors. Note the markedly delayed and reduced photopic flicker ERG (*). Flicker ERG delay indicates generalised cone system dysfunction. The rod ERGs are more severely affected than cone-derived ERGs, seen also in the DA red response (*), hence a rod-cone dystrophy. The severity of RP may not be reflected either in the fundus appearance or on structural imaging such as fundus autofluorescence (FAF) or optical coherence tomography (OCT); the ERG assists in accurate diagnosis and may provide prognostic information. Cone dystrophies have normal rod responses but abnormal cone responses, with the 30 Hz flicker response usually showing both amplitude reduction and delayed peak time, as is evident in the Fig. 11.3 (◆). Note that the DA red flash shows no

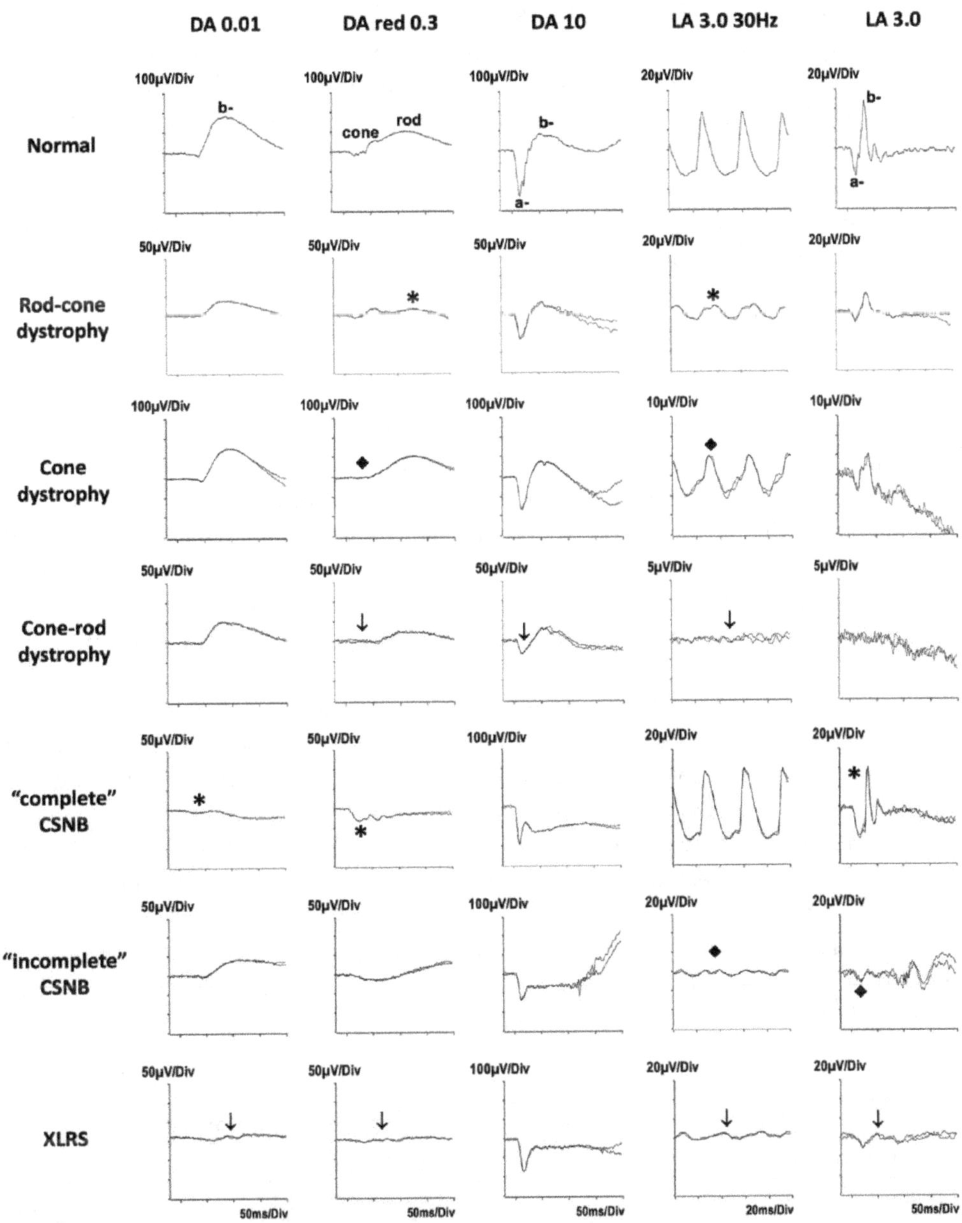

Fig. 11.3. ERGs from a variety of disorders demonstrate the ability of the ERG to localise abnormalities to the photoceptors (the upper 3 disorders) or the inner retina (the lower 3 disorders) and quantify the degree of dysfunction. See text for full details. Modified from Hathibelagal AR, Kommanapalli D, Mukherjee S, Padhy SK, Holder GE. (2024) Electroretinography. In: *Ophthalmic Diagnostics*, (eds.) Das T, Satgunam P. Springer, Singapore. https://doi.org/10.1007/978-981-97-0138-4_31 (with permission).

cone component (◆). This can be particularly useful as cone dystrophy patients are frequently photophobic and may not be able to comply with photopic testing; an undetectable cone component in the DA red ERG facilitates the diagnosis. Cone ERGs are more abnormal than rod ERGs in cone-rod dystrophy patients (↓), the degree of abnormality in the subnormal DA 10 a-wave indicating the degree of rod photoreceptor involvement (↓).

The lower 3 disorders affect the inner retina. The patient with "complete" congenital stationary night blindness (cCSNB) shows no rod system activity in the DA 0.01 response, as the underlying pathophysiology results in loss of signal transmission from all retinal photoreceptors to On-bipolar cells. The normal a-wave in the DA 10 responses confirms normal rod photoreceptor function, and the waveform, with a normal negative going a-wave but profound relative reduction in the b-wave, is an electronegative or "negative" ERG. In some cases, a minimal early deflection occurs in the DA 0.01 response (*). The early peak time excludes a rod system origin; it suggests dark-adapted cones, confirmed by the DA red flash ERG, but note the reduced positive deflection in the DA red response (*) in keeping with inner retinal cone system dysfunction. The photopic ERGs show an a-wave that commences normally (origins in photoreceptors and Off-bipolar cells); there is a broadened trough, a sharply rising b-wave lacking oscillatory potentials, and a reduced b:a ratio (*). That shape is diagnostic of loss of On-bipolar cell function but preservation of Off-bipolar cell function. The genetic variants responsible for cCSNB result in selective impairment of the function of all On-bipolar cells, both rod and cone, but spare the Off-bipolar cells. In contrast, the patient with incomplete CSNB (iCSNB) has a detectable but subnormal and delayed DA 0.01 response b-wave, but the negative waveform DA 10 response is very similar waveform to the patient with cCSNB. It is in the photopic responses that the major differences occur. Note that the 30 Hz flicker ERG is markedly subnormal and has a triphasic appearance (◆). Examination of the LA 3 response suggests the pathophysiology. The severe b-wave reduction shows that, unlike cCSNB, there must also be Off-bipolar cell involvement. There is loss of the Off-bipolar contribution to the a-wave and the very small, almost u-shaped response indicates inner retinal dysfunction involving both On- and Off- pathways (◆). Cone ERGs are far more abnormal in iCSNB than cCSNB, and this is reflected in the symptomatology; a greater proportion of iCSNB patients have nystagmus or significant visual acuity reduction, and some may even complain of photophobia rather than nyctalopia. Both On- and Off-bipolar cell pathways are affected, as the responsible genes encode proteins involved in transmission at the photoreceptor synapse, affecting both On- and Off- pathways.

Table 11.3. ERG Components and their Origins

ERG Components	Anatomical Localisation
Scotopic a-wave	Photoreceptors
Photopic a-wave	Photoreceptors and cone off-bipolar cells
Scotopic and photopic b-waves	Inner nuclear layer
Oscillatory potential (wavelets on ascending limb of b-wave)	Generated in amacrine cells. Limited clinical value

ERGs in X-linked retinoschisis (XLRS), where there is splitting of inner retinal structures, reflect inner retinal dysfunction unrelated to the blocking of specific channels. There is profound rod system abnormality in the DA 0.01 responses (↓), confirmed to be inner retinal by the negative waveform DA 10 ERG (normal a-wave = normal rod photoreceptors) and the reduction in positive components in the DA red ERG (↓). Cone flicker and single flash ERGs are subnormal and show delay and a reduced b:a ratio, but do not show (↓) the shape changes associated with the channel blocking of CSNB. Negative ERGs also occur in central retinal artery occlusion (CRAO) and various other disorders. The negative ERG in CRAO reflects the duality of the retinal blood supply, in which the photoreceptors are supplied via choroidal circulation but the inner nuclear layer, wherein lie the bipolar cells, is supplied via the CRA.

11.4 Multifocal ERG

Typical examples of multifocal ERG are shown in Fig. 11.4. It is also very useful in suspected hydroxychloroquine toxicity.

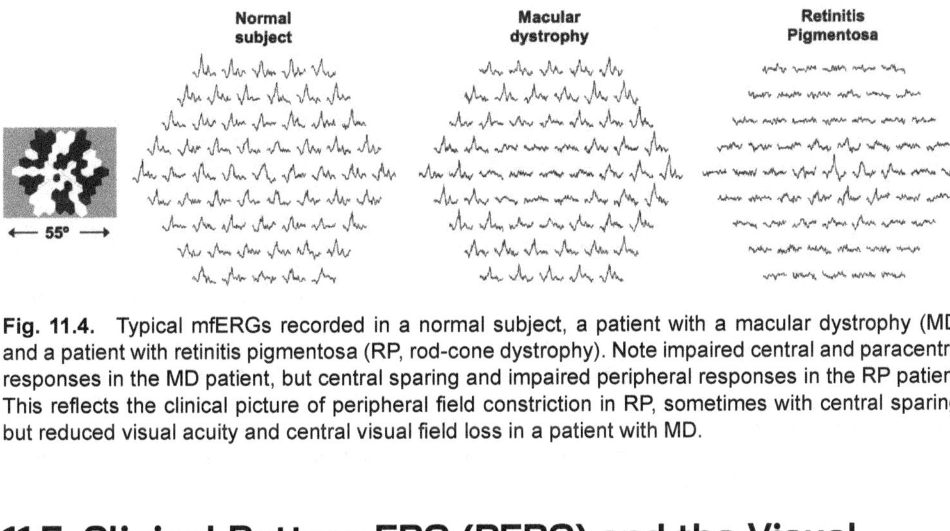

Fig. 11.4. Typical mfERGs recorded in a normal subject, a patient with a macular dystrophy (MD) and a patient with retinitis pigmentosa (RP, rod-cone dystrophy). Note impaired central and paracentral responses in the MD patient, but central sparing and impaired peripheral responses in the RP patient. This reflects the clinical picture of peripheral field constriction in RP, sometimes with central sparing, but reduced visual acuity and central visual field loss in a patient with MD.

11.5 Clinical Pattern ERG (PERG) and the Visual Evoked Potential (VEP)

Although the PERG is a macular response, and the VEP is the response of the brain to visual stimuli, extracted from the much higher amplitude background electroencephalogram (EEG) using computerised signal averaging and repetitive stimulation, in clinical practice they are often both evoked by a reversing checkerboard stimulus and PERG evidence of function at the macula may be indispensable to accurate pattern VEP interpretation. Although VEPs are a powerful and sensitive index of intracranial visual pathway dysfunction, dysfunction anywhere anterior to the cortex in the visual pathway can give an abnormal pattern VEP (e.g. the optic chiasm, optic nerve, macula, media opacity, inappropriate refraction etc.) Pattern reversal stimulation is very effective in the assessment of optic nerve function, but a diffuse flash stimulus also has clinical utility, particularly in paediatric practice.

Pattern VEPs became a prominent part of the diagnostic armamentarium in the 1970s, when it was shown that not only were they delayed in optic neuritis, a common presenting symptom of multiple sclerosis, but that they remained delayed after apparent clinical recovery, and that sub-clinical optic nerve conduction delay could be revealed by VEP in an eye with no signs or symptoms of optic nerve disease.

Fig. 11.5 shows two patients with similar presenting symptoms. They both had uniocular visual acuity reduction accompanied by retrobulbar pain made worse on eye movement, suggestive of a demyelinating retrobulbar or optic neuritis (RBN). Both had a relative afferent pupillary defect in the involved eye, a common but not diagnostic sign in optic nerve disease. Only one of the patients has optic nerve disease, demonstrating the lack of specificity of a delayed pattern VEP.

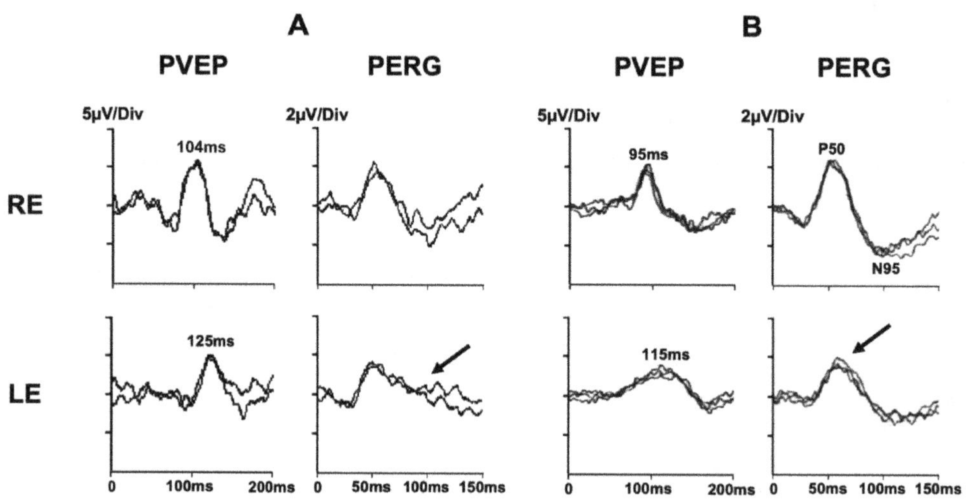

Fig. 11.5. Patient A has a relative left eye PVEP delay of 20 ms and reduction in the N95 component of the PERG in keeping with retrograde degeneration to the retinal ganglion cells from an optic nerve lesion. The changes are compatible with RBN. Patient B, referred by a neurologist for confirmation of presumed RBN, shows a similar relative VEP delay to patient A. However, there is delay in the P50 component of the PERG with associated reduction in P50 amplitude and a normal N95:P50 ratio, indicating macular dysfunction. Ophthalmological examination revealed subtle changes in keeping with posterior scleritis, which was confirmed by ultrasound. Posterior scleritis is just one of the various retinal masquerades of optic nerve disease.

To conclude, electrophysiology provides objective data about the function of the retinal and intracranial visual pathways. It is important always to remember that normal structure does not necessarily mean normal function and that optimal patient management may involve both structural and functional consideration.

Table 11.4. A Guide to Clinical Interpretation of the Different Test Types and Protocols

Test Type	Protocol	Purpose	Interpretation
Full-Field ERG (ERG)	**DA 0.01 (Dark Adapted)**	Assesses rod system sensitivity	Normal: Healthy rod function Abnormal: Rod system dysfunction but does not localise
	DA 10.0 (Dark Adapted)	Evaluates photoreceptor function, primarily rods. Specificity	Normal a-wave: Intact rod photoreceptors Reduced a-wave: Photoreceptor dysfunction Normal a-wave, reduced b:a ratio: inner retinal dysfunction
	DA 0.3 Red Flash	Differentiates rod and cone function under dark adaptation	Normal: Early cone response followed by rod response Enables assessment of dark adapted cone function and the relative degrees of rod and cone dysfunction
	30 Hz Flicker (Light Adapted)	Purely assesses cone system function	Normal: Healthy cone function Delayed: Generalised cone dysfunction Reduced amplitude, normal peak time — restricted loss of function
	LA 3.0 (Light Adapted)	Assesses cone photoreceptors and inner retinal function	Normal: Healthy a-wave and b-wave Abnormal: Cone system dysfunction. Shape important.
Pattern ERG (PERG)	**P50 Component**	Assesses macular function and central retinal ganglion cells (RGCs)	Normal: Healthy macular and RGC function Delayed/Reduced: Macular dysfunction. Can be reduced with short peak time in severe RGC loss.
	N95 Component	Reflects activity of RGCs	Reduced N95 with normal P50: RGC dysfunction. Can be primary or secondary to optic neuropathy.
Multifocal ERG (mfERG)	**Hexagonal Luminance Responses**	Spatial mapping of cone function across the central 55 degrees	Normal: Healthy central and peripheral responses Abnormal: Localised or generalised central retinal dysfunction (e.g. macular dystrophy, hydroxychloroquine toxicity)
Visual Evoked Potential (VEP)	**Pattern VEP (PVEP)**	Assesses functional integrity of the visual pathways	Normal: Intact visual pathways Delayed peak time: non-specific. Can reflect optic nerve conduction delay, e.g. optic neuritis, tumour, but delay common in maculopathy. Reduced amplitude, normal peak time: can occur in e.g. ischaemic optic neuropathy or glaucoma
	Flash VEP (FVEP)	Useful for patients unable to cooperate with pattern VEP, particularly children	Use in conjunction with PVEP. Less sensitive than PVEP but provides complimentary data.

*For accurate diagnosis and management, these interpretations should always be taken in clinical context and in conjunction with other diagnostic findings.

Take-Home Messages

Electrophysiology Enables Objective Demonstration of Function

Electrophysiological tests provide crucial objective functional assessment of the retina and intracranial visual pathways, which can significantly inform diagnosis and management.

Test Selection is Key for Accurate Diagnosis

The choice of electrophysiological test (e.g. Full-Field ERG vs. Pattern ERG) is guided by the clinical presentation; different tests provide information about different aspects of visual pathway function.

Interpreting Results Requires Clinical Context

Electrophysiological data are rarely diagnostic in isolation, and must always be taken in clinical context.

Standardisation Important

Adherence to standardised testing protocols, such as those set by the International Society for Clinical Electrophysiology of Vision (ISCEV), is critical for obtaining meaningful and reproducible results. The role of well-trained technical staff in obtaining high quality data cannot be over-emphasised.

Electrophysiological Patterns Can Reveal Specific Disorders

ERG findings can localise retinal dysfunction to specific cell types or layers, and in inherited retinal diseases can assist with diagnosis, prognosis, and the objective monitoring of disease progression. Objective assessment of treatment efficacy in inflammatory disease can guide management decisions.

References

1. Holder GE. (2001) The pattern electroretinogram and an integrated approach to visual pathway diagnosis. *Prog Ret Eye Res* **20**:531–561. PMID: 11390258.
2. Holder GE, Celesia GG, Miyake Y, *et al.* (2010) International Federation of Clinical Neurophysiology: Recommendations for Visual System Testing. *Clin Neurophysiol* **121**:1393–1409. PMID: 20558103.
3. The ISCEV Standards for electrophysiological testing can be found at www.iscev.org.

Chapter 12

BASIC STATISTICS FOR THE CLINICIAN: AN APPROACH TO DATA ANALYSIS

Lingam Gopal

Learning Objectives

1. Type of studies.
2. Understanding the data in terms of categorical or numerical; outcome and independent variables, potential confounders, etc.
3. Importance of normal distribution, or a lack of it.
4. Grouping the data.
5. Descriptive statistics.
6. Measures.
7. Univariate analysis.
8. Multivariate analysis.
9. Concept of statistical significance.
10. Common pitfalls.

12.1 Introduction

Data is the information collected while conducting a study. The raw data is then analysed to give useful information, such as the description of incidences/prevalences, cause-effect relationships, etc.

Types of Studies

With respect to the timing of data collection:

- Retrospective: Data that is collected are from events that have occurred before the study was planned — i.e. the exposure and outcome have already occurred
- Prospective: The exposure and the outcome have not occurred at the time of initiation of the study
- Ambispective: Has components of prospective and retrospective studies. In most cases, the exposure has already occurred, but the outcome has not

With respect to the frequency of data collection:

- Cross-section studies: One-time collection of data
- Cohort studies: Collection of data multiple times over a specified period
- Case control studies: Cases (with the outcome of interest) are recruited, and data collected retrospectively. Matched controls (usually age and sex

matched) are selected who do not have the outcome of interest, and various variables are compared between the two groups to understand cause and effect relationships.

- Intervention studies: Where two groups are selected, with one receiving intervention and the other serving as the control. Data is collected prospectively according to a set protocol.

12.2 Game Plan for Analysis

1. *Defining the outcome variables*: Depends on the primary and secondary objectives of the study.
2. *Defining the independent variables*: These are various factors that individually or cumulatively can affect the outcome variable of interest.
3. *Identifying potential confounders*: These are factors that are associated with both the independent variable and outcome variable and hence can confuse the interpretation. True association can be brought out by adjusting for the confounder using statistical tools.
4. *Effect modifiers*: Unlike the confounders, effect modifiers have a true relationship with the outcome variable and modify the influence of the independent variable.
5. *Identifying collinearity*: When two variables, very closely associated with each other, are included in a model, they independently cannot predict the outcome variable. Hence, one of them has to be dropped in the final model.
6. *Defining the type of variables*:
    - Qualitative (categorical): Can be binary (e.g. Gender), Unordered (e.g. Nationality) or ordered (e.g. Degree of pain). Ordered variables do not have true measured value (unlike height or weight, etc.) but roughly indicate the magnitude and direction.
    - Quantitative (numerical): Can be discrete (e.g. Number of children); continuous (e.g. Weight, Height, BP, etc.)

12.3 Data Management Before Analysis

1. *Transfer of data from source to proforma*:
    - Data to be copied as it is and not reduced: E.g. blood pressure — actual figures to be noted, rather than reducing it to less than 120; more than 120, etc. This avoids the loss of information.
    - Double entry helps avoid errors
    - Patient identity is to be removed at this stage with the help of a master chart that is preserved password-protected in a secure location
2. *Transfer of raw data into an Excel sheet*: Importance of avoiding wrong entries cannot be overemphasised.

3. *Data cleaning*:
   - Check for errors in entry — in doubt, verify with raw data
   - Look for plausibility — the entry should make sense, e.g. if the entry shows the age of 200 years, date of birth later than the date of surgery, etc. — there is an obvious error in the entry. Histograms can be generated for each variable and outliers can be identified and rechecked.
   - Look for consistency: e.g. pregnancy entries for a male, etc.
4. *Testing for normality*: Continuous variables should be tested for normality of distribution.
   - Looking at a histogram/scatter plot: normally distributed data will have a pattern resembling the normal curve
   - One can apply formal testing for normality using the Shapiro-Wilk test
   - If normally distributed — one can apply usual tests, such as t test, paired t test, etc.
   - If not normally distributed
     - One can use nonparametric tests
     - One may be able to convert the non-normal data to normal data by transformation (e.g. logarithm of the data)
5. *Data reduction*:
   - Categorical variables:
     - In addition to numbering the categories in a variable, grouping is done to reduce the number of categories to manageable levels. E.g. diabetic medication can be reduced to 1 — insulin, 2 — oral hypoglycaemic agents, 3 — both and 0 — none.
   - Numerical variables:
     - E.g. Age can be reduced to decade-wise grouping, etc.
     - Binarisation can be done using the ROC curve
     - Knowledge-based grouping can be done based on the objectives of the study
6. *Principles in data reduction of numerical variables*:
   - Can be in equal intervals or unequal intervals
   - If unequal intervals are chosen, there should be a rationale based on the objectives of the study
   - No overlaps between the intervals are permitted
   - Terminal intervals can be collapsed if the number of values is likely to be few

12.4 Statistical Analysis

1. *Descriptive statistics*:
   - Basic data is described in terms of measures of central distribution (such as mean/mode or median), range, etc.

- One can use tables, bar graphs, histograms, pie graphs, box and whisker plots, etc., to present the information
- Descriptive statistics helps familiarise oneself with the data to facilitate more advanced analysis

2. *Measures that can be used to express the data*:
   - Disease frequency — Incidence, Prevalence
   - Measures of central tendency (average): Mean, Mode, Median
   - Measures of variation: Standard deviation, Variance, Range
   - Measures of association or effect: Risk ratio, Odds ratio, Risk difference
   - Measures of impact: Attributable risk, Population attributable risk

Table 12.1. Measures of Outcome and Effect

Type of Analytical Study	Measure of Outcome (Disease Occurrence)	Measure of Effect (Exposure)
Ecological	Rate, risk, prevalence, mean or median	Correlation coefficient, Regression coefficient
Cross sectional	Prevalence, odds, means or median	Prevalence ratio, Prevalence difference, Odds ratio, Difference of means or medians
Cohort	Rate, risk, odds, means or median	Rate ratio, Risk ratio, Odds ratio, Rate difference, Risk difference, Vaccine efficacy, Difference between means or medians
Case control	None	Odds ratio, Vaccine efficacy
Interventional	Rate, risk, odds, means or median	Rate ratio, Risk ratio, Odds ratio, Rate difference, Risk difference, Vaccine efficacy, Difference between means or medians

3. *Univariate analysis*: Outcome variable is tested for association with each one of the independent variables — this is called "crude association", since it ignores the influence of confounding.
4. *Multivariate analysis*: The true association between two variables is only known when it is adjusted for other variables that have been tested. This is possible with regression analysis. Typically, linear regression is used for continuous variables, although categorical variables can be added to the model. Logistic regression can be used for both categorical and continuous independent variables. The outcome variable has to be binary — i.e. dichotomous (yes or no).
5. *Basic statistical tests*:

Table 12.2. Basic Statistical Tests

<table>
<tr><th colspan="4">Association Between Continuous and Categorical Variable</th></tr>
<tr><td rowspan="4">Continuous variable vs. Categorical variable with two levels</td><td rowspan="2">Unpaired data</td><td>Parametric test</td><td>t test</td></tr>
<tr><td>Non-parametric test</td><td>Wilcoxon's rank sum test, Mann-Whitney U test, Kendall's S test</td></tr>
<tr><td rowspan="2">Paired data</td><td>Parametric test</td><td>Paired t test</td></tr>
<tr><td>Non-parametric test</td><td>Wilcoxon's signed rank test</td></tr>
</table>

<table>
<tr><th colspan="4">Association Between Continuous and Categorical Variable</th></tr>
<tr><td rowspan="2">Continuous variable vs. Categorical variable with two or more levels</td><td rowspan="2"></td><td>Parametric test</td><td>ANOVA</td></tr>
<tr><td>Non-parametric test</td><td>Kruskal Wallis one way analysis of variance</td></tr>
<tr><th colspan="4">Association Between Two Continuous Variables</th></tr>
<tr><td colspan="4">Linear regression, Pearson's coefficient (parametric test), Spearman's coefficient or Kendall's rank correlation (non-parametric test)</td></tr>
<tr><th colspan="4">Association Between Two Categorical Variables</th></tr>
<tr><td colspan="3">Total number more than 40</td><td rowspan="2">Chi square test</td></tr>
<tr><td colspan="3">Total number 20–40 but expected number per cell more than 5</td></tr>
<tr><td colspan="3">Total number less than 20</td><td rowspan="2">Fisher's exact test</td></tr>
<tr><td colspan="3">Total number 20–40 but expected number per cell less than 5</td></tr>
<tr><th colspan="4">Regression Analysis</th></tr>
<tr><td colspan="2">Linear regression</td><td colspan="2">• Predominantly for continuous variables
• Can also have categorical variable</td></tr>
<tr><td colspan="2">Logistic regression</td><td colspan="2">• Categorical + continuous variables
• Outcome variable should be binary (dichotomous)</td></tr>
<tr><td colspan="3">Conditional logistic regression</td><td>Matched studies</td></tr>
<tr><td colspan="3">Poisson regression</td><td>Rates</td></tr>
<tr><td colspan="3">Cox's regression (of proportional hazards)</td><td>Survival data</td></tr>
</table>

12.5 Statistical Significance

P Value

Most statistical tests give out a p value to grade the level of significance that can be attached to a described association. P = <0.05 means the chances that a difference as large as the observed difference can occur by chance is less than 5%. Effectively, it means the association is significant.

Confidence Interval

Another way of expressing the level of significance is the confidence interval. A 95% confidence interval means:

- Sample estimate +/– 1.96 * Standard Error ($=sd/\sqrt{n}$)
- Sample estimate can be mean, difference of means, difference of proportions, etc.
- Interpretation: What is the confidence with which we can state that the sample drawn from the population contains the mean of the true population?
- The narrower the interval, the more reliable are the results
- If the confidence interval straddles the null point, it also indicates the lack of significance of the result

Interpretation

A significant association with $P < 0.05$ noted in the study could mean:

- True association
- Chance (due to sampling variation)
- Confounding
- It is important that scientific knowledge is used to provide a sensible explanation for the significant associations that are found

Common Pitfalls in Statistical Analysis

1. Data dredging: Searching for all possible associations with the outcome variable can lead to dramatic but spurious results since, at a 5% significance level, a one in 20 times chance significance can be seen.
2. Subgroup analysis: Be cautious of finding subgroups with significant association when the main analysis was not significant. The study may not be powered to answer this question.

Conclusions

1. The quality of data that is input decides the output as well. Hence, errors should be corrected before analysis.
2. Getting familiar with the data is important before applying statistical tests.
3. Avoid loss of information during analysis. Grouping the data is appealing but tends to lead to a loss of information.
4. Normal distribution of data should be assessed before choosing the correct type of statistical test.
5. Univariate analysis should be followed by multivariate analysis in order to get at the true associations while adjusting for other variables.
6. Data presentation in correctly labelled tables is as important as the analysis.
7. Inferences are drawn from the analysis based on scientific knowledge and appropriateness of the findings. Remember that even a significant association at a 0.05 level can still be by chance, although that likelihood is low (5%).

Chapter 13

CLINICAL APPROACHES

13.1 Approach to Leukocoria

HISTORY

Presenting Complaint:
- Age of onset
  - Bilateral RB → 1 year
  - Unilateral RB → 2 years
- Duration of white reflex
  - From birth → congenital causes, e.g. PFV
  - Acquired later on e.g. RB
- Other symptoms
  - Pain, redness → RB with anterior segment involvement
  - Strabismus → RB, cataract

Past Medical/ocular History:
- Premature birth → ROP
- Trauma → cataract
- Infections, e.g. TORCH → Toxoplasmosis, cataract
- Exposure to pets → Toxoplasmosis

Family History:
- Present → RB, FEVR, coloboma

WHITE PUPILLARY REFLEX noticed on:
- Flash photography
- Observation by family members
- Examination of the red reflex

CLINICAL EXAMINATION

CHARACTERISTICS

Laterality:
- Unilateral → RB, Coats', PFV, toxocariasis
- Bilateral → RB, FEVR, ROP

Colour of reflex:
- White → RB
- Yellow→ exudates, RD, Coats'
- Blue/Grey → cataract

IOP:
- High IOP → could be secondary to anterior segment neovascularisation in RB/Coats'
- Strabismus present?
- Commonly present in RB, cataract

ANTERIOR SEGMENT
- Small eye with shallow AC → PFV
- Iris coloboma → choroidal coloboma
- Inflammation or neovascularisation in AC → RB, Coats', longstanding RD
- Crystalline cholesterol deposits in AC → Coats'
- Lens opacity → cataract, PFV

POSTERIOR SEGMENT
- Vitreous —
  - Seeding → RB
  - Vitritis → Toxocariasis
  - Persistent hyaloid canal → PFV
- Optic disc –
  - Excavation → morning glory disc anomaly, optic disc coloboma
  - Bergmeister papilla → PFV
- Blood vessels
  - Uniformly dilated/tortuous → RB
  - Irregular saccular dilation → Coats'

INVESTIGATIONS
- B scan ultrasonography
  - Low reflectivity → Coats', RD, toxocariasis
  - High internal acoustic reflectivity → RB (due to calcium)
  - Persistent hyaloid remnants → PFV
- Fundus fluorescein angiography (FFA)
  - Retinal telangiectasia "light bulbs" → Coats'
  - Rapid homogenous hyperfluorescence → RB
  - Reticular hyperfluorescence → toxocariasis
  - Peripheral avascular zone → ROP, FEVR
- Magnetic resonance imaging (MRI)
  - RB → evaluate pineal gland
- Blood serology
  - Toxocariasis, TORCH infections
- Genetic testing
  - Important for genetic counselling in patients with RB, FEVR, Coats'

Legend: AC = anterior chamber; FEVR = familial exudative vitreoretinopathy; IOP = intraocular pressure; PFV = persistent foetal vasculature; RB = retinoblastoma; ROP = retinopathy of prematurity; RD = retinal detachment; TORCH = toxoplasmosis, other (syphilis, Varicella zoster, parvovirus B19), rubella, cytomegalovirus, herpes infections.

13.2 Clinical Pathway for Chronic Visual Loss

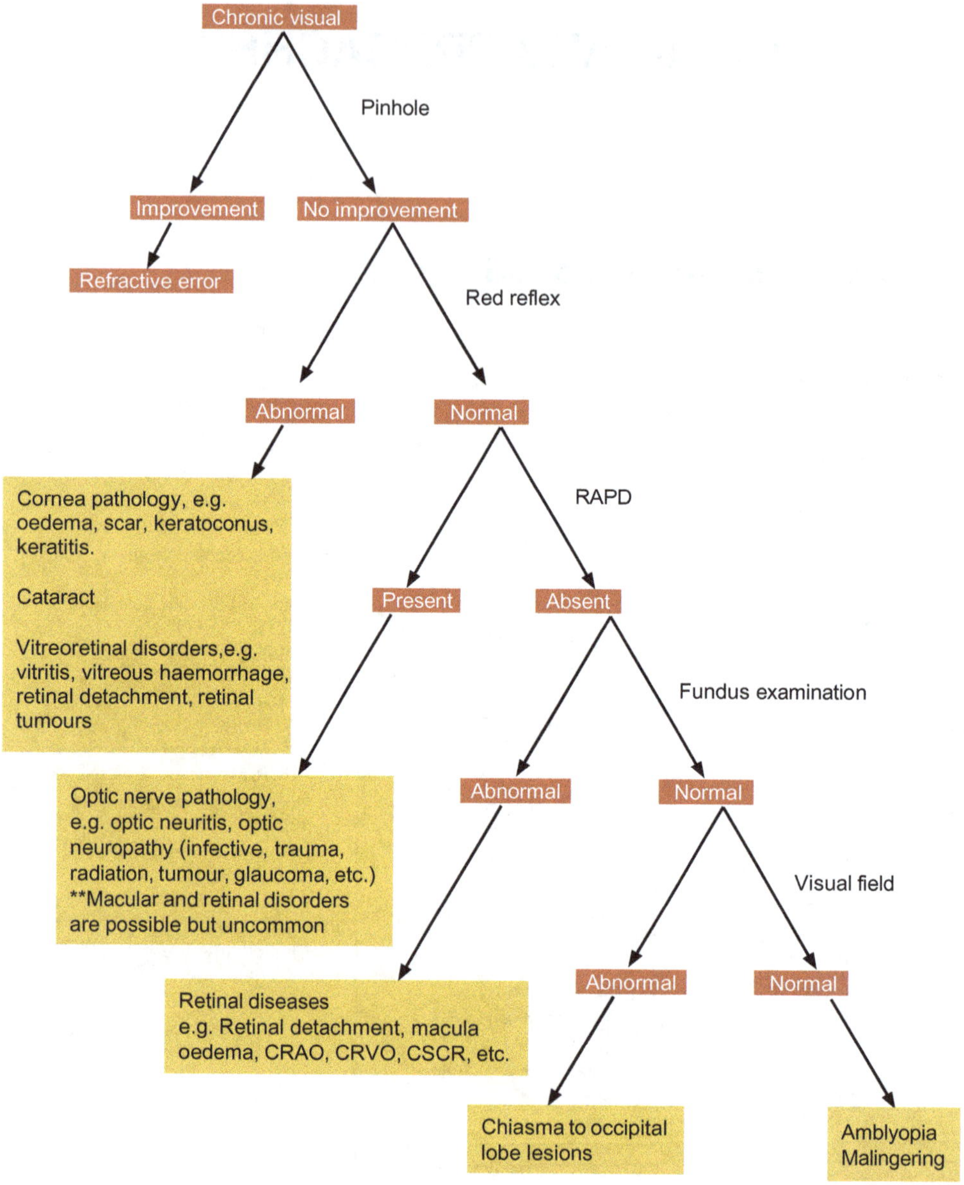

Abbreviations:
RAPD – Relative Afferent Pupillary Defect
CRAO – Central Retinal Artery Occlusion
CRVO – Central Retina Vein Occlusion
CSCR — Central Serous Chorioretinopathy

13.3 Clinical Pathway for Acute Visual Loss

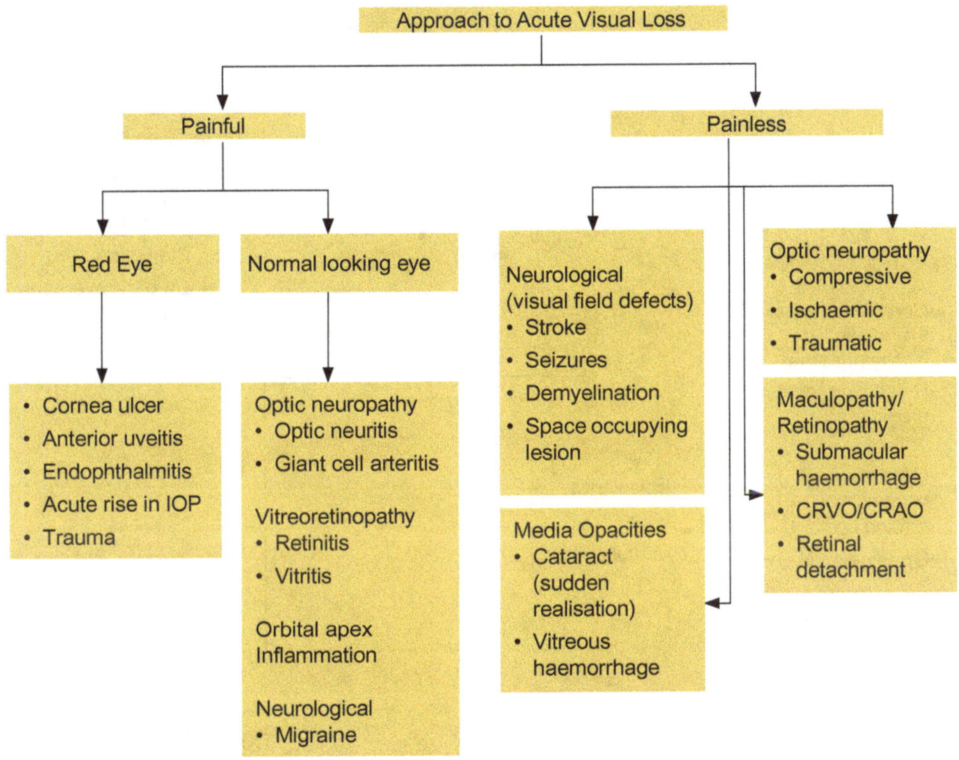

13.4 Diagnostic Flowchart in an Acute Red Eye

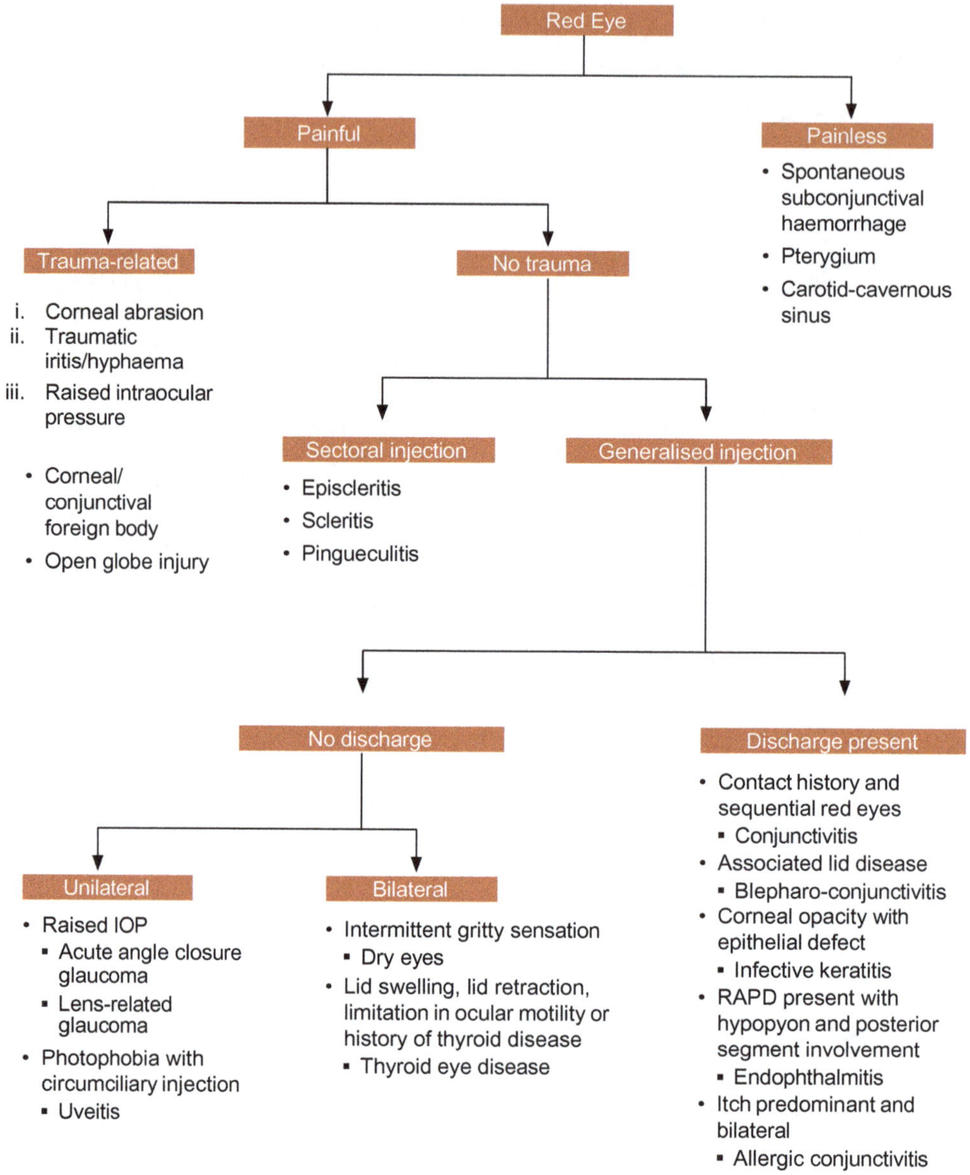

13.5 Neuro-ophthalmology Approaches

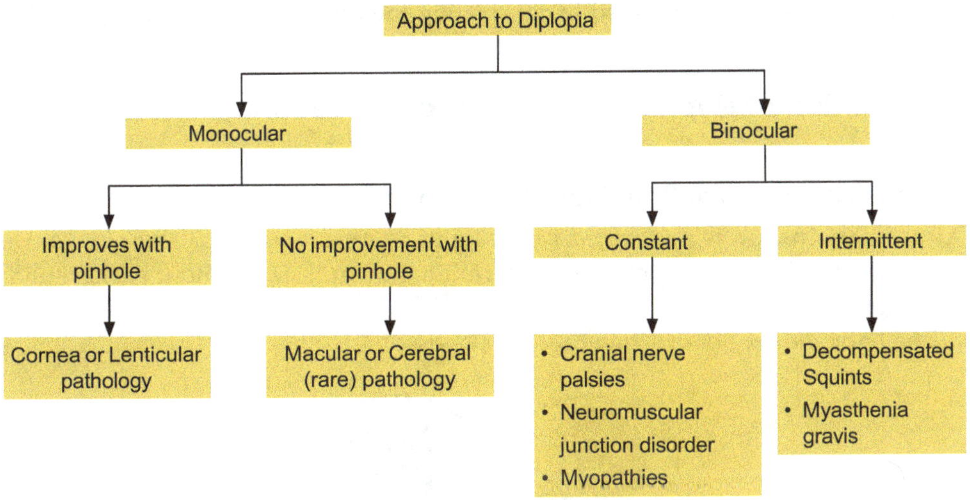

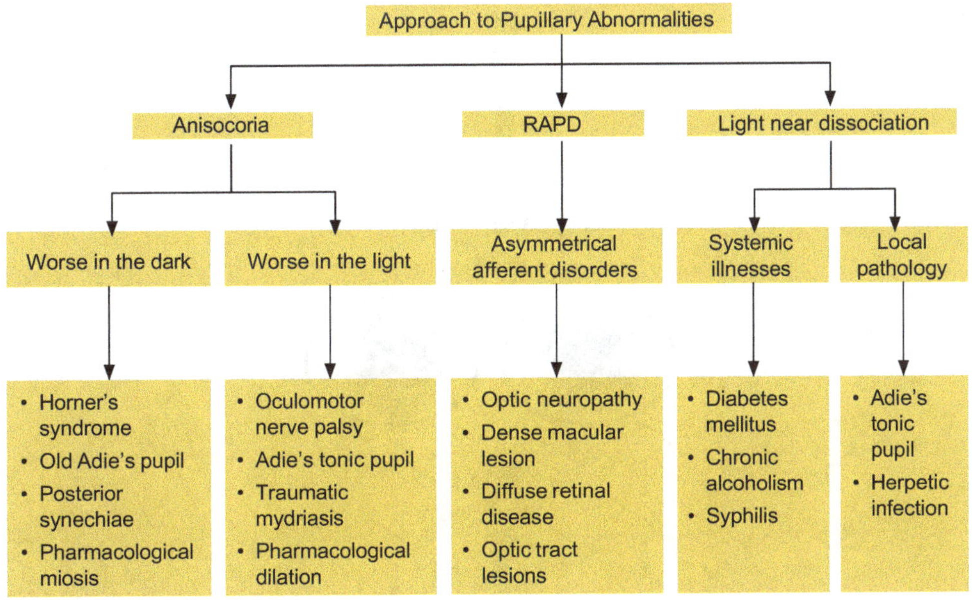

13.6 Pupil Examination

There are several steps involved in completing the pupil examination (Figs. 13.1a and 13.1b).

Examination of Pupil Size (Testing for Anisocoria) (Figs. 13.1a and 13.1b)

Diffuse Illumination of Both Eyes With a Torch

Diffuse illumination is performed in the light, as Asian eyes typically have dark iris, making it difficult to accurately determine the pupil size without background illumination.

The light should not obstruct the visual axis.

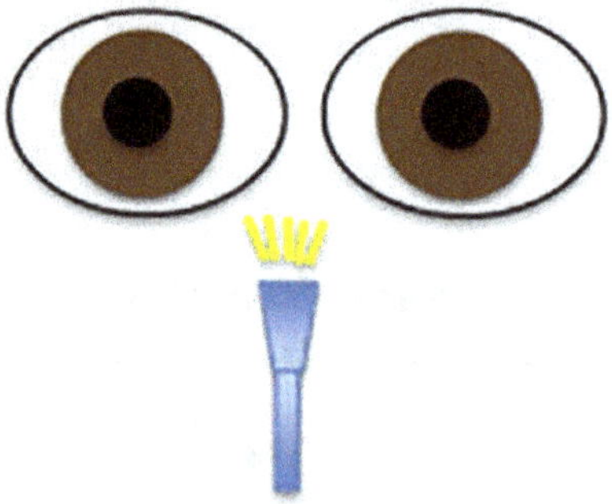

(a)

Fig. 13.1a. In light.

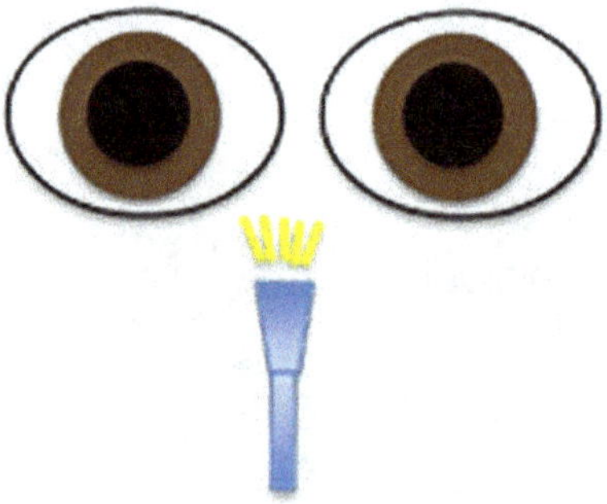

(b)

Fig. 13.1b. In the dark.

Direct and Consensual Light Reflex (Figs. 13.1c-i to 13.1c-iii)

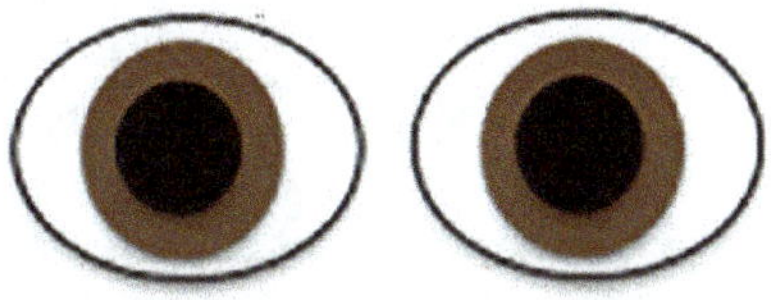

(c-i)

Fig. 13.1c-i. Demonstrates normal pupils in the dark.

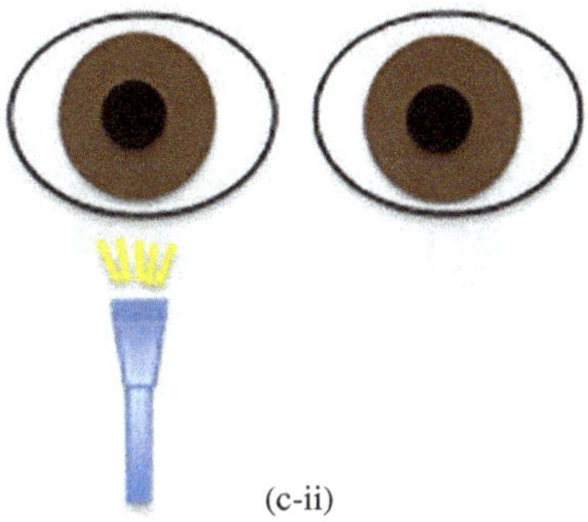

(c-ii)

Fig. 13.1c-ii. On direct stimulation of a normal pupil, with a bright, focussed light source, the pupil constricts briskly.

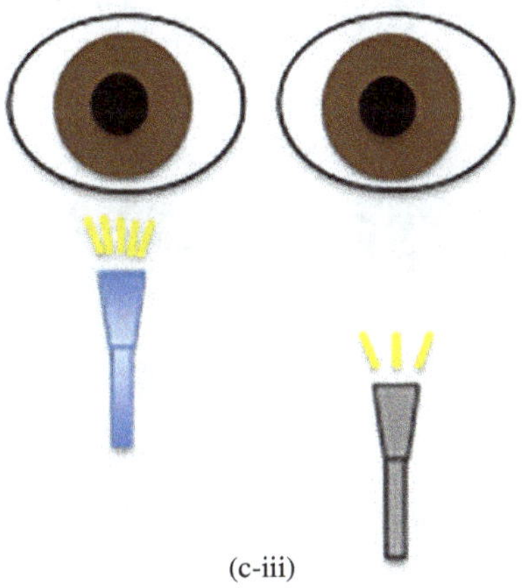

(c-iii)

Fig. 13.1c-iii. Using a dim light (grey torch), the other pupil can be seen to react briskly as well, owing to a normal consensual light response.

Swinging Torchlight Test (Figs. 13.1d-i to 13.1d-iv Demonstrate how a Relative Afferent Pupillary Defect is found on this test)

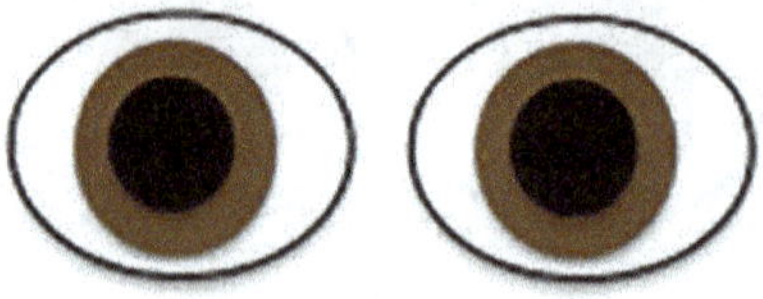

(d-i)

Fig. 13.1d-i. Demonstrates normal pupils in the dark.

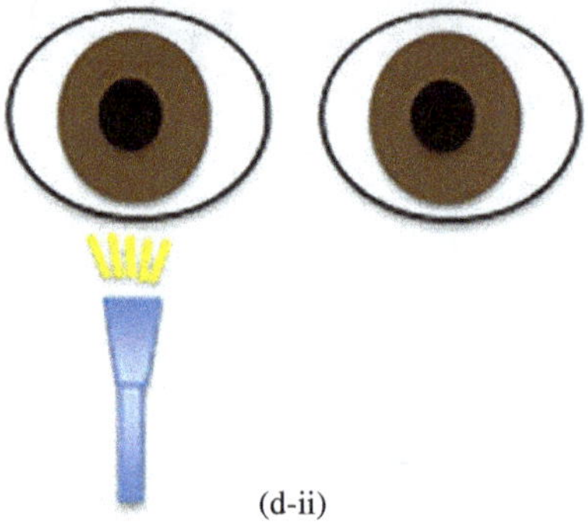

(d-ii)

Fig. 13.1d-ii. On direct stimulation of a normal pupil, with a bright, focussed light source, the pupil constricts briskly.

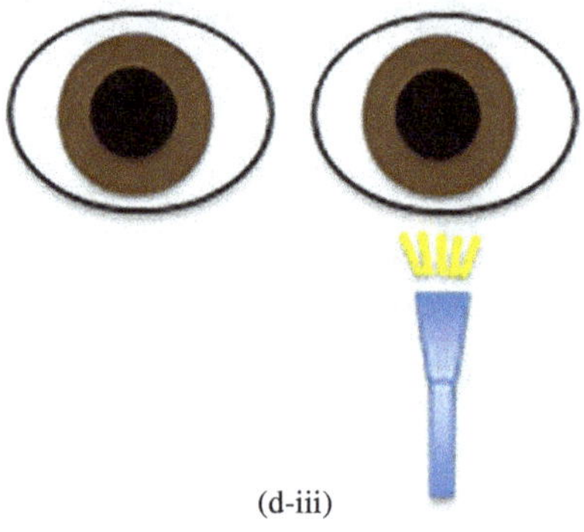

(d-iii)

Fig. 13.1d-iii. The torch should be swung rapidly to stimulate the other pupil, which will show mild dilation.

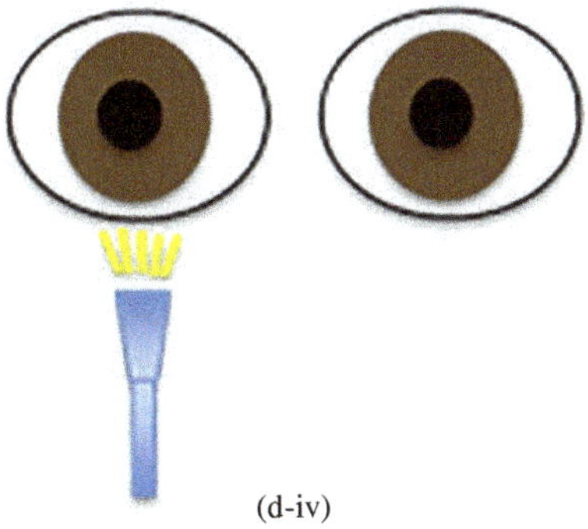

(d-iv)

Fig. 13.1d-iv. Swinging the torch back to the normal pupil will elicit a brisk response.

Light-Near Dissociation (Figs. 13.1e-i and 13.1e-ii)

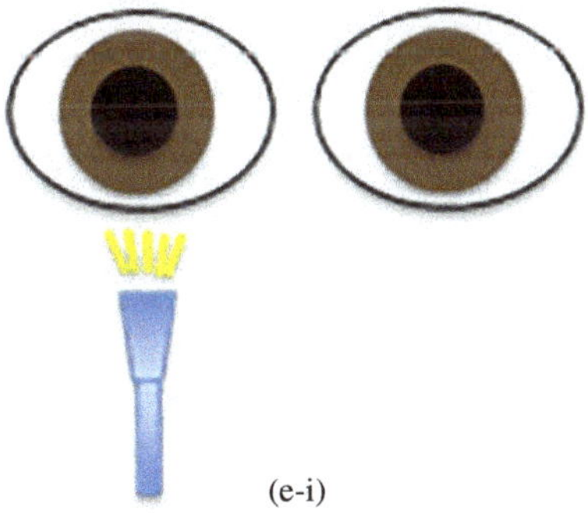

(e-i)

Fig. 13.1e-i. Direct light reflex is sluggish.

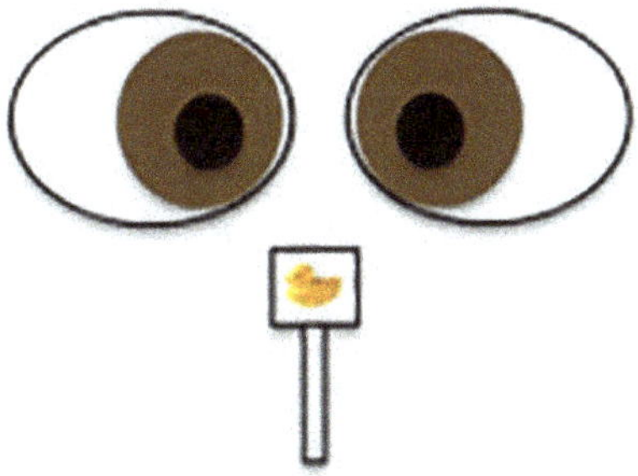

(e-ii)

Fig. 13.1e-ii. Using an accommodative target, the subject demonstrates a better "near" response.

Chapter 14

CLINICAL EXAMINATION

14.1 Approaches to Visual Acuity

Learning Objective

- Assessment of visual acuity is the first mandatory step to any ophthalmic evaluation.

Flowchart

Visual Acuity Checking

Equipment	• Check that the correct equipment is available • Snellen/ETDRS chart • Occluder and pinhole (Fig. 14.1)
UCVA	• Check and record the patient's uncorrected visual acuity (UCVA) • People who normally wear glasses must be tested with glasses • Place the patient 3 or 6 metres from the chart, depending on the chart • Use adequate illumination • One eye should be checked each time while occluding the fello w eye (with an occluder or palm of hand) • Ask the patient to read each consecutive line from the top of the chart • Record the line containing the smallest letters that can be read correctly by the patient
Pinhole	• Place a pinhole over the tested eye while occluding the fellow eye • Check and record the patient's visual acuity with a pinhole with the same technique as for UCVA testing • If there is an improvement compared to UCVA, this is indicative of a refractive error

Measurements in Patients with Poor Visual Acuity

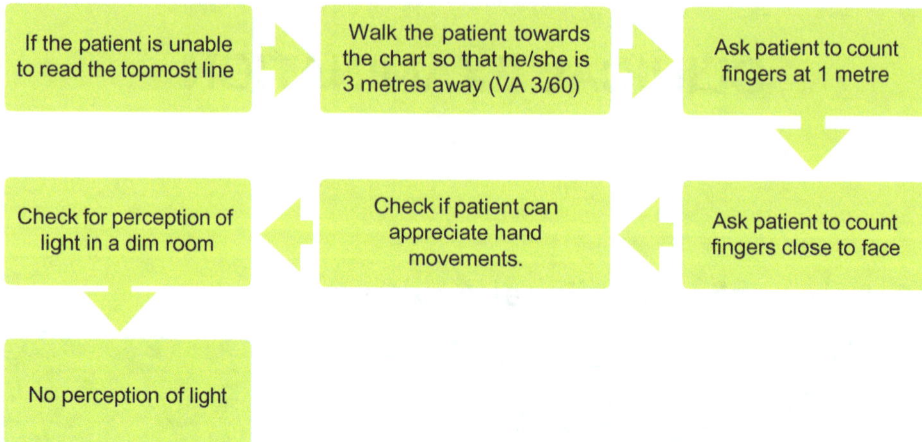

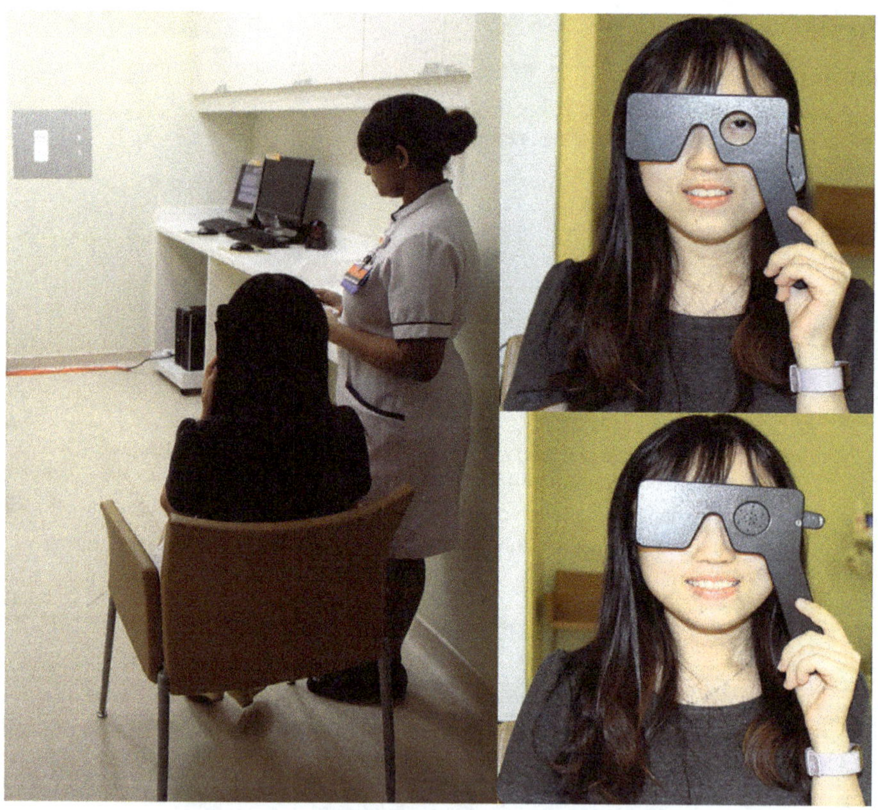

Fig. 14.1. The picture on the left shows the proper set up for visual acuity measurement. The pictures on the right show the proper way of holding the occluder without the pinhole first (top-right) and then with the pinhole (bottom-right) while checking visual acuity for the left eye.

Take Home Messages

- Make sure the patient sits at a correct distance.
- Patient's other eye must be occluded properly.

14.2 Cover Test

Learning Objective

To evaluate a patient presenting with/suspected to have an ocular deviation.

Pre-requisites for Cover Test

- Eye movement capability
- Image formation and perception
- Foveal fixation in each eye
- Attention and cooperation

3 Types of Cover Test

- Cover-uncover test (steps of this will be covered here only)
  - Detects the presence of manifest strabismus
  - Differentiates heterophoria from heterotropia
- Alternate cover test (with or without prisms)
  - Measures total deviation, regardless of whether it is latent or manifest
  - Does not specify how much of each type of deviation is present
- Simultaneous prism cover test
  - Determines actual heterotropia when both eyes are uncovered
  - Performed by covering the fixating eye at the same time the prism is placed in front of the deviating eye, using increasing prism powers until the deviated eye no longer shifts

Cover tests should be performed with fixation at distance and at near, with and without glasses (if present).

Cover-Uncover Test

1. Inspect (Fig. 14.2)
   - Ask the patient to fixate on a distant (or near) target
   - Look for any glasses present

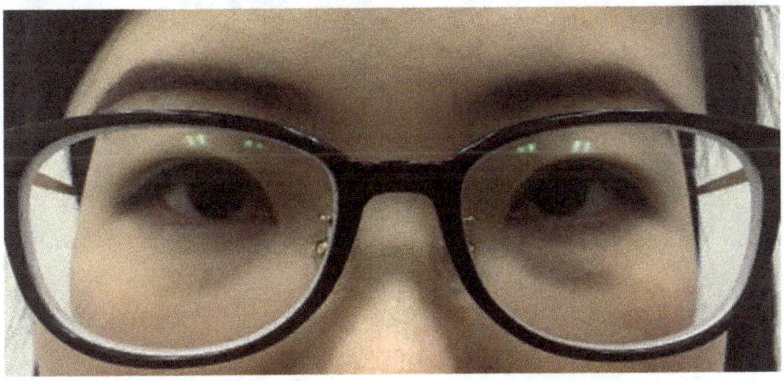

Fig. 14.2. Fixating on a distant/near target.

i. Can provide clues to the type of refractive error (myopia or hyperopia) and type of deviation (hyperopia associated with esotropia)

- Look for any abnormal head posture (AHP), tilt, ptosis, ocular deviation

  i. Can provide clues to the underlying condition, e.g. ptosis could suggest III nerve palsy, Horner's syndrome

- If ocular deviation is present, confirm with Hirschberg corneal light reflex

2. Cover fixating eye first (Fig. 14.3)

   - Comment on the deviation of the uncovered eye (if there is movement or if it maintains/takes up fixation)
   - Comment on the eye underneath the cover

     i. Any dissociated vertical deviation (DVD)

     ii. Any latent nystagmus

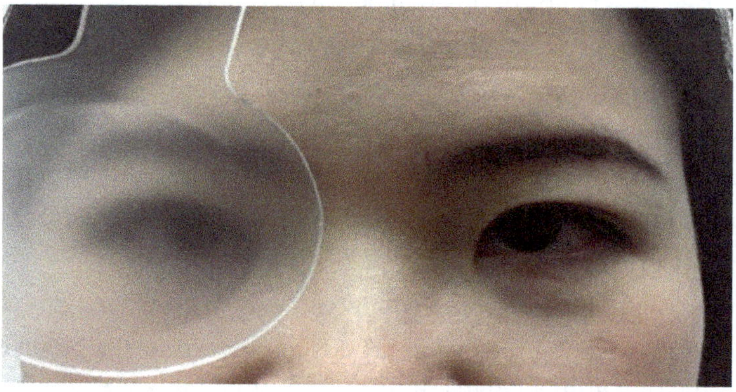

Fig. 14.3. Cover test — on covering the right eye, comment on the deviation of the uncovered eye as well as the eye underneath the cover.

3. Cover the other eye now (Fig. 14.4)

   Comment on both the uncovered and covered eye (as per step 2 above)

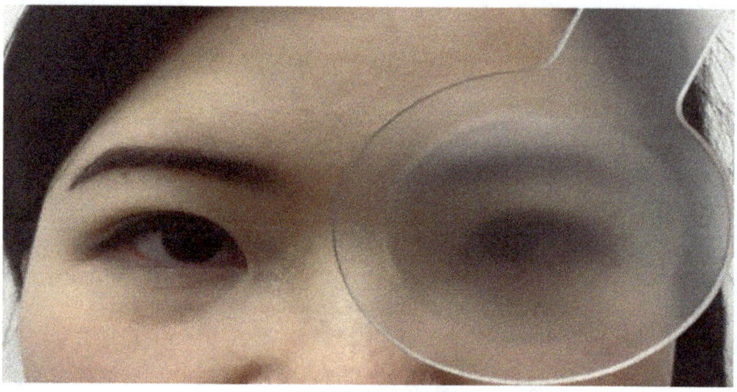

Fig. 14.4. Cover test on the other eye.

Take Home Message

A meticulously performed cover test differentiates different types of ocular deviation.

14.3 Normal Fundus Examination

Learning Objectives

- Understanding the normal fundus examination.
- Recognise key structures in the fundus.

Tools for Fundus Examination

The examination of the fundus can be done in various ways. Options include the direct ophthalmoscope, slit lamp with condensing lenses, binocular indirect ophthalmoscope (BIO), fundus cameras, etc.

The main differences between the different devices are the field of view, as well as the magnification of the image received. The handheld direct fundoscope has the smallest field of view amongst all the options mentioned.

Method of Examination

With the direct ophthalmoscope, the examiner is presented with a small field of view. A systematic examination must be done to examine the optic disc, vessels and macula.

General tips

- Examine the patient in a darkened room

Red reflex

- Ask the patient to look at the light of the fundoscope to examine the red reflex
- Use the brightest illumination

Fundus examination

- Ask the patient to fixate on a distant target to reduce eye movement
- Reduce the illumination of your direct ophthalmoscope when examining the fundus so as to improve patient comfort and allow better fixation/reduced eye movements
- Go as close to the patient's eye as possible to get a wider field of view

Components of Direct Fundoscope

- Lens wheel (Fig. 14.5)
- Filter selection (Fig. 14.6)
- Aperture selection (Fig. 14.7)

Lens Wheel

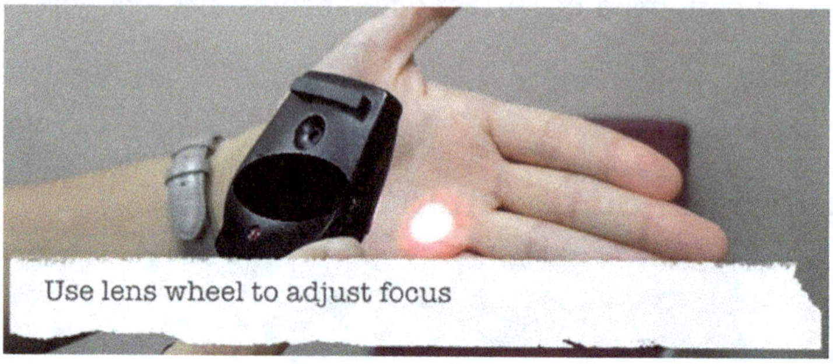
Use lens wheel to adjust focus

Fig. 14.5. Lens wheel.

Filter Selection

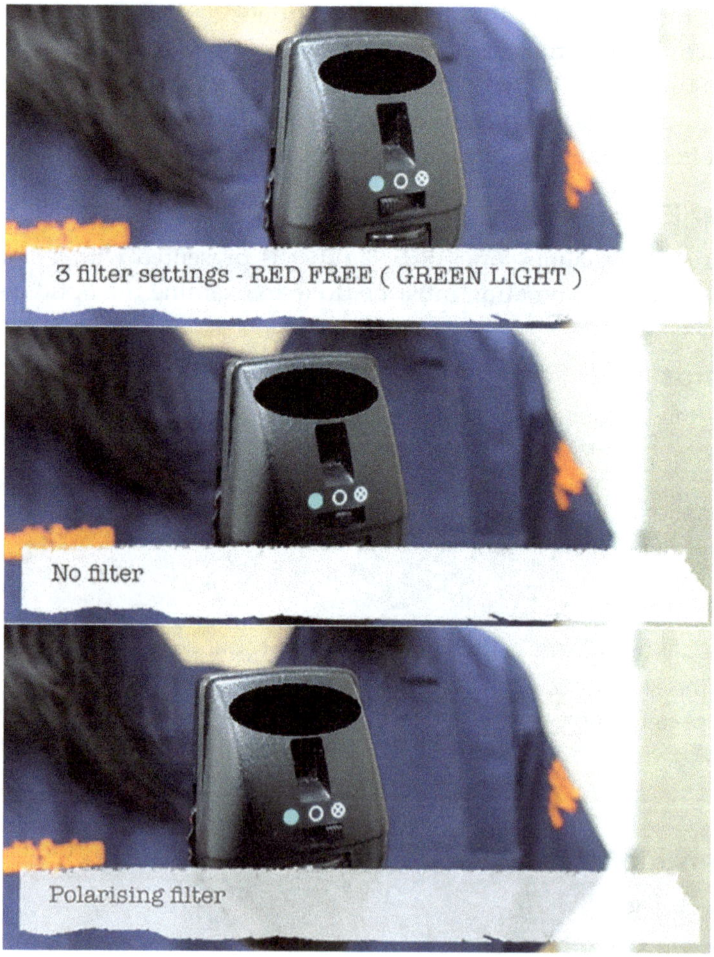
3 filter settings - RED FREE (GREEN LIGHT)
No filter
Polarising filter

Fig. 14.6. Filter selection.

Aperture Selection

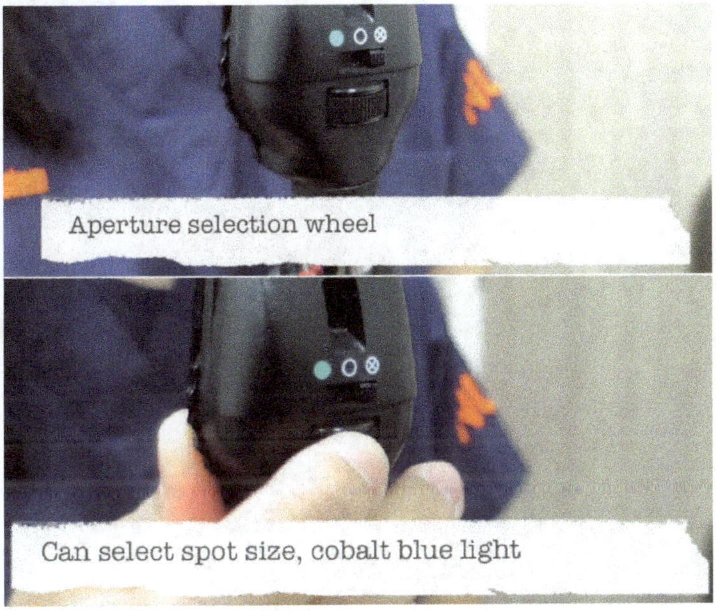

Fig. 14.7. Aperture selection.

Steps in Direct Fundoscopy

- Start with a red reflex to assess for media opacities (usually due to a cataract)
- Ask the patient to focus at a distant target (Fig. 14.8)
- Dial the lens wheel till a clear image of the retina is obtained
- Examine the optic disc, vessels, peripheral retina and macula (Fig. 14.9)

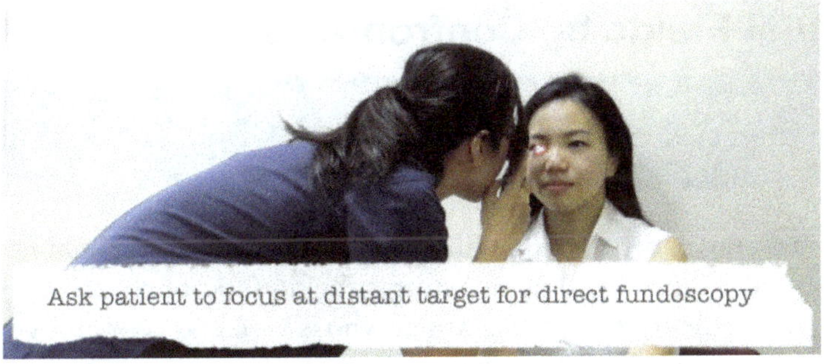

Fig. 14.8. Patient focus for direct fundoscopy.

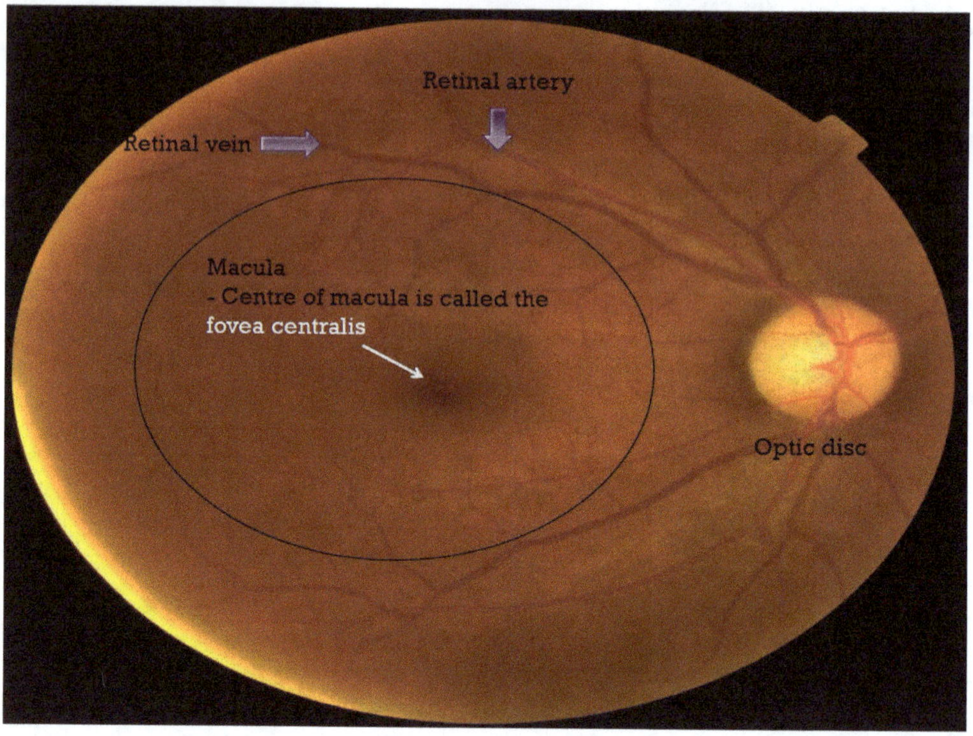

Fig. 14.9. Overview of anatomical structures in the retina.

> **Take Home Messages**
> - It is important to recognise a normal retinal anatomy.
> - Examine the macula last as this is very sensitive to light.

14.4 Visual Fields by Confrontation

> **Learning Objective**
> To be able to perform confrontation visual field.

When examining the patient, confrontational visual field testing should be performed and documented. Figure 14.10 demonstrates the method of checking visual fields by confrontation. Subsequently, in a patient who is well and cooperative, perimetry (either static or kinetic) should be used to document the visual field defect, which is useful for diagnosis and subsequent management.

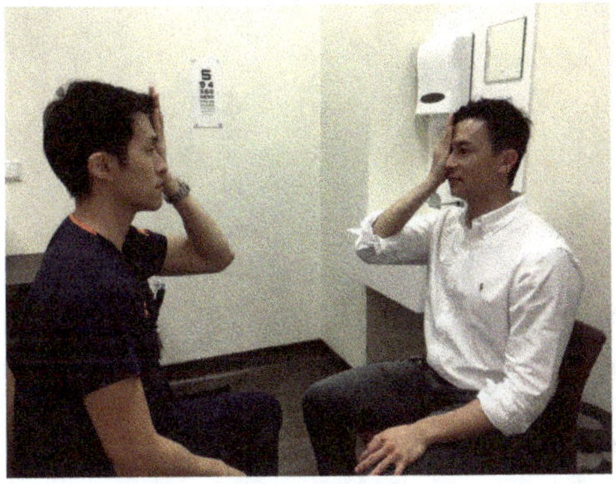

Fig. 14.10A. Both the patient and the examiner should be at eye level, and each eye is tested individually.

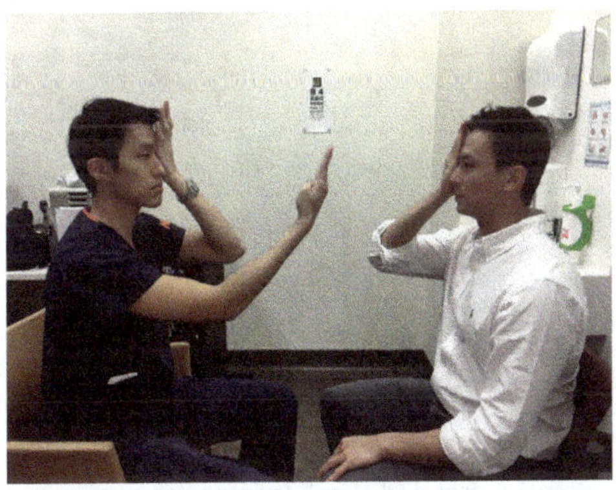

Fig. 14.10B. Start by testing the central VF, with fingers placed equidistant between the patient and the examiner.

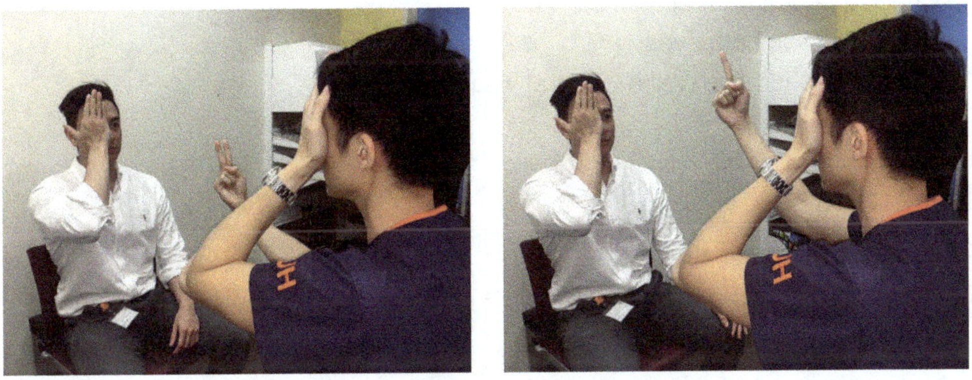

Fig. 14.10C–D. Subsequently, test the patient's ability to count his fingers in the para-central VF (4 quadrants); with hands placed approximately a shoulder width apart.

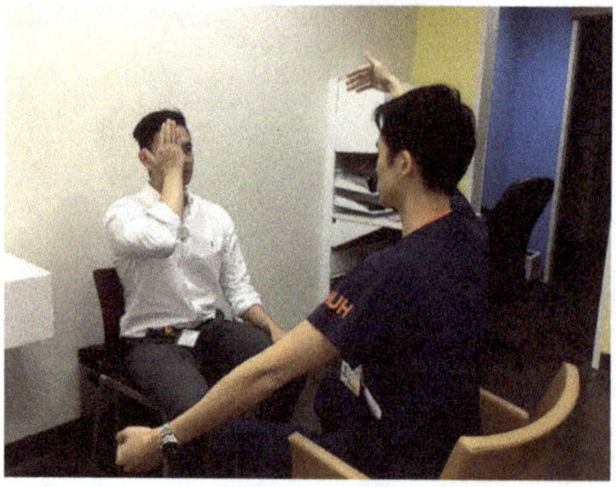

Fig. 14.10E. Check peripheral vision by hand movement.

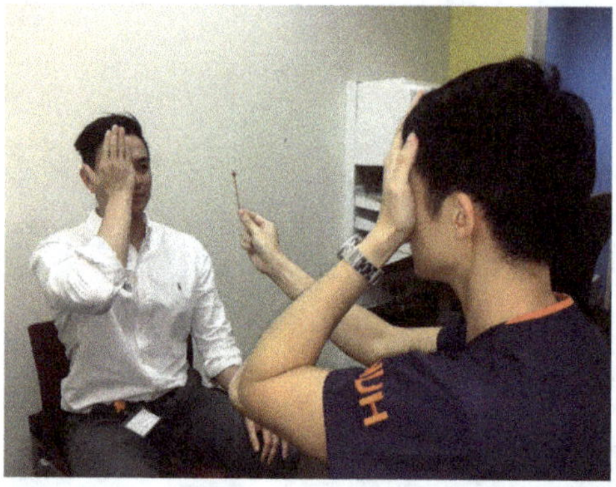

Fig. 14.10F. Delineate VF defect and check for macular involvement with a red hatpin.

Take Home Messages

- Check one quadrant at a time.
- Check fields in both eyes.
- Check peripheral as well as central visual fields.

References

1. Cover tests. www.aao.org.
2. Wilson FM. *Practical Ophthalmology — A Manual for Beginning Residents,* 4th ed.

Chapter 15

END OF POSTING TESTS (EOPT)

Learning Objectives

- EOPTs are scenario-based multiple essay questions (Total 10 marks)
- These tests evaluate the theoretical knowledge gained during the ophthalmology rotation, covering various topics
- Successful completion of the end-of-posting test is often a requirement for progressing to the next stage of medical training or to ensure that a student is competent in ophthalmology before moving on to other specialties

15.1 Basic Anatomy of the Eye

<u>Question 1</u>

This is a bony structure of orbit.

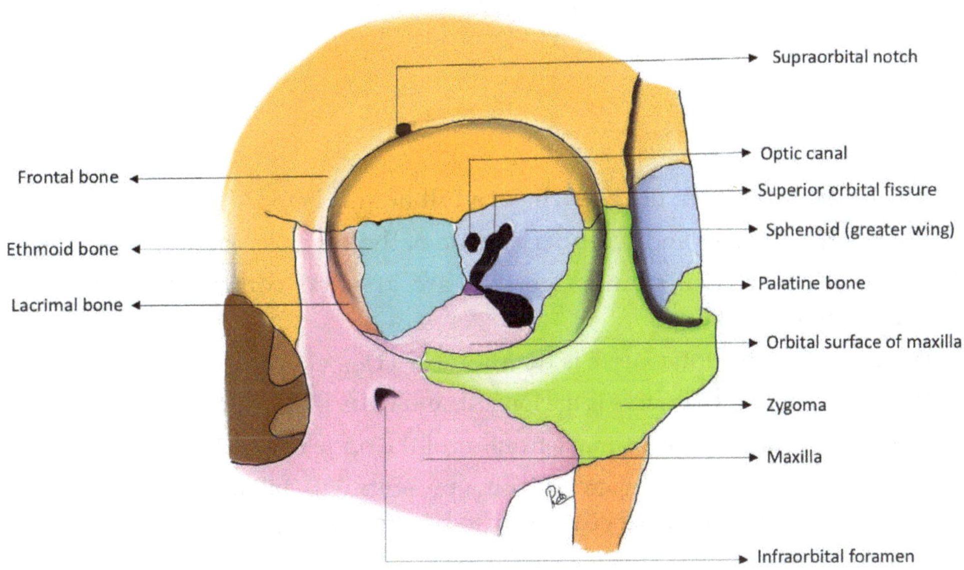

1. Which bones make up the floor of the orbit? (3)
2. Name 3 major nerves that pass through the superior orbital fissure. (3)
3. Which structure of the orbit transmits ophthalmic artery? (1)
4. Why do some patients develop infraorbital anaesthesia after orbital floor fracture? (2)
5. What is the slit between the greater wing of the sphenoid and maxilla called? (1)

Answers

1. Maxilla, orbital plate of zygomatic bone and palatine bone
2. (Any 3) Trochlear, oculomotor, abducent, lacrimal and frontal
3. Optic canal
4. Involvement of infraorbital branch of maxillary nerve
5. Inferior orbital fissure

Question 2

This is a cross-section of orbit and orbital content.

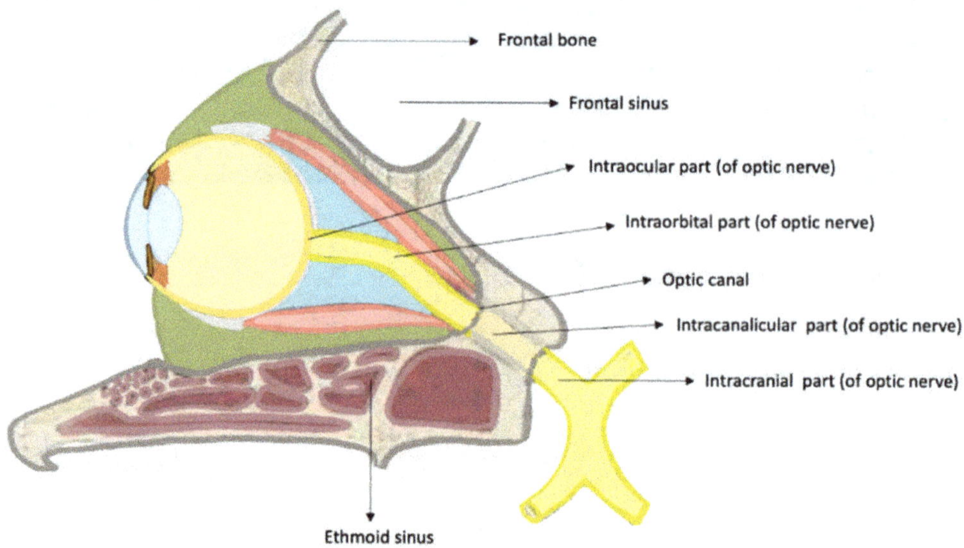

1. What is the volume of the globe in an adult human being? (1)
2. What is the primary and secondary action of the superior oblique muscle? (2)
3. Name two extraocular muscles that are affected commonly in thyroid ophthalmopathy. (2)
4. Which part of the optic nerve is the shortest? (1)
5. Which part of the optic nerve is the longest, and what is the approximate length? (2)
6. What is the commonest primary tumour of the optic nerve? (1)
7. A patient with pituitary macroadenoma presents with bitemporal hemianopia. Which part of the optic nerve is likely to be affected? (1)

Answers

1. Approximately 6.5 mL.
2. Primary: intorsion; Secondary: depression.

3. Any muscles can be involved but the most common are the inferior rectus and the medial rectus (in that order).
4. Intraocular part is shortest (approximately 1 mm).
5. Intraorbital segment of the optic nerve, approximate length 25 mm.
6. Optic nerve glioma.
7. Optic chiasm.

15.2 Cornea and External Eye Diseases

Question 3

A 30-year-old lady presents with 2 days' history of right eye redness and pain.

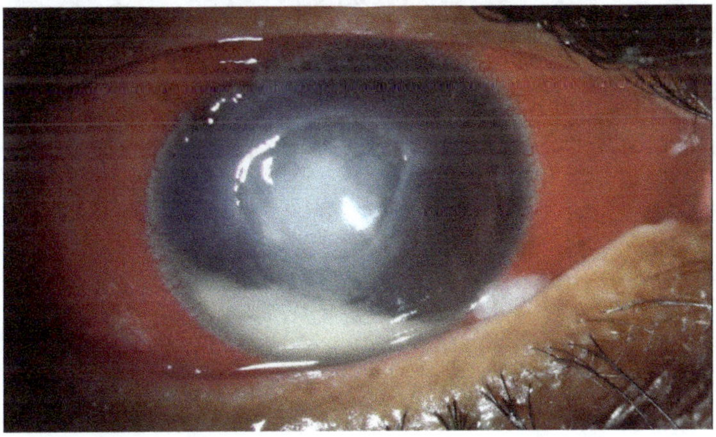

1. What is the most likely diagnosis? (1)
2. Describe the clinical signs seen in this photo. (3)
3. Name 3 risk factors. (3)
4. How will you manage the patient? (3)

Answers

1. Infectious keratitis.
2. Diffuse conjunctival injection, central large epithelial defect with infiltration, hypopyon.
3. Contact lens wear, trauma, history of recurrent corneal erosion.
4. Corneal scraping to send for aerobic, anaerobic and fungal culture. Start hourly fortified broad spectrum topical antibiotics and topical cycloplegia. Trace the cultures and titrate the antibiotics according to sensitivity results and the clinical response.

Question 4

A 60-year-old gentleman notices a growth at the corner of his eye over many years.

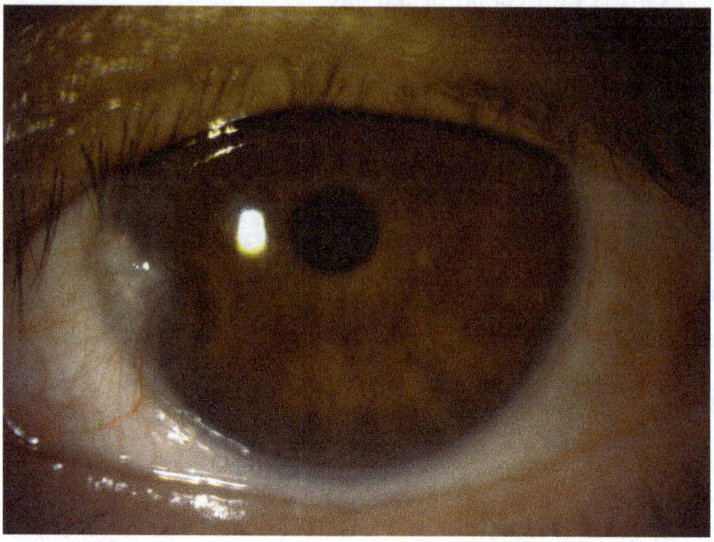

1. What is the diagnosis? (1)
2. What are the possible symptoms? (3)
3. What is the main risk factor? (1)
4. How will you manage this patient? (2)
5. When will you consider surgical removal? (3)

Answers

1. Pterygium.
2. Eye irritation, blurring of vision, change in refractive error.
3. Ultraviolet exposure from sunlight.
4. Conservative with lubricating eye drops.
   If symptomatic, for surgical excision with conjunctival autograft.
5. Pterygium crossing the visual axis, high induced astigmatism, persistent eye irritation, concerns related to cosmesis.

Question 5

11-year-old boy who presents with persistently itchy eyes with discharge.

1. What clinical sign is shown here? (1)
2. What is the most likely diagnosis? (1)
3. What other medical history will you ask the patient for? Name 2. (2)
4. What are the other clinical signs you will look for in the eye? (3)
5. How will you manage this patient? (3)

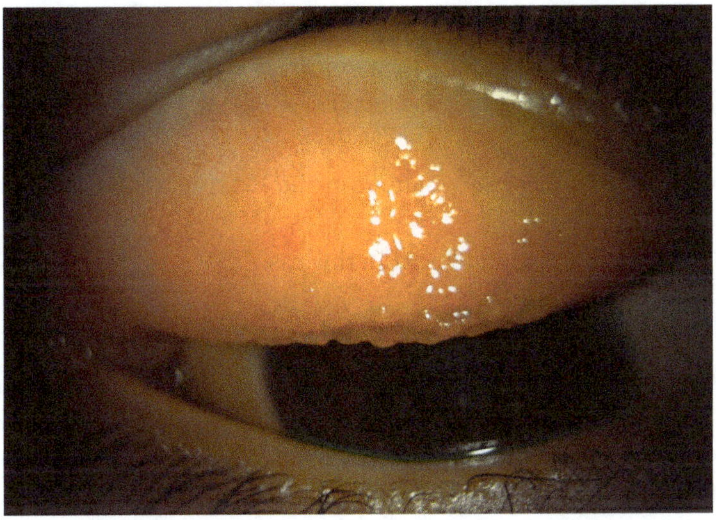

Answers

1. Cobblestone papillae.
2. Vernal keratoconjunctivitis.
3. History of allergic rhinitis, eczema, asthma.
4. Conjunctival injection, Horner Trantas dots, corneal epithelial erosions, shield ulcer.
5. Allergen avoidance, topical mast-cell stabilisers, topical anti-histamine, topical steroids, lubricating eye drops.

Question 6

A 43-year-old man was hit in the right eye by a sharp object while working on a construction site and complains of severe pain along with an acute loss of vision immediately after.

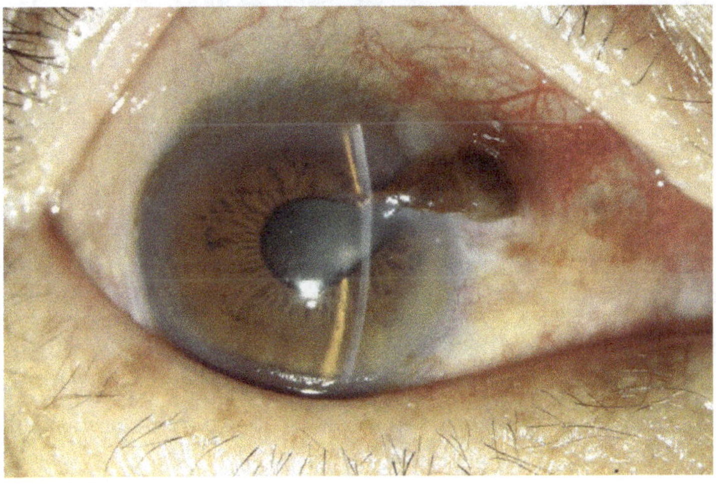

1. What is your diagnosis? (1)
2. Describe the clinical findings in the anterior segment photo. (3)
3. What radiological examination should be ordered in the Emergency Department and why? (2)
4. How would you manage this patient in the Emergency Department prior to surgery? (3)
5. What is the definitive management in this case? (1)

Answers

1. Right eye globe rupture.
2. Corneal laceration, scleral laceration, prolapsed iris, subconjunctival haemorrhage, distorted pupil.
3. CT orbits to rule out intraocular foreign body.
4. Nil by mouth, intravenous antibiotics, shield eye, anti-tetanus toxoid (any 3, 3 marks).
5. Repair of laceration.

Question 7

A construction worker was mixing cement when it splashed and entered his left eye. This is the photo of his left eye.

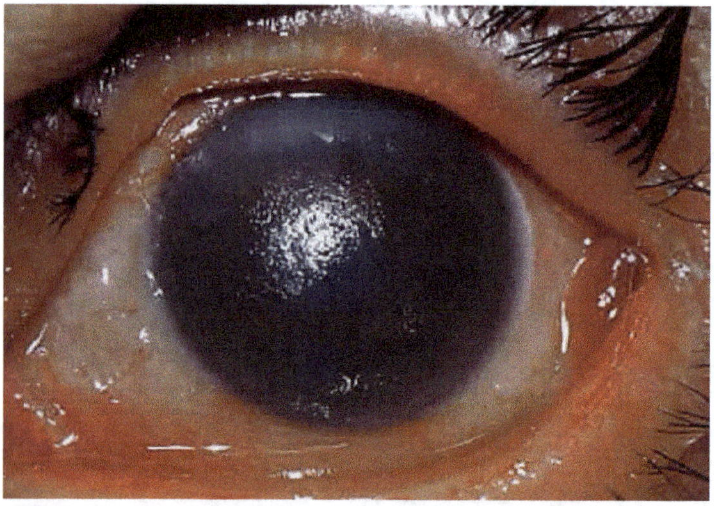

1. What injury did he sustain? (1)
2. Is cement alkaline or acidic? Which is more toxic to the eye? (2)
3. Describe what you see in this clinical picture. (2)
4. What 2 immediate measures should be performed when you see him at A&E? (2)
5. Provide 3 possible complications that this patient may have in the future. (3)

Answers

1. Chemical injury.
2. Alkaline, alkaline.
3. Hazy cornea, conjunctival injection, limbal ischaemia.
4. Irrigate, look for particles by everting the lid.
5. Persistent epithelial defect, limbal stem cell deficiency, symblepharon or ankyloblepharon, glaucoma, cataracts, corneal decompensation, dry eyes, corneal opacification.

15.3 Cataract

Question 8

A 60-year-old taxi driver came for her routine eye examination. Her uncorrected visual acuity was 6/24, which improves to 6/18 with glasses. Her intraocular pressure was 15 mm Hg. There is no relative afferent pupillary defect. Her dilated fundus examination is unremarkable.

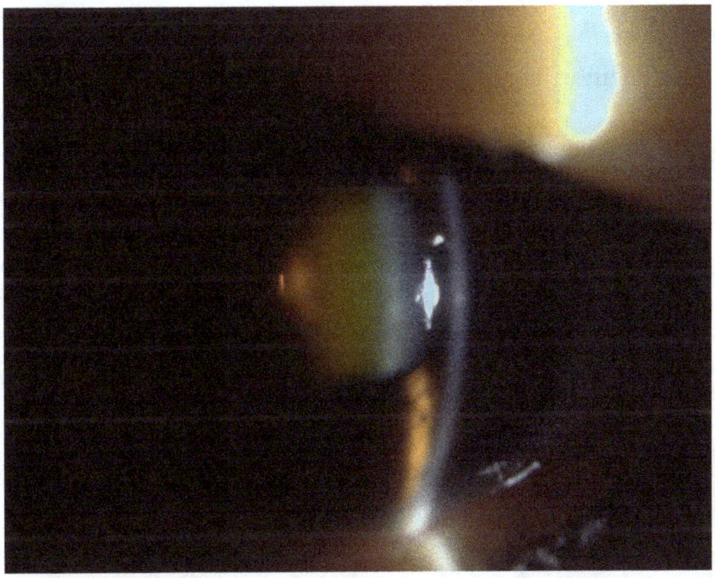

1. Her dilated anterior segment photo is shown. What is the most likely type of cataract she has? (1)
2. Name two other morphological types of cataracts you know. (2)
3. How would you immediately manage this patient? (3)
4. Name different techniques of cataract surgery. (2)
5. Name two intraoperative complications of cataract surgery. (2)

Answers

1. Nuclear sclerosis/nuclear sclerotic cataract.
2. Any two: Cortical cataract, posterior subcapsular cataract, posterior polar cataract.
3. Any of the following (up to 3 marks):

   Advise her to stop vocational driving immediately.

   Prescribe glasses for best correction.

   Arrange cataract surgery for her at the earliest availability.

   Issue extended medical certificate until vision recovers to vocational driving requirements.
4. Any two of the following:

   Phacoemulsification

   Extracapsular cataract surgery

   Small incision cataract surgery

   Intracapsular cataract surgery
5. Any two of the following:

   Posterior capsular rupture

   Nuclear drop

   Expulsive haemorrhage

Question 9

An 85-year-old patient with dementia and previously treated proliferative diabetic retinopathy is having his routine eye examination. His best corrected visual acuity is hand movement bilaterally. Examination of the anterior segment shows a shallow anterior chamber with bilateral dense cataracts. His intraocular pressure is 20 mmHg bilaterally. There is no relative afferent pupillary defect. However, on dilated fundus examination, the retina was not visible. This is the picture of one of the eyes.

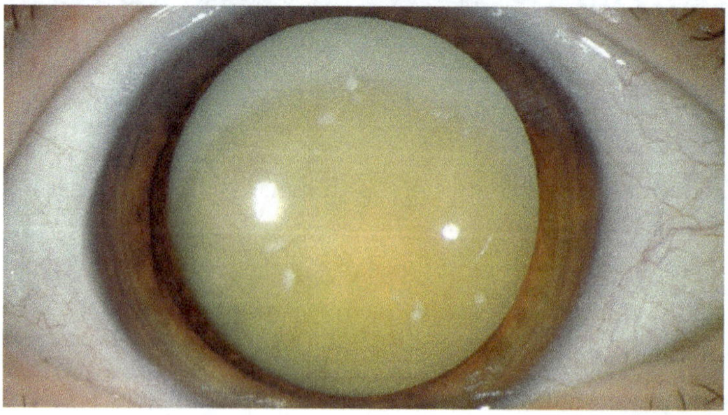

1. Identify the type of cataract. (1)
2. How will you counsel this patient regarding his cataract surgical outcome? (2)
3. Please identify four risk factors for this patient undergoing phacoemulsification. (4)
4. What kind of anaesthesia would you like to advise for this patient? (1)
5. Please identify two potential postoperative complications for this patient after uneventful phacoemulsification. (2)

Answers

1. Hypermature Morgagnian cataract.
2. The prognosis remains poor in view of the old patient, dense cataract and unknown status of the retina.
3. Any four of the following:

   Elderly patient with zonular weakness.

   Poor cooperation due to dementia.

   Dense cataract.

   Shallow anterior chamber.

   Poor pupillary dilation due to diabetes.
4. I would prefer general anaesthesia as the patient has dementia.
5. Any of the following (up to 2 marks):

   Persistent corneal oedema/corneal decompensation/pseudophakic bullous keratopathy.

   Pseudophakic cystoid macular oedema/diabetic macular oedema/Irvine-Gass syndrome.

   Exogenous endophthalmitis.

   Persistently raised intraocular pressure.

   Zonular dialysis.

Question 10

A 64-year-old taxi driver presents to your clinic with progressive blurring of vision over the last two years. He has had cataract surgery 8 years ago, which significantly improved his vision. However, as of late, he reports the presence of a misty-like vision with associated glare when driving at night. You notice the following findings while examining him:

1. What is the diagnosis? (1)
2. How would you manage this? (2)
3. The patient is interested to find out more about the procedure. How would you explain this to the patient? (3)
4. What are the possible complications of this procedure? (4)

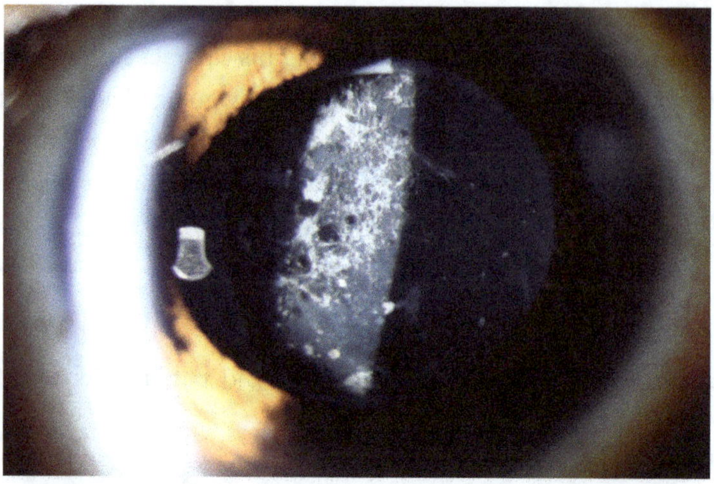

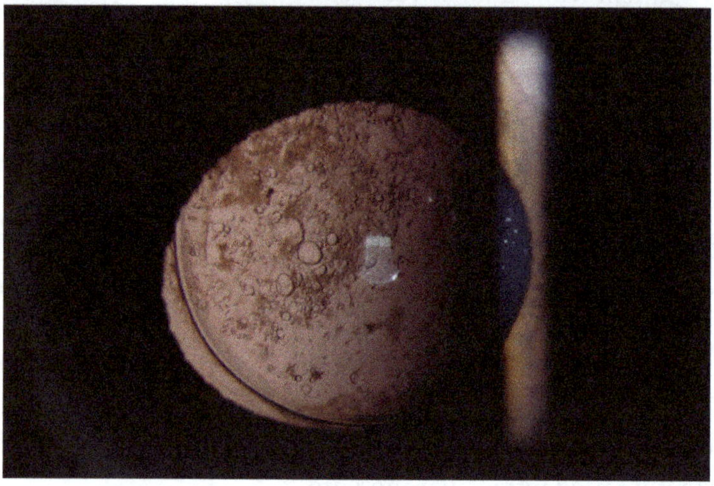

Answers

1. Posterior capsule opacification.
2. Posterior capsule opacification is a common occurrence after cataract surgery. This is typically managed in a clinical setting by performing a laser procedure, termed a YAG posterior capsulotomy.
3. A YAG posterior capsulotomy is a laser procedure used to treat posterior capsule opacification (PCO), a common complication following cataract surgery. This clouding posterior capsule can impair vision similarly to a cataract. The procedure involves the application of a specialised Nd YAG laser to create a small opening in the cloudy posterior capsule. The entire procedure usually takes a few minutes and is typically painless. As the cloudy layer is removed, light passes through the lens implant unobstructed, and this results in significant improvement in vision.
4. Rare complications include increased intraocular pressure (IOP), retinal detachment, cystoid macular oedema, damage to the intraocular lens (IOL) and corneal oedema.

<u>Question 11</u>

A 54-year-old gentleman with a known history of diabetes presents at your clinic reporting the presence of decreased visual acuity associated with glare and halos, particularly at night. When examining him in your clinic you notice the following findings:

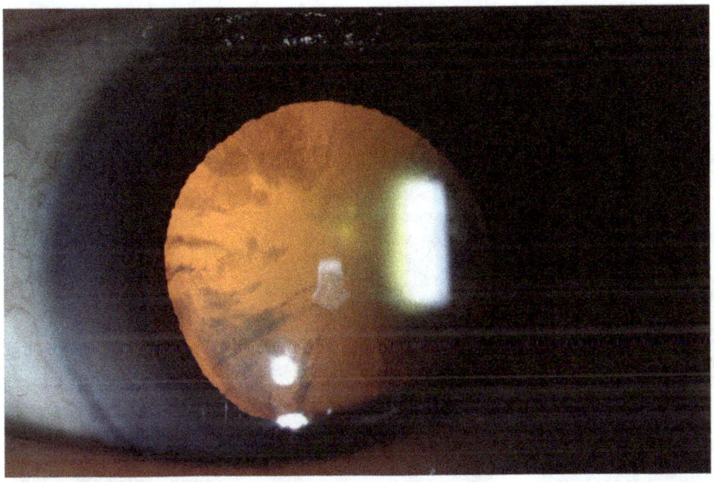

1. What is the most likely cause of his symptoms? (1)
2. What symptoms do patients typically report with cortical cataracts? (3)
3. This patient would like to consider cataract surgery, and he has heard from his friends that multifocal intraocular lenses are an option that will allow him to be completely free of glasses. On further questioning, you note that he loves driving on long trips, which frequently involves overnight driving. Do you think that he be a suitable candidate? (1)

   Please justify your answer (3)
4. What other categories of intraocular lenses are available? (2)

<u>**Answers**</u>

1. The presence of a cortical cataract.
2. Patients with cortical cataracts typically report the presence of glare, particularly at night, given that the cortical spokes tend to involve the periphery of the crystalline lens. As the pupil is dilated in dim conditions, patients are typically more symptomatic from the cortical component of cataracts during this period, although these can subsequently progress to involve the central aspect of the lens and the visual axis. Other common symptoms that patients with cataracts report include decreased visual acuity and decreased contrast sensitivity.
3. No.

   Justification: While multifocal intraocular lenses confer an increase in the range of vision, they are also associated with a range of adverse visual effects, such as glare and halos. These may be more prominent at night. Other disadvantages of multifocal intraocular lenses include a decrease in contrast sensitivity and poorer vision in dimly lit environments, amongst others. This patient is unlikely to be a suitable candidate for a multifocal lens. Other options should be explored.

4. Monofocal (and monodical plus) lenses, and extended depth of focus (EDOF) lenses.

Question 12

A 20-year-old gentleman presents to your clinic reporting the presence of progressive blurring of vision involving his right eye, associated with increased sensitivity to bright lights. He finds that his vision is worse in the daytime, compared to the evenings. On examination of the patient, you identify the following findings:

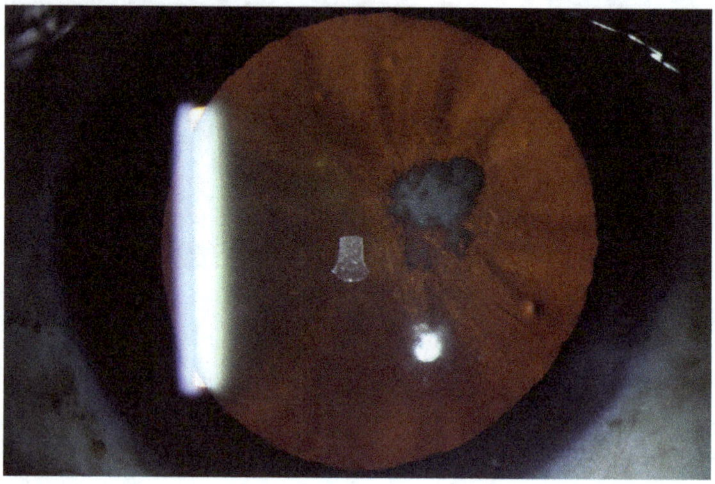

1. What is your diagnosis? (1)
2. What are the common causes of this type of cataract? (4)
3. On further questioning, he recalls an incident where he had gotten into a fist fight and had been punched in the face. What other findings would you be considering in your examination of this patient? (3)
4. Why is identification of these important? (2)

Answers

1. There is the presence of a cataract with an anterior subcapsular component.
2. Trauma, ocular inflammation, keratitis, use of medications such as amiodarone.
3. Assessing for the presence of other concomitant ocular injuries. These include corneal and scleral wounds, iris damage, zonular status, and damage to the retina or optic nerve.
4. These injuries may result in a more complex and complicated surgery and affect the final visual prognosis.

15.4 Glaucoma

Question 13

A 69-year-old gentleman defaulted his diabetic retinopathy screen and presented a year later in the clinic with raised intraocular pressure (30 mmHg).

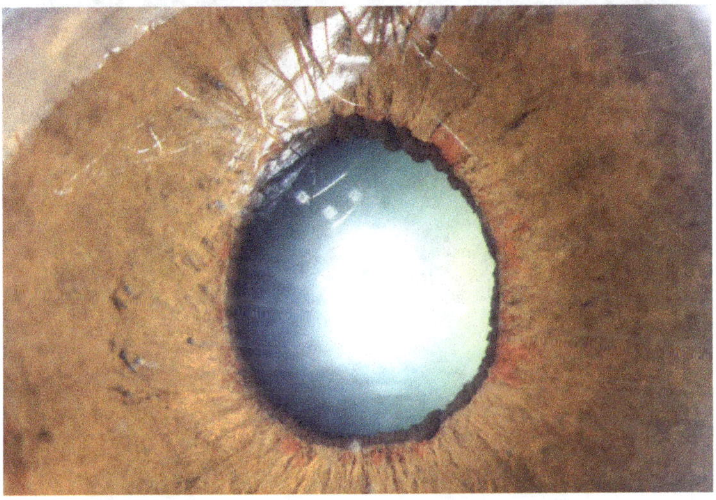

1. Describe the key clinical finding in the photo. (1)
2. Name the type of glaucoma that he is likely to have. (1)
3. Name 3 ocular conditions that predisposes the patient to this type of glaucoma. (3)
4. How do you manage this condition? (5)

Answers

1. Rubeosis iridis.
2. Neovascular glaucoma.
3. Any 3: Proliferative diabetic retinopathy, ocular ischaemic syndrome, retinal vein occlusion, chronic uveitis, chronic retinal detachment, ocular tumours.
4. Control vascular risk factors (1), Manage the underlying ischaemic process (e.g. PRP/intravitreal anti-VEGF) (1), Manage the raised IOP with glaucoma medications (1), and if the patient still has raised IOP despite maximum tolerable medications, can consider laser (TCP/MPTCP) (1) or surgery (1).

Question 14

A 70-year-old gentleman went for a yearly diabetic retinopathy eye screen and was noted to have this finding during examination:

1. Describe the finding as highlighted by the white arrow. (1)
2. Name the eye condition that is often described together with this eye finding. (1)
3. Describe 2 other optic disc findings in the photo. (2)
4. Name 3 risk factors for this condition. (3)
5. Name 3 investigations that can be carried out for this condition. (3)

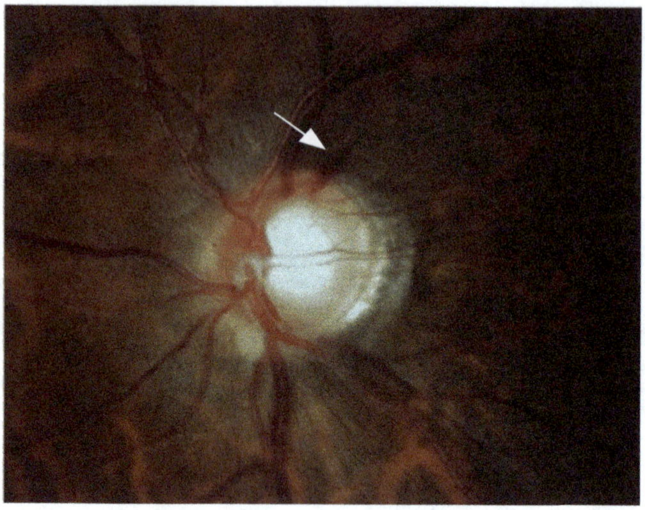

Answers

1. Drance haemorrhage.
2. Normal tension glaucoma.
3. Any 2: Optic disc cupping, thin inferior rim, bayoneting of vessels, nasalisation of vessels.
4. Any 3: Migraine, sleep apnoea, Raynaud's syndrome, previous history of significant blood loss, family history of glaucoma.
5. Any 3: Humphrey visual fields, OCT RNFL, CCT, stereo-disc photos, OCTA.

Question 15

A 74-year-old lady had a history of right eye trabeculectomy done 12 years ago. She complains of right eye redness, blurring of vision and pain for the past 3 days.

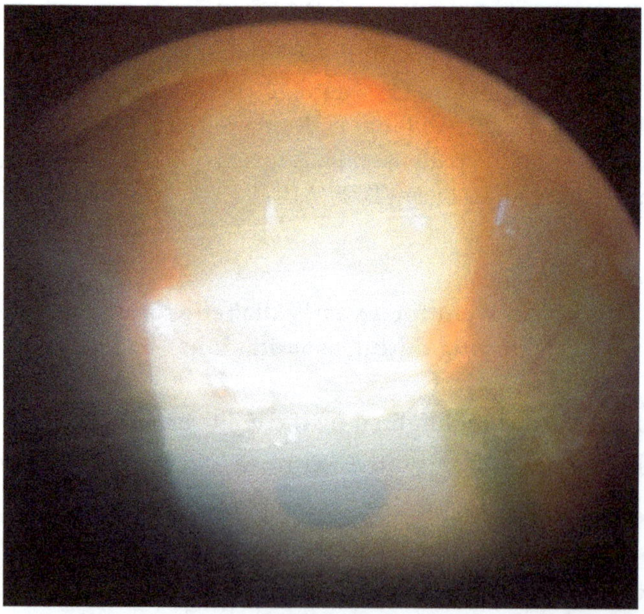

1. Describe what you see in the photo. (3)
2. What examination findings will suggest endophthalmitis in this case? (3)
3. What is the diagnosis? (1)
4. Name 3 other complications associated with trabeculectomies. (3)

Answers

1. Cystic avascular bleb, surrounding conjunctival injection, fluid within bleb looks turbid.
2. Any 3: Presence of RAPD, hypopyon, vitritis, loss of red reflex.
3. Right blebitis.
4. Any 3: Suprachoroidal haemorrhage, malignant glaucoma, wipe out/blindness, raised IOP, hypotony, endophthalmitis, hyphaema, overfiltration, wound leak, pupil block, scleral perforation, cataract progression.

Question 16

This is a 76-year-old Indian lady who presented with painful red eye and an intractable headache.

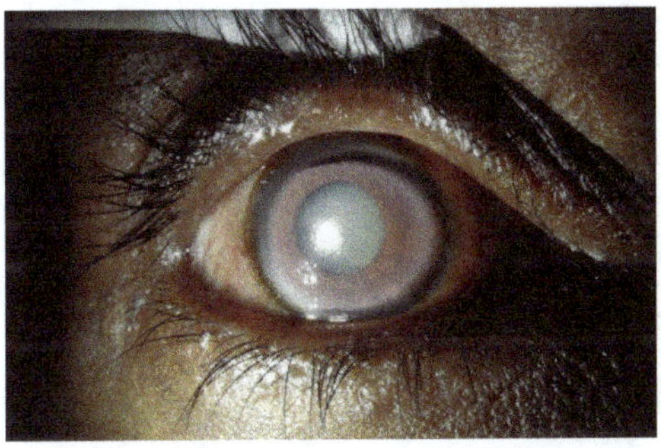

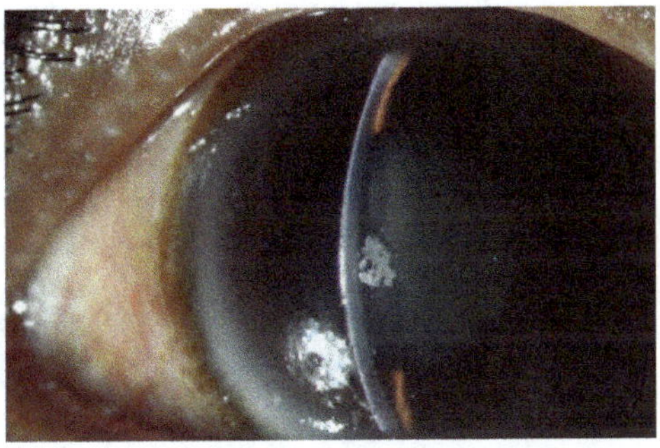

1. Describe what you see in these photos (3).
2. What are the other symptoms and signs she may have? (5)
3. What is the immediate treatment? (2)

Answers

1. Hazy cornea, mid-dilated pupil, conjunctival injection and shallow anterior chamber depth.
2. Symptoms — nausea/vomiting, glares and haloes and blurred vision. Signs — raised intraocular pressure, glaukomflecken, closed angles on gonioscopy in the affected and fellow eye.
3. Reduce intraocular pressure (medically followed by relieving the pupil block by performing a laser peripheral iridotomy).

Question 17

This is an ophthalmic investigation:

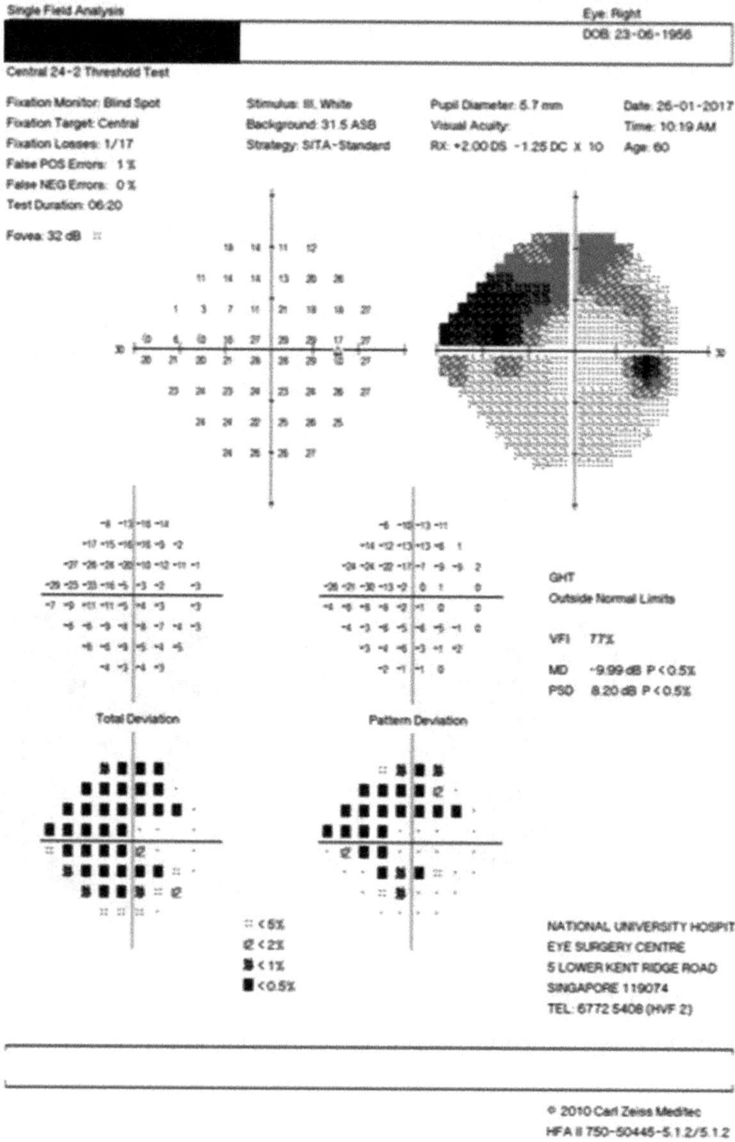

1. Describe this investigation and what are the indications? (4)
2. How is the reliability of this test determined? (3)
3. Describe the defect shown in this investigation and what are the possible diagnoses? (3)

Answers

1. Static automated perimetry.

   Common indications include diagnosis and monitoring of eye and neurological conditions, such as glaucoma, maculopathy, optic neuropathy and intracranial pathology.

2. This is a subjective test, and the reliability indices include fixation losses, false positive and false negative catch trials.
3. Superior arcuate defect in the right eye. Possible diagnosis includes glaucoma and retinopathy involving the inferior retina.

15.5 Uveitis

<u>Question 18</u>

A 6-year-old female complains of left eye pain for the past one week.

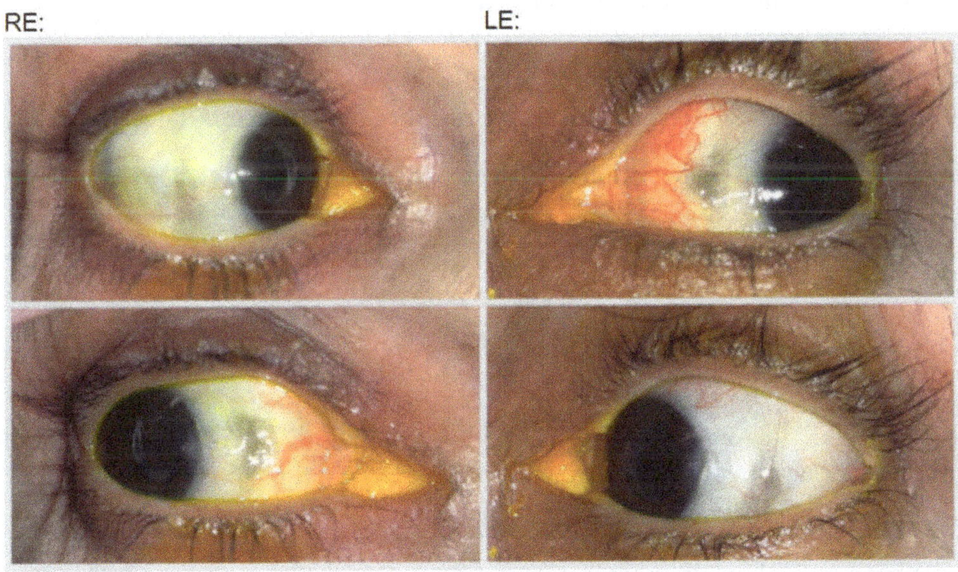

Image 1

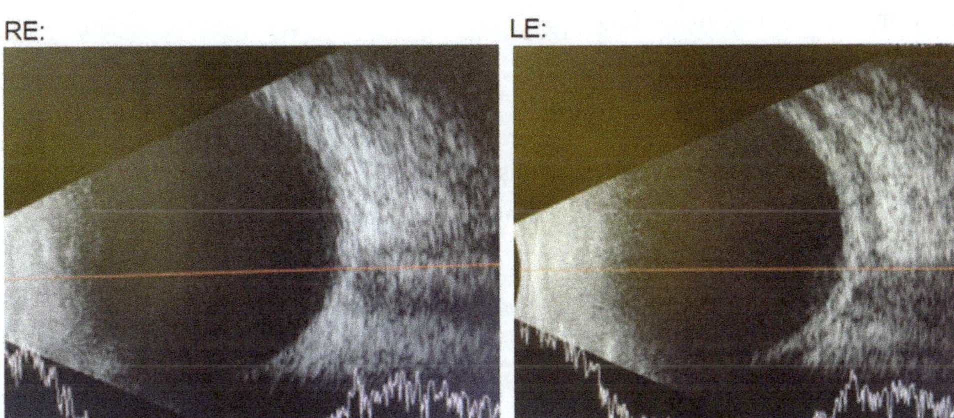

Image 2

1. Describe the clinical signs in Image 1. (2)
2. What is the imaging test shown in Image 2? (1)
3. What is the sign shown in Image 2, and what does it imply? (2)

4. What is the diagnosis? (2)
5. How would you investigate the patient? (3)

Answers

1. Left eye scleral injection, both eyes scleromalacia.
2. B-scan ultrasonography.
3. T-sign, fluid in the subtenon space.
4. Left eye posterior scleritis.
5. Blood investigations: Rheumatoid Factor, anti-neutrophil cytoplasmic antibody (ANCA), TB quantiferon, anti-ENA panel.

Question 19

A 27-year-old female presented with recurrent redness in her left eye

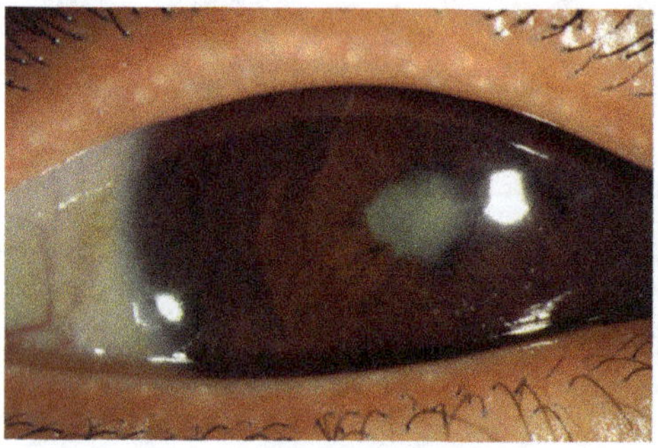

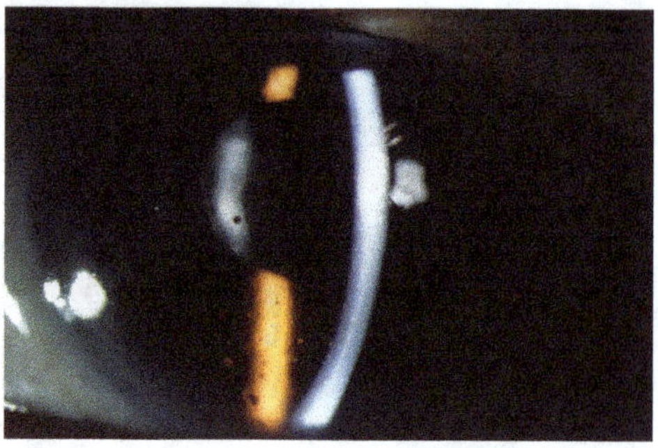

1. Describe the clinical signs. (4)
2. What could other symptoms be apart from red eye? (2)
3. Name a possible diagnosis. (1)
4. Name 3 possible causes. (2)

Answers

1. (Any 4) Posterior synechia, peripheral anterior synechia, white cataract, keratic precipitate, neovascularisation of iris, iris nodules.
2. Recurrent eye pain, blurring of vision.
3. Chronic anterior uveitis.
4. TB, sarcoidosis, syphilis, infiltrative.

15.6 Vitreo-retina

Question 20

A 50-year-old man presents with right eye blurring of vision for the last 1 month.

1. Describe the abnormalities in this fundus photograph. (2)
2. What is the diagnosis? (1)

3. What are the risk factors? (3)
4. The patient has reduced vision. What are the possible causes? (2)
5. What are the pharmacotherapeutic options for the treatment of cystoid macular oedema? (2)

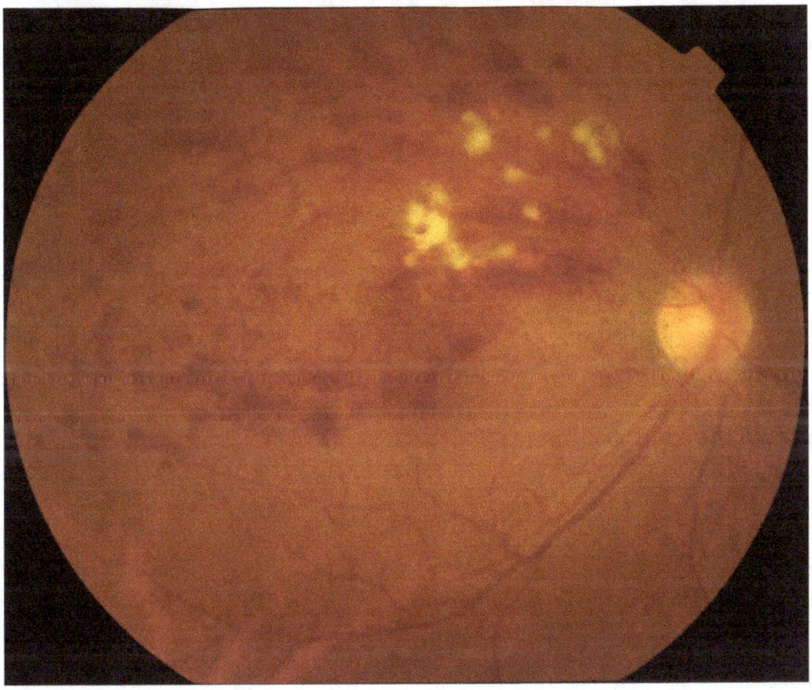

Answers

1. Flame-shaped haemorrhage, dot and blot haemorrhage involving the macula, cotton wool spots.
2. Right eye branch retinal vein occlusion.
3. Hypertension, hyperlipidaemia, diabetes.
4. Macular oedema, macular ischaemia.
5. Intravitreal anti-vascular endothelial growth factor, intravitreal corticosteroid.

Question 21

A 40-year-old patient presents with right eye blurring of vision for the last 3–4 months. He mentions he has been seeing a GP periodically and has been on metformin for the last 15 years.

1. What is the diagnosis? (1)
2. What systemic disease can give rise to this ocular complication? (1)
3. What is the eye screening recommendations for patients with diabetes? (4)
4. What is the management for patients with proliferative diabetic retinopathy? (2)

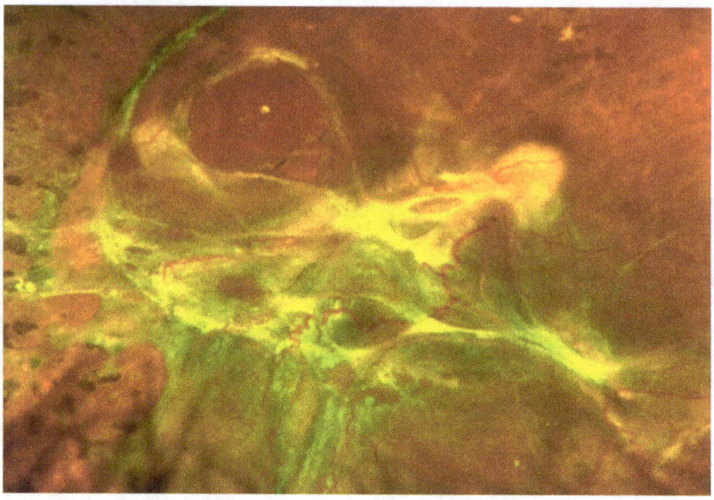

Answers

1. Tractional retinal detachment.
2. Diabetes mellitus.
3. T1DM: 5 years after diagnosis, then annually. T2DM: upon diagnosis, then annually.
4. Systemic: optimise glycaemic control; Ocular: pan-retinal photocoagulation.

Question 22

A 60-year-old lady presents with blurring of vision in both eyes for 6 months. She says she underwent some treatment at a private eye clinic 1 month ago for both eyes.

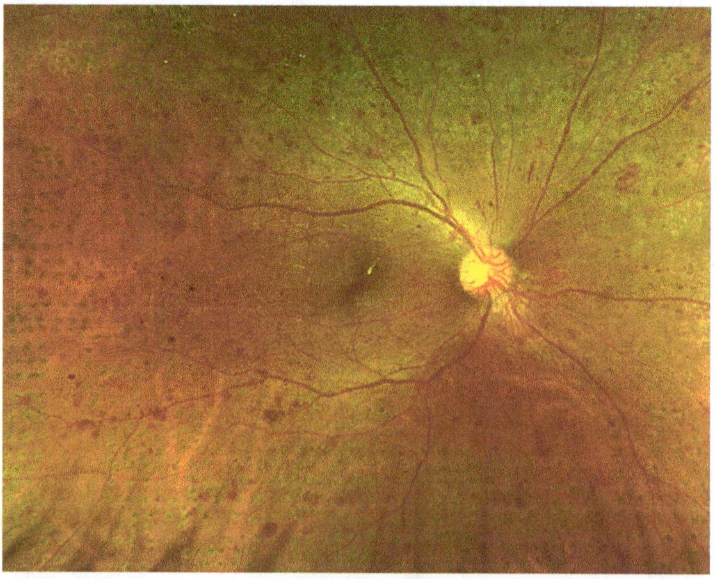

1. Describe features present in this fundus photograph. (3)
2. What is the diagnosis? (1)
3. What other ocular complications can develop? (4)

Answers

1. Laser photocoagulation scars, neovascularisation of the disc, blot haemorrhages/venous beading.
2. Proliferative diabetic retinopathy.
3. Diabetic macular oedema, vitreous haemorrhage, tractional retinal detachment, neovascular glaucoma.

Question 23

A 42-year-old patient with a history of diabetes reports blurring of vision in one eye for the last 2 months.

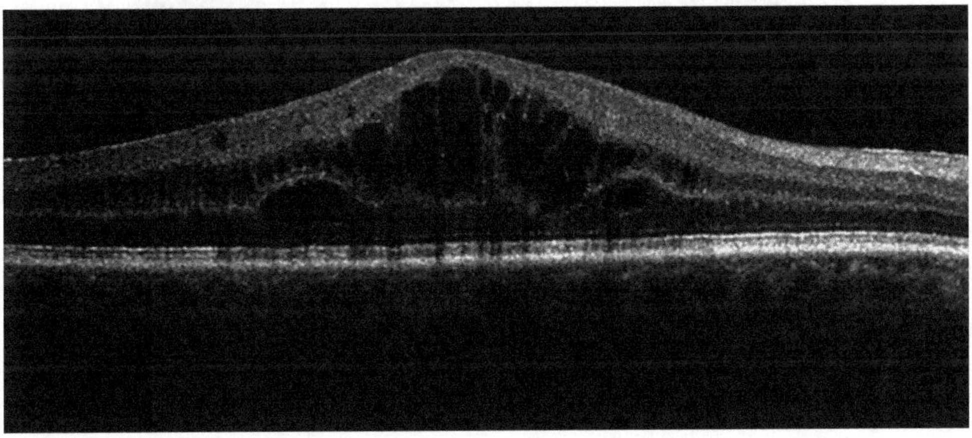

1. What are the possible causes for his blurring of vision? (3)
2. What is the name of this investigation? (2)
3. What does this image show? (1)
4. What are the ocular treatment options? (3)
5. What else is important in the management of this patient? (1)

Answers

1. Diabetic macular oedema, vitreous haemorrhage, retinal detachment, cataract.
2. Macular optical coherence tomography.
3. Diabetic macular oedema.
4. Intravitreal anti-vascular endothelial growth factor, intravitreal corticosteroids, focal/grid laser.
5. Optimising glycaemic control.

Question 24

A 40-year-old man with a history of poorly controlled diabetes presents with eye pain and redness.

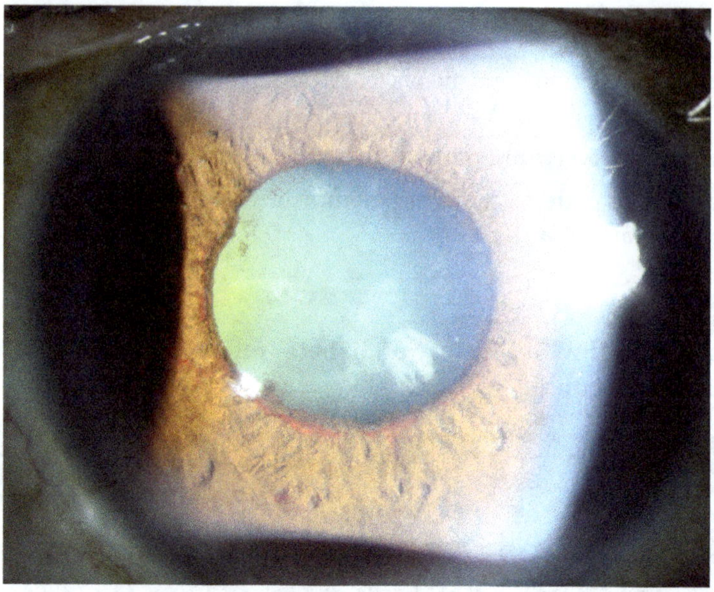

1. Describe the abnormalities in this anterior segment photograph. (2)
2. What other examination should be performed? (2)
3. What is the diagnosis if the intraocular pressure is elevated? (1)
4. What are possible causes for this? (2)
5. How do you manage such cases? (3)

Answers

1. Neovascularisation of the iris, cataract.
2. Measurement of the intraocular pressure, gonioscopy, retinal fundus examination.
3. Neovascular glaucoma.
4. Proliferative diabetic retinopathy, ischaemic central retinal vein occlusion, ocular ischaemic syndrome.
5. Anti-glaucoma eye drops, intravitreal injection of anti-VEGF, pan-retinal photocoagulation, glaucoma surgery if IOP is not controlled with eye drops.

Question 25

An 80-year-old gentleman with a history of smoking reports seeing distorted vision and a dark spot in his right eye.

1. Describe the abnormality on this fundus photograph. (2)
2. What is the likely diagnosis? (2)
3. Name two investigations you would like to perform. (2)
4. What is the management for this patient? (3)

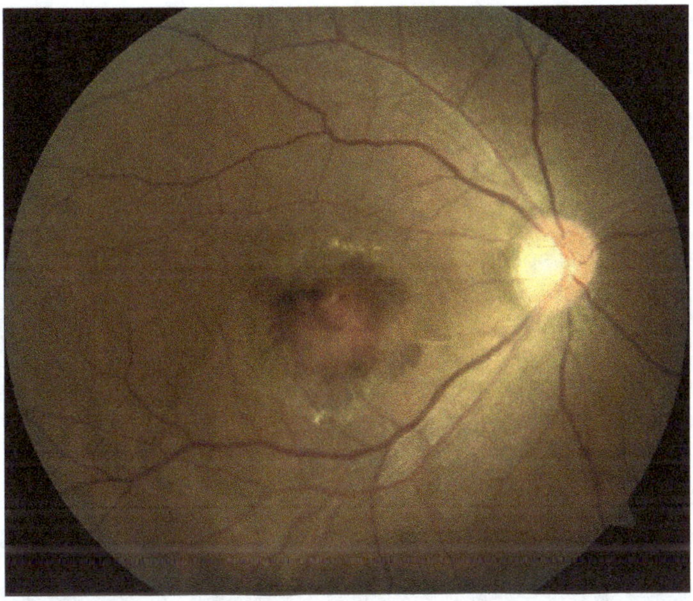

Answers

1. Subretinal haemorrhage involving macular and perimacular region, few drusens.
2. Neovascular/wet, age-related macular degeneration.
3. (Any 2): Optical coherence tomography, OCT angiography, fundus fluorescein angiography, indocyanine green angiography.
4. Intravitreal injection of anti-vascular endothelial growth factor, smoking cessation, antioxidant/AREDS supplementation.

Question 26

A 60-year-old lady presents to the A&E with a complaint of sudden painless loss of vision in one eye.

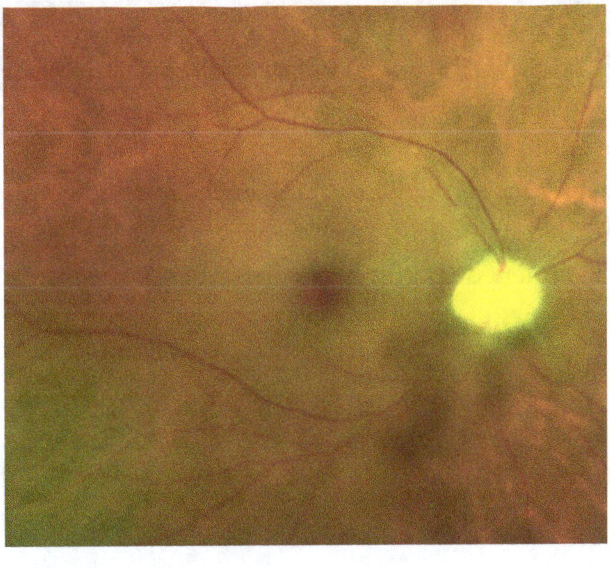

1. Enumerate the clinical findings seen in this fundus photo. (3)
2. What is the likely diagnosis? (1)
3. What are the systemic risk factors for this condition? (3)
4. How do you manage this patient in an emergency? (3)

Answers

1. Pale disc, cherry red spot, vascular attenuation, pale retina.
2. Central retinal artery occlusion.
3. Hypertension, hyperlipidaemia, carotid artery stenosis, cardiac emboli.
4. Ocular massage, IV acetazolamide/IOP lowering eye drops, anterior chamber paracentesis.

Question 27

This is the fundus photograph of a patient with blurring of vision in his right eye:

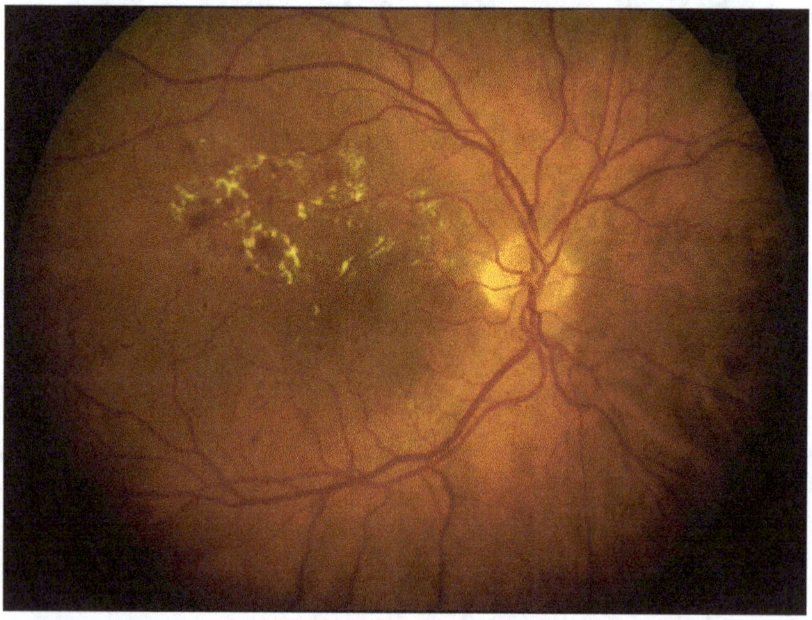

1. Name three signs in the photograph. (3)
2. What abnormality in this photograph might explain his symptoms? (1)
3. What underlying condition is this patient likely to have? (1)
4. What ocular treatment does this patient require? (2)
5. What would he benefit from in terms of systemic treatment? (2)
6. What would happen if he refused treatment? (1)

Answers

1. Hard exudates close to macula, dot haemorrhage, blot haemorrhage.
2. Maculopathy/clinically significant macular oedema.

3. Diabetes mellitus.
4. Macular laser/focal laser, intravitreal injection of anti-VEGF.
5. Control DM, control other co-morbidities such as HPT, lipids, renal failure if any.
6. Visual loss from maculopathy/retinopathy.

15.7 Oculoplastics

Question 28

A 68-year-old male presents with a change in his appearance over the past 3 months. This is associated with palpitations as well as a noted increase in irritability and anxiety. He has reported heat intolerance and an increase in appetite but a loss of weight.

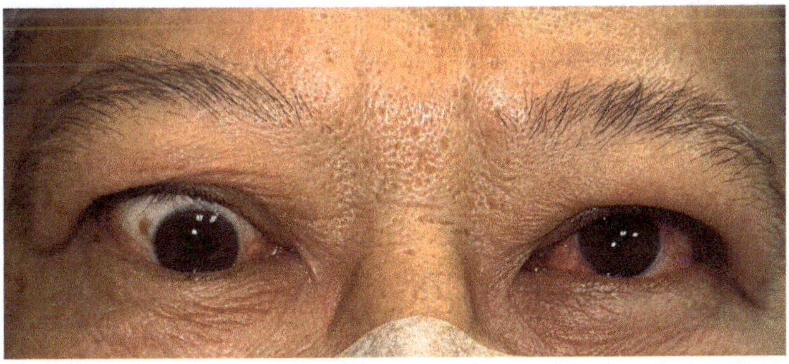

1. Describe what do you see here? (2)
2. What signs and symptoms do you think would be worrying here? (2)
3. What is the diagnosis? (2)
4. What can increase the risk of severe disease? (2)
5. How would you treat his condition? (2)

Answers

1. Puffy erythematous eyelids, conjunctival injection, right upper eyelid retraction, left chemosis, ocular misalignment.
2. Drop in vision, white corneal infiltrate, double vision, lagophthalmos, conjunctival injection.
3. Active severe thyroid eye disease.
4. Smoking, old age, poor control of thyroid status, high TSH receptor-binding antibody (TRAb) or thyroid-stimulating immunoglobulin (TSI) levels, hypertension/diabetes, male gender.
5. Multidisciplinary management to optimise his thyroid status, optimise his risk factors, lubricating eye drops, systemic immunosuppression, orbital decompression surgery.

Question 29

An 8-year-old boy presents with nausea and vomiting after he was hit in the left eye whilst playing soccer. His heart rate was noted to drop to 40 beats per minute when looking up.

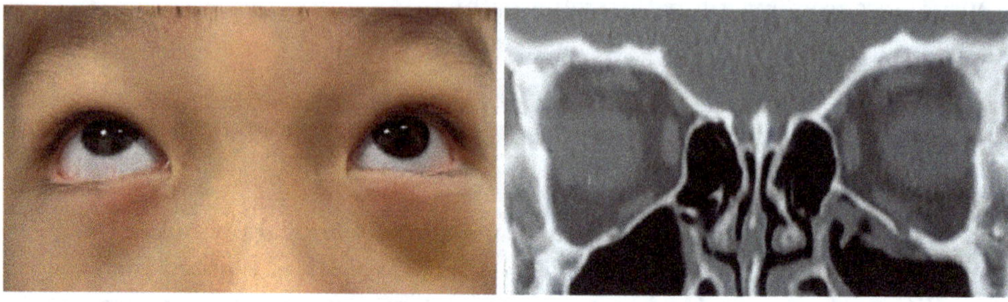

1. What do you see here? (2)
2. What do you think has caused this? (1)
3. What do you think has caused his signs and symptoms? (3)
4. What investigation is shown here? (1)
5. How would you manage him? (3)

Answers

1. Left infraorbital ecchymosis, left hypotropia.
2. Left orbital floor fracture with possible entrapment.
3. Greenstick fracture/trapdoor fracture with extraocular muscle-intermuscular septum complex (EOM-IMS complex) entrapment, resulting in bradycardia and nausea on up-gaze.
4. Orbital imaging with computed tomography.
5. This is an ophthalmic emergency. I would admit the patient and arrange for a release of the trapdoor fracture with repair of the orbital floor as soon as possible.

Question 30

A 6-year-old boy presents with worsening right upper eyelid swelling and pain over 2 days duration. He denies any eyelid injury or any insect bite. He remained afebrile on presentation to the emergency department.

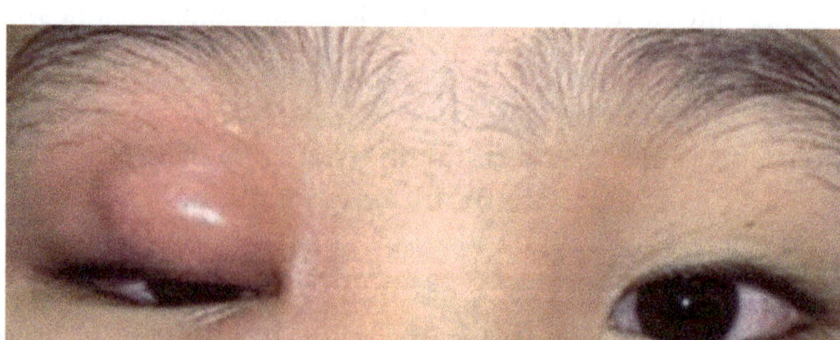

1. What do you see here? (2)
2. What do you think this is? (2)
3. What would you do for this patient? (2)

   Two days later he returns for a review, and you note that he has worsened clinically:

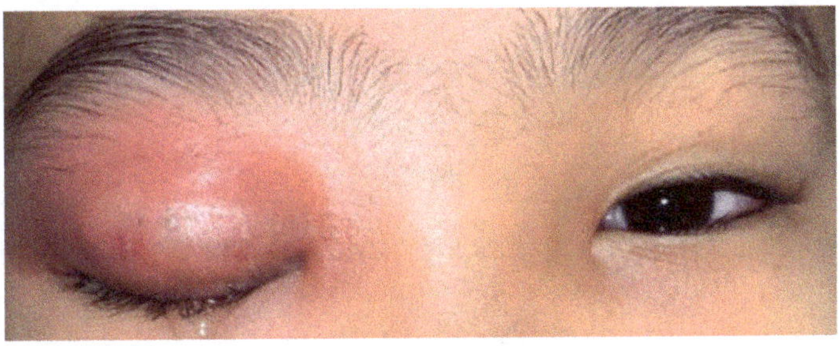

4. What are you worried about here? (2)
5. What would you do for this patient? (2)

<u>Answers</u>

1. Right upper eyelid swelling and erythema that is obscuring the visual axis. The eye remains white.
2. Right preseptal cellulitis, probably from an infected internal hordeolum.
3. Admit to commence broad spectrum systemic intravenous antibiotics, warm compresses, monitor closely for clinical signs of orbital cellulitis, consider incision and drainage when an abscess develops.
4. Orbital cellulitis with an abscess that can lead to blindness or death. I am unable to assess the underlying eye condition.
5. Admit immediately — this is an ophthalmic emergency. Start intravenous antibiotics, perform urgent contrast-enhanced orbital imaging via computed tomography or magnetic resonance imaging to look for signs of orbital cellulitis, subperiosteal abscess and paranasal sinusitis or orbital tumours. Keep patient nil by mouth to prepare for incision and drainage of the orbital abscess with appropriate smears and cultures.

15.8 Paediatric Ophthalmology and Strabismus

<u>Question 31</u>

An 8-year-old girl was noted by her schoolteacher to be having difficulty reading off the screen in class.

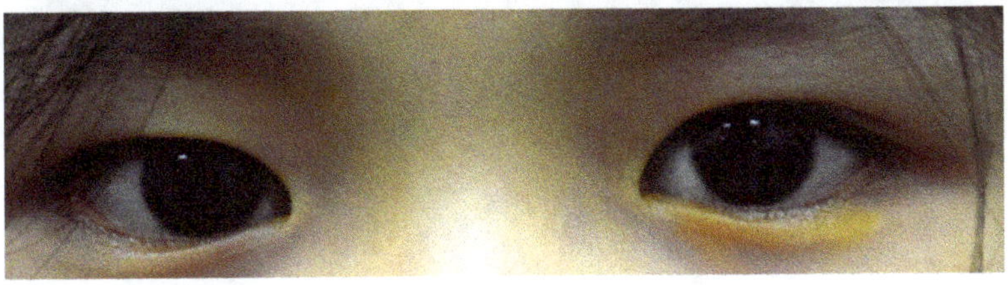

Fig. 15.1

Time	Right					Left				
	Distance		Pinhole		Near	Distance		Pinhole		Near
	W Glasses	W/O Glasses	W Glasses	W/O Glasses		W Glasses	W/O Glasses	W Glasses	W/O Glasses	
11:18	6/18-1					6/24				

Remarks Snellen (singles)
Tested w/ trial frames

Fig. 15.2.

Type	Post Op	Right						Left			
		Sph	Cyl	Axis	VA	Add	NVA	Sph	Cyl	Axis	VA
Cyclorefraction		+2.00	-3.75	175	6/12			+2.00	-3.50	170	6/9

Fig. 15.3.

1. What eyelid sign do you see in the first photograph? (1)
2. You checked her vision subjectively and noted her vision (Fig. 15.2). You therefore decided to proceed with a cycloplegic refraction and noted the above (Fig. 15.3). Interpret the results as shown in Figs. 15.1 and 15.2. (2)
3. What else would you examine for in a child with this eyelid condition? (2)
4. How would you manage her? (3)
5. What complications are you worried about? (2)

Answers

1. Bilateral lower eyelid epiblepharon.
2. Meridional astigmatism with poor best-corrected vision in both eyes.
3. Fluorescein staining of her cornea to look for keratopathy.
4. Commence lubrication with preservative free eye drops and gels. Offer surgery and correction of her lower eyelid epiblepharon. Commence her on full corrective spectacle wear.
5. Corneal scarring and amblyopia.

Question 32

A 3-month-old infant was brought in by her parents for concerns of a weird appearance of her eyes when taking photos. This is her picture as shown.

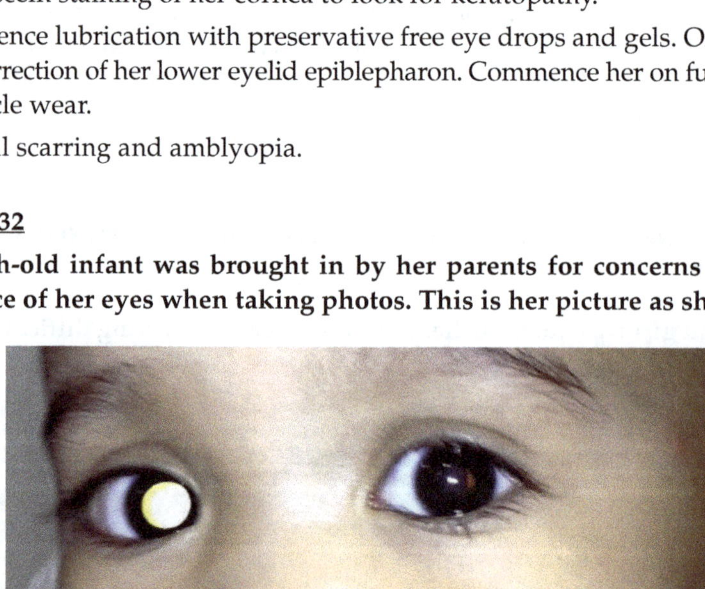

1. Name the clinical sign shown here. (1)
2. Name 3 causes of leukocoria. (3)
3. Name any 2 types of treatment options in the management of retinoblastoma. (2)
4. What are the principles of management in retinoblastoma? (4)

Answers

1. Leukocoria/white pupillary reflex.
2. (Any 3) Retinoblastoma, congenital cataracts, persistent foetal vasculature (PFV), retinopathy of prematurity (ROP), Coat's disease, congenital infections (toxoplasmosis, toxocara), optic disc anomalies.
3. (Any 2) Enucleation, transpupillary thermal therapy, intra-arterial/intravitreal/systemic chemotherapy, cryotherapy.
4. Save life, save globe/eye, save vision, manage any complications.

Question 33

1. Name 3 causes of amblyopia. (3)
2. How can you manage/treat amblyopia? (2)
3. This boy is brought in by his parents after his school vision assessment. This is his refraction as shown. What is the diagnosis? (3)

RIGHT eye				LEFT eye			
Sph	Cyl	Axis	VA	Sph	Cyl	Axis	VA
–1.00	–0.50	180	6/6	–5.00	–0.50	180	6/15

4. How would you manage this child's condition? (2)

Answers

1. Refractive/anisometropia, strabismus, vision deprivation.
2. Optimise vision with glasses as needed, commence part-time patching of the better-seeing eye to treat amblyopia, consider atropine penalisation if the child is unable to comply with patching treatment.

   Depending on the cause of the amblyopia, the following can be done:

   i. Cataracts — remove the cataracts by surgery.
   ii. Anisometropia — provide full-time glasses wear.
   iii. Strabismus — consider patching the fixating eye and/or strabismus surgery.
3. Left eye anisometropic amblyopia.
4. Prescribe him full-time glasses wear to optimise his vision. Review in 3 months to see if there is any improvement to his vision in the left eye. If his left eye is still amblyopic despite full-time glasses wear, consider part-time patching of the right eye.

Question 34

A 3-day-old infant was brought to the Emergency Department for concerns of tearing from both his eyes.

1. What are the sight-threatening causes of tearing in an infant? (2)
2. You notice that the infant has sticky yellowish purulent discharge. What condition are you worried about? (1)
3. Name 3 infective causes of purulent discharge in this child. (3)
4. How would you manage this child? (4)

Answers

1. Congenital glaucoma, ophthalmia neonatorum.
2. Ophthalmia neonatorum.
3. *Neisseria gonorrhoea*, *Chlamydia trachomatis*, Herpes simplex virus.
4. (Any 4): Admit the child if noted to be septic, and investigate for the cause of the tearing by sending conjunctival scrapings for microbiological diagnosis. Co-manage the patient with a paediatrician. Counsel the parent about the need to start topical broad-spectrum antibiotics. Teach the parent to perform hourly eye toileting. Review the child daily until cultures are available. Tailor the treatment according to the culture results/sensitivity.

Question 35

1. What is the most common form of strabismus? (2)
2. What is the most feared consequence of a constant manifest strabismus in a child? (2)
3. A four-year-old girl was brought in for a second opinion for the inward deviation of her right eye. She is wearing glasses of a high plus power. With glasses, she does not appear to have any eye deviation at all. Name this condition. (2)
4. Describe the principles of strabismus management. (4)

Answers

1. Intermittent exotropia.
2. Strabismic amblyopia.
3. Fully accommodative esotropia.
4. Prescribe glasses as needed, treat any strabismic amblyopia with part-time patching as needed, consider orthoptic exercises, e.g. in IXT, prisms may be prescribed to relieve diplopia if needed, consider strabismus surgery.

Question 36

This baby was brought in by her parents:

1. Describe what you see. (3)
2. What possible complications can result from this condition? (2)

3. What can be done to manage the ptosis in this child? (2)
4. If the ptosis occurred in the presence of heterochromia iridis, what is your likely diagnosis, and what are the other signs of this condition? (3)

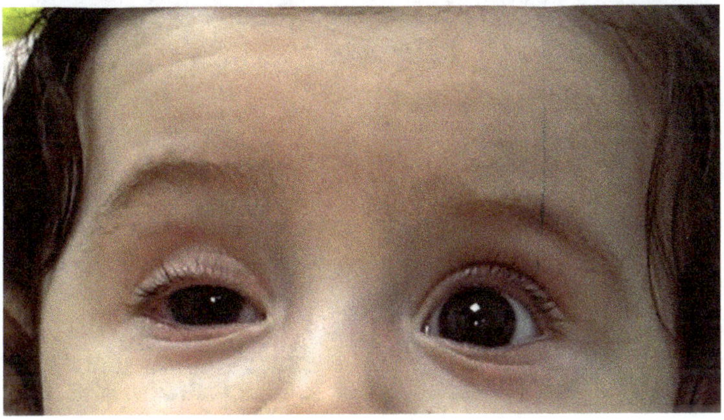

Answers

1. Right side partial congenital ptosis that does not appear to obscure the visual axis. There is overaction of the frontalis muscle on the right side.
2. Right amblyopia if the visual axis is obscured or if there is significant astigmatism in the right eye compared to the left (meridional amblyopia).
3. Conservative management — tape up the eyelid; if the child is older and glasses are required, can consider eyelid crutches attached to the glasses. Consider ptosis repair surgery when the child is older: mild ptosis — levator aponeurosis repair; severe ptosis — consider frontalis sling or frontalis flap.
4. Right Horner's syndrome, anisocoria that is worse in the dark, anhidrosis, reverse ptosis.

15.9 Neuro-ophthalmology

Question 37

A 31-year-old lady presents with acute onset right-sided blurring of vision for 2 days. This is the fundus photograph of the right eye:

1. Describe the significant findings in the fundus picture above. (2)
2. What possible pupillary abnormality would you expect to find? (1)
3. Other than pupil examination, what else can you do to assess optic nerve function? (3)
4. What are possible differential diagnoses? (2)
5. How would you investigate this patient? (2)

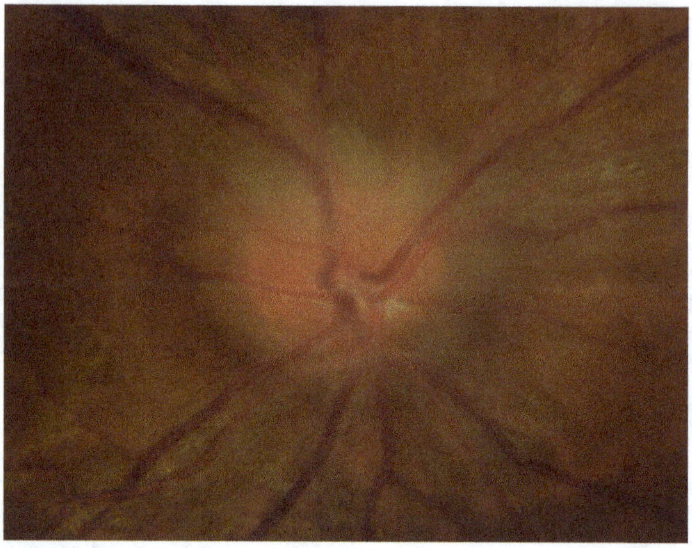

Answers

1. (Any 2) Blurred disc margin, swollen disc, obliterated cup.
2. Relative afferent pupillary defect.
3. Visual acuity, colour vision, visual fields by confrontation.
4. (Any 2) Optic neuritis, compressive lesions, idiopathic intracranial hypertension, malignant hypertension.
5. (Any 2) Check BP, lumbar puncture, MRI brain.

Question 38

A 59-year-old woman presented with sudden-onset painless blurring of vision in the right eye upon waking up. On examination, vision in the right eye was 6/30 with altitudinal visual field defect and the following optic disc appearance:

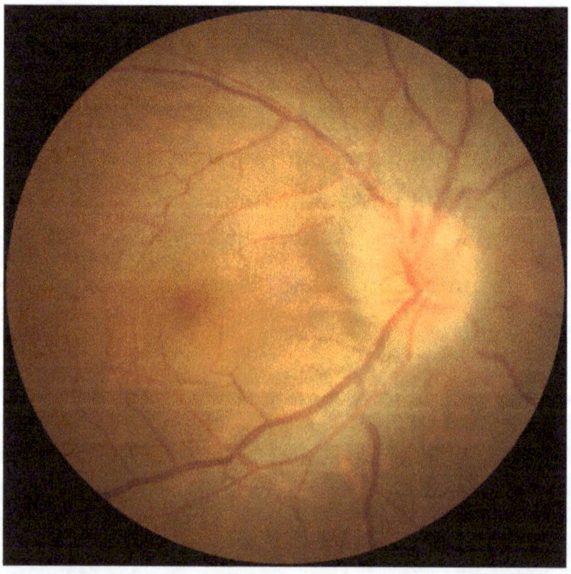

1. Name 2 features of the optic disc seen in the photograph. (2)
2. What other signs might be present? (2)
3. What is the most likely diagnosis? (1)
4. What are the known risk factors? (3)
5. How would you manage the patient? (2)

Answers

1. (Any 2) Blurred disc margin, disc haemorrhage, obliterated disc cup.
2. Loss of colour vision, RAPD.
3. Ischaemic optic neuropathy.
4. (Any 3) Vascular risk factors such as hypertension, diabetes, dyslipidaemia and smoking, crowded disc.
5. (Any 2) Take further history for symptoms suggestive of giant cell arteritis (jaw claudication, scalp tenderness, myalgias, headache); send blood for ESR, CRP, platelets; optimise vascular risk factors, stop smoking, prevent nocturnal hypotension.

Question 39

A 71-year-old man had presented with headache and transient visual obscuration. This is the fundus picture:

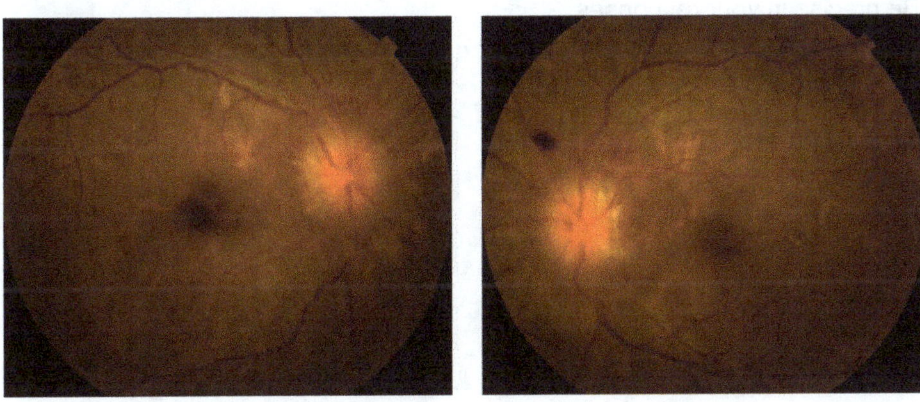

1. Name 3 clinical signs visible on the photographs. (3)
2. What 2 other ophthalmic clinical signs might be detected on examination? (2)
3. What life-threatening causes do you need to rule out? (2)
4. What investigations would you perform? (3)

Answers

1. (Any 3) Blurred disc margin, obscuration of optic disc cup, bilateral swollen optic disc, disc hyperaemia, peripapillary and disc haemorrhage.
2. Enlarged blind spot, cranial nerve palsy (false localising sign).
3. Malignant hypertension, raised intracranial pressure from infection or SOL.
4. Check BP, neuroimaging of the brain (MRI), lumbar puncture to look for opening pressure and evidence of infection.

15.10 Principles and Practice of Low Vision

Question 40

1. What is the functional definition of low vision? (3)
2. What is functional vision? (1)
3. Name 3 functional impacts of low vision. (3)
4. Describe 2 functional implications of peripheral field defect. (2)
5. What chart is used in a low vision evaluation? (1)

Answers

1. Best-corrected visual acuity of worse than 6/12 in the better eye and/or with contrast sensitivity loss, scotoma or field loss.
2. A person's ability to integrate aspects of vision to perform a task.
3. Cloudy media, central field defect and peripheral field defect.
4. Navigation, mobility and locating objects.
5. ETDRS chart.

Take Home Messages

- Read the scenario carefully and look at the mark distribution in each question before answering.
- Be precise in your responses.
- Students are typically tested with six questions in the Ophthalmology EOPT (Total 60 marks).

GLOSSARY

1. AAU: Acute Anterior Uveitis
2. AC: Anterior Chamber
3. ACE: Angiotensin Converting Enzyme
4. AION: Anterior Ischaemic Optic Neuropathy
5. AKC: Atopic Keratoconjunctivitis
6. AMD: Age Related Macular Degeneration
7. ANA: Antinuclear Antibodies
8. ANCA: Anti-neutrophil Cytoplastic Antibodies
9. APAC: Acute Primary Angle Closure
10. AREDS: Age-related Eye Disease
11. AS-OCT: Anterior Segment Optical Coherence Tomography
12. BCC: Basal Cell Carcinoma
13. BCNS: Basal Cell Nevus Syndrome
14. BCVA: Best-corrected Visual Acuity
15. BIO: Binocular Indirect Ophthalmoscope
16. BRAO: Branch Retinal Artery Occlusion
17. BRVO: Branch Retinal Vein Occlusion
18. CACG: Chronic Angle Closure Glaucoma
19. CB: Ciliary Body
20. CCF: Carotico-cavernous Fistula
21. CME: Cystoid Macular Oedema
22. CMV: Cytomegalo Virus
23. CN: Cranial Nerve
24. CNVM: Choroidal Neovascular Membrane
25. CPEO: Chronic Progressive External Ophthalmoplegia
26. CRAO: Central Retinal Artery Occlusion
27. CRVO: Central Retinal Vein Occlusion
28. CSCR: Central Serous Choroidoretinopathy
29. CSF: Cerebrospinal Fluid
30. CSME: Clinically Significant Macular Oedema
31. CSNB: Congenital Stationary Night Blindness
32. CT: Computer Tomography
33. DCR: Dacryocystorhinostomy

34. DM: Diabetes Mellitus
35. DRP: Diabetic Retinopathy Photograph
36. DVD: Dissociated Vertical Deviation
37. ECCE: Extracapsular Cataract Extraction
38. ELDR: Endoscopic Lacrimal Ductal Recanalization
39. ERG: Electrophysiology
40. ESR: Erythrocyte Sedimentation Rate
41. ETDRS: Early Treatment Diabetic Retinopathy Study
42. EUA: Examination Under Anaesthesia
43. FAF: Fundus auto fluorescence
44. FB: Foreign Body
45. FBC: Full Blood Count
46. FDDT: Fluorescein Dye Disappearance Test
47. FEVR: Familial Exudative Vitreoretinopathy
48. FFA: Fundus Fluorescein Angiogram
49. FPL: Forced Preferential Looking
50. GHT: Glaucoma Hemifield Test
51. GO: Grave's Orbitopathy
52. GPA: Glaucoma Progression Analysis
53. GPC: Giant Papillary Conjunctivitis
54. HAART: Highly Active Antiretroviral Therapy
55. HIV: Human Immunodeficiency Virus
56. HLA: Human Leucocytic Antigen
57. HM: Hand Movement
58. HRT: Heidelberg Retinal Tomography
59. HSV: Herpes Simplex Virus
60. HTN: Hypertension
61. HZO: Herpes Zoster Ophthalmicus
62. HZV: Herpes Zoster Virus
63. IAM: Internal Acoustic Meatus
64. ICCE: Intracapsular Cataract Extraction
65. ICE Syndrome: Irido-corneal-endothelial Syndrome
66. ICG: Indocyanine Green
67. ICP: Intracranial Pressure
68. IIH: Idiopathic Intracranial Hypertension
69. IOL: Intraocular Lens
70. ION: Ischaemic Optic Neuropathy
71. IOP: Intraocular Pressure
72. IRMA: Intraretinal Microvascular Anomaly

73. IRU: Immune Reconstitution Uveitis
74. ISCEV: International Society for Clinical Electrophysiology of Vision
75. IVDU: Intravenous Drug Users
76. JIA: Juvenile Idiopathic Arthritis
77. JRA: Juvenile Rheumatoid Arthritis
78. KPs: Keratic Precipitates
79. LPS: Levator Palpebrae Superioris
80. MD: Mean Deviation
81. mfERG: Multifocal ERG
82. MG: Myasthenia Gravis
83. MRD: Margin-reflex Distance
84. MRI: Magnetic Resonance Imaging
85. MRSA: Methicillin Resistant *Staphylococcus Aureus*
86. MSS: Moh's Micrographic Surgery
87. NAAION: Non-arteritic Anterior Ischaemic Optic Neuropathy
88. NLDO: Nasolacrimal Duct Obstruction
89. NMO: Neuromyelitis Optica
90. NMOSD: NMO Spectrum Disorder
91. NPDR: Non-proliferative Diabetic Retinopathy
92. NSAID: Non-steroidal Anti-inflammatory Drugs
93. NVA: Neovascularisation of the Angle
94. NVD: Neovascular Disc
95. NVE: Neovascular Elsewhere
96. NVG: Neovascular Glaucoma
97. OCP: Ocular Cicatricial Pemphigoid
98. OCT: Optical Coherence Tomography
99. OKN: Optokinetic Nystagmus
100. OSNM: Optic Nerve Sheath Meningioma
101. PAC: Primary Angle Closure
102. PACG: Primary Angle Closure Glaucoma
103. PAS: Peripheral Anterior Synechia
104. PCR: Polymerase Chain Reaction
105. PDR: Proliferative Diabetic Retinopathy
106. PDT: Photodynamic Therapy
107. PERG: Pattern ERG
108. PFV: Persistent Foetal Vasculature
109. PNET: Primitive Neuroectodermal Tumour
110. POAG: Primary Open Angle Glaucoma
111. PORT: Punctate Outer Retinal Toxoplasmosis

112. PRP: Panretinal Photocoagulation
113. PSD: Pattern Standard Deviation
114. PTC: Pseudotumour Cerebri
115. PXF: Pseudoexfoliation Syndrome
116. RAPD: Relative Afferent Pupillary Defect
117. RB: Retinoblastoma
118. RD: Retinal Detachment
119. RF: Rheumatoid Factor
120. RFNL: Retinal Nerve Fibre Layer
121. ROP: Retinopathy of Prematurity
122. RP: Retinitis Pigmentosa
123. RPE: Retinal Pigment Epithelium
124. SCC: Squamous Cell Carcinoma
125. SGC: Sebaceous Gland Carcinoma
126. SINS: Surgically-induced Necrotising Scleritis
127. SITA: Swedish Interactive Threshold Algorithm
128. SJS: Stevens Johnson Syndrome
129. SO: Silicone Oil
130. SOF : Superior Orbital Fissure
131. SUN: Standardisation of Uveitis Nomenclature
132. TB: Tuberculosis
133. TCP: Transscleral Cytophotocoagulation
134. TED: Thyroid Eye Disease
135. TM: Trabecular Meshwork
136. TORCH: Toxoplasma, Rubella, CMV, Herpes
137. TRD: Tractional Retinal Detachment
138. UBM: Ultrasound Bio-microscopy
139. UCVA: Uncorrected Visual Acuity
140. VCC: Variable Corneal Compensator
141. VEGF: Vascular Endothelial Growth Factor
142. VEP: Visual Evoked Potential
143. VF: Visual Fields
144. VFI: Visual Field Index
145. VKC: Vernal Keratoconjunctivitis
146. VKH: Vogt-Koyanagi-Harada
147. XLRS: X-linked retinoschisis
148. YAG: Yttrium Aluminium Garnet

INDEX

www.ingramcontent.com/pod-product-compliance
Lightning Source LLC
LaVergne TN
LVHW081936200926
848484LV00009B/2443

* 9 7 8 9 8 1 9 8 0 3 5 4 5 *